THE NEIGHBORHOOD: FACULTY NAVIGATION GUIDE

THE NEIGHBORHOOD: FACULTY NAVIGATION GUIDE

JEAN FORET GIDDENS, RN, PhD
Professor, College of Nursing
University of New Mexico
Albuquerque, New Mexico

Pearson

Boston   Columbus   Indianapolis   New York   San Francisco   Upper Saddle River
Amsterdam   Cape Town   Dubai   London   Madrid   Milan   Munich   Paris   Montreal   Toronto
Delhi   Mexico City   Sao Paulo   Sydney   Hong Kong   Seoul   Singapore   Taipei   Tokyo

Publisher: Julie Levin Alexander
Publisher's Assistant: Regina Bruno
Editor-in-Chief: Maura Connor
Executive Acquisitions Editor: Pamela Fuller
Editorial Assistant: Jennifer Aranda
Managing Production Editor: Patrick Walsh
Production Liaison: Cathy O'Connell
Production Service: Elm Street Publishing Services
Manufacturing Manager: Ilene Sanford
Art Director: Maria Guglielmo
Interior Design: Elm Street Publishing Services
Cover Design: Mary Siener
Director of Marketing: Karen Allman
Marketing Specialist: Michael Sirinides
Marketing Assistant: Crystal Gonzalez
Digital Media Product Manager: Travis Moses-Westphal
Media Project Manager: Rachel Collett
Composition: Integra Software Services Pvt. Ltd.
Printer/Binder: Courier/Kendallville
Cover Printer: Lehigh-Phoenix/Hagerstown

Notice: Care has been taken to confirm the accuracy of information presented in this book. The authors, editors, and the publisher, however, cannot accept any responsibility for errors or omissions or for consequences from application of the information in this book and make no warranty, express or implied, with respect to its contents.

The authors and publisher have exerted every effort to ensure that drug selections and dosages set forth in this text are in accord with current recommendations and practice at time of publication. However, in view of ongoing research, changes in government regulations, and the constant flow of information relating to drug therapy and drug reactions, the reader is urged to check the package inserts of all drugs for any change in indications of dosage and for added warnings and precautions. This is particularly important when the recommended agent is a new and/or infrequently employed drug.

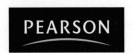
www.pearsonhighered.com

ISBN-10:   0-13-504998-9
ISBN-13: 978-0-13-504998-3

ABOUT THE AUTHOR

Jean Foret Giddens

Jean Foret Giddens, RN, PhD, is Professor and Senior Associate Dean at the College of Nursing, Health Sciences Center, University of New Mexico. A nurse educator for more than 25 years, she is considered an expert in curriculum, conceptual learning, educational research, and innovative teaching strategies. She has authored and contributed to several nursing textbooks and media products and written more than 20 peer-reviewed journal articles. In addition, Dr. Giddens has extensive experience as a nursing education consultant and has presented her work at multiple national and international meetings. She initially developed *The Neighborhood* for students attending the University of New Mexico nursing program.

ACKNOWLEDGMENTS

The Neighborhood represents the efforts of numerous individuals, including the nursing faculty who provided ideas for the stories, the nursing faculty and nurse clinicians who reviewed the stories for accuracy, and the numerous individuals who served as characters for the stories. A special thanks to Jon Sibray, Alex Roessner, and John Giddens, the systems support staff at the University of New Mexico College of Nursing; their efforts and support made this project possible.

CONTENTS

SECTION I INTRODUCTION

Getting Started: Technical Information   2
  System Requirements   2
  Access and Registration   2
Navigating *The Neighborhood*   2
  Moving Between Seasons   2
  Character Stories   2
  Newspaper   3
  Community Facts   3
Technical Support   3
Description of *The Neighborhood*   3
  Theoretical Linkage and Basis for Learning   4
    Storytelling   4
    Longitudinal Case Study   5
    Interpretive Pedagogy   5
    Standardized Patients   5
Features   5
  Featured Characters   5
    Biography and Stories   6
    Content Links   6
    Photographs and Video Vignettes   6
    Medical Records   6

    Supporting Characters   6
    Newspaper   6
    Community Facts   7
Visual Map of *The Neighborhood* Characters   7
Instructional Tips and Techniques   9
Exemplary Teaching Strategies   10
  Featured Character Case Study   10
  Role-Play   10
  Simulation   11
    Concept or Topic Analysis   11
    Games   11
    Comparing and Contrasting   11
    Policy Analysis   12
    Family History/Genogram   12
    Concept Map   12
    Small Group Discussion   12
    Developing a Care Plan or Teaching Plan   12

SECTION II SPECIALTY COURSE USE AND SUGGESTED CHARACTERS

Course Use Overview   38
Nursing Fundamentals—Basic Nursing Skills   38
  Fundamental Concepts   38
  Basic Nursing Skills   42
  Newspaper Links to Fundamental
    Concepts and Basic Skills   43
Adult Health Nursing   44
  Respiratory System   44
  Cardiovascular System   44
  Neurologic System   45
  Musculoskeletal System   45
  Gastrointestinal System   46
  Urologic System   46
  Metabolic System and Nutrition   46
  Immune System   47
  Acid Base/Fluid Electrolyte Disturbances   47
  Visual and Auditory Systems   47
  Neighborhood Hospital Links   47
  Newspaper Links to Adult Health Nursing   47
Maternity and Women's Health   48
  Pregnancy   48
  Women's Health Issues   49
  Newspaper Links to Maternity and Women's
    Health   49

Pediatric and Family Nursing   49
  Health Promotion and Wellness   50
  Health-Related Problems   50
  Family and Social Issues   52
  School Nurse Topics   52
  Newspaper Links to Pediatric and Family
    Nursing   53
Mental Health Nursing   53
  Psychotic Disorders   54
  Cognitive Disorders   54
  Mood Disorders   54
  Other Mental Health Issues   54
  Newspaper Links to Mental Health
    Nursing   55
Geriatric Nursing   55
  Health-Related Conditions   55
  Family and Social Issues   57
  Senior Center Nurse Topics   58
  Newspaper Links to Geriatric
    Nursing   59
Community Health   59
  Common Community Health Topics   59
  Newspaper Links to Community
    Health   60

Nursing Leadership and Professional Concepts
   Course 61
     Professional Practice Issues 61
     Roles of the Professional Nurse 63
     Newspaper Links to Nursing Leadership and
       Professional Concepts 65

Health Promotion 65
   Character Stories 65
   Newspaper Links to Health
     Promotion 67

SECTION III   FEATURED CHARACTER OVERVIEWS AND STORIES

HOUSEHOLD CHARACTERS 70

Allen Household 70
  Clifford Allen 71
    Season 1 71
    Season 2 72
    Season 3 74
  Pamela Allen 76
    Season 1 76
    Season 2 78
    Season 3 80
  Gary Allen 82
    Season 1 82
    Season 2 83
    Season 3 85
Bley Household 87
  Jimmy Bley 87
    Season 1 87
    Season 2 89
    Season 3 91
  Cecelia Bley 93
    Season 1 93
    Season 2 95
    Season 3 97
James Household 99
  Norma James 99
    Season 1 99
    Season 2 102
    Season 3 104
Johnson Household 107
  Yvonne Johnson 107
    Season 1 107
    Season 2 109
    Season 3 112
  Randall Johnson 114
    Season 1 114
    Season 2 115
    Season 3 117
Martin Household 119
  Gilbert Martin 121

    Season 1 121
    Season 2 122
    Season 3 125
  Helen Martin 127
    Season 1 127
    Season 2 129
    Season 3 131
  Mary Martin 133
    Season 1 133
    Season 2 135
    Season 3 137
  Anthony Martin 139
    Season 1 139
    Season 2 140
    Season 3 142
  Kristina Martin 144
    Season 1 144
    Season 2 145
    Season 3 147
  Tracie Ames 149
    Season 1 149
    Season 2 150
    Season 3 152
  Mark Martin 153
    Season 2 153
    Season 3 155
  Tyler Martin 157
    Season 2 157
    Season 3 158
Ocampo Household 160
  Danilo Ocampo 160
    Season 1 160
    Season 2 163
  Lydia Ocampo 164
    Season 1 164
    Season 2 166
    Season 3 168
Reyes Household 169
  Angelo Reyes 169

    Season 1 169
    Season 2 172
    Season 3 174
  Rachel Reyes 176
    Season 1 176
    Season 2 178
    Season 3 180
  Peter and Marissa Reyes 182
    Season 3 182
Evelyn Riley Household 184
  Evelyn Riley 184
    Season 1 184
    Season 2 186
    Season 3 189
  Jenna Riley 190
    Season 1 190
    Season 2 192
    Season 3 193
  Jason Riley 196
    Season 1 196
    Season 2 198
    Season 3 199
**Riley and Holmes
Household 201**
  Jessica Riley 202
    Season 1 202
    Season 2 204
    Season 3 207
  Casey Holmes 209
    Season 1 209
    Season 2 211
    Season 3 212
  Ryan Riley 214
    Season 1 214
    Season 2 215
    Season 3 216
  Carrie Holmes 218
    Season 2 218
    Season 3 218

Ross and Jaramillo Household   220
  Greg Ross   220
   Season 1   *220*
   Season 2   *222*
   Season 3   *224*
  Benito Jaramillo   226
   Season 1   *226*
   Season 2   *227*
   Season 3   *229*
Young Household   231
  Steve Young   232
   Season 1   *232*
   Season 2   *233*
   Season 3   *235*
  Angie Young   236
   Season 1   *236*
   Season 2   *238*
   Season 3   *241*
  Kelsey Young   243
   Season 1   *243*
   Season 2   *244*
   Season 3   *246*
  Marcus Young   247
   Season 1   *247*
   Season 2   *248*
   Season 3   *250*
  Eric Young   251
   Season 2   *251*
   Season 3   *252*

NURSE CHARACTERS   254

Neighborhood Hospital   254
  Kate Swanson   255
   Season 1   *255*
   Season 2   *256*
   Season 3   *257*

Patrick Richman   258
  Season 1   *258*
  Season 2   *260*
  Season 3   *261*
Bobby Schofield   262
  Season 1   *262*
  Season 2   *263*
  Season 3   *264*
Neighborhood Senior Center Nursing Clinic   266
  Karen Williams   266
   Season 1   *266*
   Season 2   *268*
   Season 3   *269*
Neighborhood Women's Health Specialists   272
  Carol Ramsey   272
   Season 1   *272*
   Season 2   *274*
   Season 3   *276*
Neighborhood Public Schools   278
  Violet Brinkworth   278
   Season 1   *278*
   Season 2   *280*
   Season 3   *281*
Neighborhood Newspaper   284
  Season 1   284
  Season 2   293
  Season 3   301
References   309
Subject Index   310

CONTENTS

Ross and Jaramillo Household 220
  Cruz Ross 220
    Season 1 220
    Season 2 223
    Season 3 224
  Rachel Jaramillo 225
    Season 1 226
    Season 2 227
    Season 3 229
Young Household 231
  Steve Young 232
    Season 1 232
    Season 2 233
    Season 3 235
  Anne Young 236
    Season 1 236
    Season 2 238
    Season 3 240
  Kelsey Young 243
    Season 1 243
    Season 2 244
    Season 3 246
  Marcus Young 247
    Season 1 247
    Season 2 248
    Season 3 250
  Eric Young 251
    Season 1 252
    Season 3 253

NURSE CHARACTERS 254

Neighborhood Hospital 254
  Rae Swanson 254
    Season 1 255
    Season 2 256
    Season 3 257

Patrick Bachman 258
    Season 1 258
    Season 2 260
    Season 3 261
Bobby Schofield 261
    Season 1 262
    Season 2 264
    Season 3 265
Neighborhood Senior Center Nursing Clinic 266
  Karen Williams 266
    Season 1 266
    Season 2 268
    Season 3 269
Neighborhood Women's Health Specialists 272
  Carol Ramsey 272
    Season 1 272
    Season 2 274
    Season 3 276
Neighborhood Public Schools 278
  Violet Brinkworth 278
    Season 1 278
    Season 2 280
    Season 3 281
Neighborhood Newspaper 284
    Season 1 284
    Season 2 285
    Season 3 301
References 309
Subject Index 319

INTRODUCTION

Welcome to *The Neighborhood,* an online virtual community that supports learning throughout the nursing program. This Faculty Navigation Guide introduces you to *The Neighborhood* and provides suggestions for incorporating this new way of learning into the nursing curriculum and your classroom.

Please access *The Neighborhood* at www.pearsonneighborhood.com.

GETTING STARTED: TECHNICAL INFORMATION

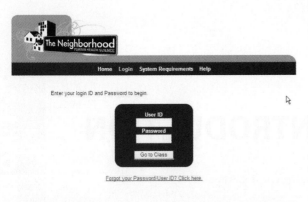

System Requirements

For detailed and up-to-date system requirements, please visit *The Neighborhood* home page at http://www.pearsonneighborhood. com. Click the "Support" link at the top of the page, then select "System Requirements".

Access and Registration

Schools must designate an administrator who will be trained to set up *The Neighborhood* for the program's courses and will work with Pearson to register faculty and student with their personal accounts.

Details for institutional purchase and administrator training are available through your sales representative and through *The Neighborhood* home page under the "Support" link.

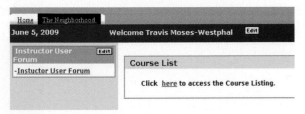

Login:

Here's how you log in to *The Neighborhood*:

1. Go to *The Neighborhood* home page. The URL is: www.pearsonneighborhood.com
2. Click the Login button on the top right corner of the screen.
3. Enter the username and password you received from your program administrator to log in.
4. After you log into *The Neighborhood*, you will be taken to your campus home page. From there, you can access all the stories by clicking on the course your school is using. You can also access the Instructor User Forum and Customer Technical Support from the site.

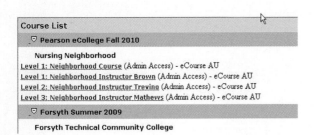

NAVIGATING THE NEIGHBORHOOD

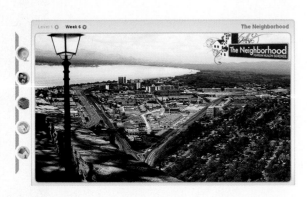

Moving Between Seasons

From the home page, instructors can navigate among seasons (Season 1, Season 2, and Season 3) by clicking on the *Season* link located in the upper left corner of the screen. Students' ability to access different seasons depends on the season of access assigned to the student.

Character Stories

The household and nurse characters are accessed by clicking on the ***HOUSEHOLDS*** and ***HEALTH CARE SETTINGS*** links on the left of the page. All characters who live in a household or work in a community health-care facility can be found using these links. Within the households or nurse characters, users can navigate between episodes using the drop-down menu in the upper left of the screen.

To go back to the home page, click on the bottom button with the house icon on it.

Some of the character stories include video clips in a given episode. To play the video, click on the **VIDEO** link, and then click on the icon to play. Make sure your computer speakers are turned on with sufficient volume to hear the audio portion of the video.

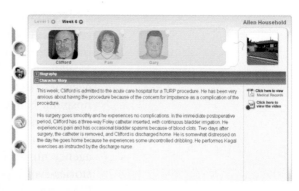

Newspaper

The Neighborhood Newspaper is accessed from the home page on the **NEIGHBORHOOD INFORMATION** icon on the left-hand side of the screen redundant. As with the character stories, users can navigate among episodes to which they have access by using the drop-down menu at the top left-hand side of the screen. To go back to the home page, click on the home button.

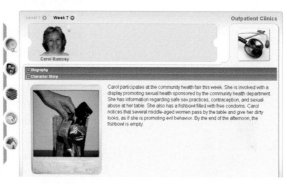

Community Facts

The Neighborhood has a Community Facts link that acts as a community home page. This link is found under the **NEIGHBORHOOD INFORMATION** icon on the left-hand side of the screen.

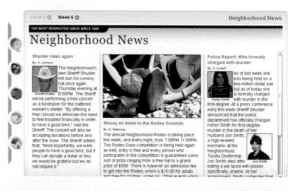

TECHNICAL SUPPORT

A full-time Web programmer ensures ongoing site maintenance of *The Neighborhood*. Date progression (for episode story updates) is automated, and dates are adjusted each semester by the program administrator. A clearly marked icon located within the site allows users to access technical support if needed. On the Personal Homepage/Portal, a help button is located in the upper right-hand corner. In addition, when you are in *The Neighborhood* Season/Course, a help button is located in the upper right-hand corner there as well.

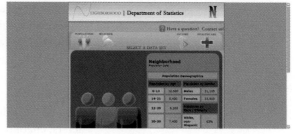

Requests for technical support are sent directly to *The Neighborhood* Web programmer to ensure immediate attention.

DESCRIPTION OF *THE NEIGHBORHOOD*

The Neighborhood, a virtual community specifically designed to enhance nursing education, represents a paradigm shift in teaching and learning. This Web-based community features 11 households and several community agencies. Interacting within the households and community agencies are 40 featured characters, representing individuals from various cultural groups across the age, health-illness, and socioeconomic spectrums.

Health-related issues are depicted through the household characters and represent acute and chronic biophysical and psychosocial problems correlating to the incidence and prevalence in population groups. Health care is represented in *The Neighborhood* across multiple environments, including the home, community agencies (such as schools and a senior center), outpatient offices, clinics, and a hospital. Nurse characters featured in the community agencies depict personal and professional issues faced by nurses in a variety of roles, including hospital nurse, nurse manager, advanced practice nurse, school nurse, and community agency nurse. *The Neighborhood* is presented in the context of a story; character stories evolve per episode over three academic terms and are supplemented with biographical information, photographs, video clips, medical records, and related newspaper articles. Students see the stories as they unfold based on their access season. Specifically, students with Season 1 access only see Season 1 stories up to the current episode of the term; students with Season 2 access can review all of the Season 1 stories and only Season 2 stories up to the current episode of the term; and students with Season 3 access can view all Season 1 and Season 2 stories, and only Season 3 stories up to the current episode of the term. Faculty and students with Season 4 access can see all stories. This is important for faculty to keep in mind when planning learning activities using *The Neighborhood* stories and events.

Students may well be exposed to concepts within the stories before formally studying them in didactic courses or encountering them in the clinical setting. Students can draw on these virtual experiences, thus enhancing didactic and clinical learning. Because the virtual community links to all courses, students and faculty have a shared experience through the stories, enabling them to link within and between courses.

Theoretical Linkage and Basis for Learning

Virtual communities represent an emerging technological application for nursing education. Although many computer-based learning programs exist, there are no direct comparisons with *The Neighborhood*. *The Neighborhood* is significantly different pedagogically in focus, depth, scope, function, and application. It has strong links to several well-founded teaching strategies: storytelling, longitudinal case study, interpretive pedagogy, and standardized patients. These strategies represent multicontextuality (Iberra, 2001), as well as constructivist, humanistic, and neurophysiologic learning theories.

Storytelling.   The primary basis of learning in *The Neighborhood* is through character stories. Storytelling in this context focuses on the lived experiences of the characters, enabling students to gain an appreciation for personal issues and competing variables that are often not captured by journal articles and textbooks. *The Neighborhood* stories have the potential to grab and hold the interest and attention of students in a way that is similar to a good novel or television series. Milton (2004) describes storytelling as a "coming-to-know process" that provides a mechanism for learning concepts in a meaningful context. The multiple benefits of storytelling as a teaching strategy are described in the literature, including role modeling and enhancement of cultural sensitivity, empathy, ethical insight, self-esteem, critical thinking, and communication (Charon, 2004; Davidhizar & Lonser, 2003; Durgahee, 1997; Hodge, Pasqua, Marquez, & Geishirt-Cantrell, 2002; Milton, 2004).

Longitudinal Case Study.   Case study involves the analysis of a clinical situation or incident. This widely used teaching strategy includes the presentation of a patient (usually in a clinical context) with specific questions or problems for learners to analyze and address. Case-based learning has been used in nursing education for several years in a variety of applications and educational settings, including the traditional classroom, Web-based courses, clinical courses, and simulations. Benefits of case-based learning include acquisition of skills in critical thinking, clinical reasoning, organization and interpretation of information, and enhancement of student confidence (Thomas, O'Connor, Albert, Boutain, & Brandt, 2001).

The Neighborhood represents a unique form of case-based learning. The longitudinal application (over three academic terms), the interrelationship among the characters and community, and the fact that cases are told from the perspective of the characters represent significant differences from the traditional case-based approach.

Interpretive Pedagogy.   *Interpretative pedagogy* is a process of drawing meaning from situations or experiences through reflection. In nursing education, interpretive pedagogy stimulates and develops thinking and cultivates a deep understanding of the lived experiences of individuals (Diekelmann, 2005; Ironside, 2005). The character stories provide a virtual experience that enables students to think critically and analyze circumstances in the context of realistic situations, thus enhancing affective learning. These opportunities are extended to all students, as opposed to a select few students who might encounter such experiences in a clinical setting.

Standardized Patients.   Standardized patients are paid individuals who assume the identity of patients and accurately portray these patients in specific clinical scenarios (Ebbert & Connors, 2004). Standardized patients have been successfully used in medical education as well as graduate nursing education, particularly advanced practice education, for several years. The reported benefits of standardized patients include improvement of assessment and communication skills, knowledge development, and cultural competency (Ebbert & Connors, 2004; Rutledge, Garzon, Scott, & Karlowicz, 2004; Seibert, Guthrie, & Adamo, 2004; Vessey & Huss, 2002). The use of standardized patients has also been reported as a way to measure learning outcomes through performance of assessment and differential diagnosis (Shawler, 2008).

The Neighborhood essentially incorporates the use of standardized patients, but in a virtual context. Although there is no direct interaction between the student and the characters, all students and faculty are exposed to the same experiences through the character stories, providing for many of the same benefits (knowledge development, assessment skills, and cultural competency) and remaining accessible at all times—unlike traditional standardized patients.

FEATURES

Featured Characters

There are 40 characters who live and work in *The Neighborhood*. Featured characters include several elements within the Web site: biography and stories, photos and video vignettes, medical records, and content links.

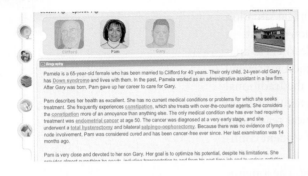

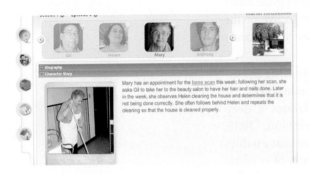

Biography and Stories.   Each featured character is introduced by a brief biography, followed by episode stories that evolve over three academic terms (or 45 episodes). It is important to note that *The Neighborhood* does not correlate to real time; that is, the time frame between story updates might represent one or more episodes. In most cases, the stories in each episode are limited to one paragraph, so students will not feel overwhelmed by keeping up with the stories. However, when a major event occurs, the episode story is longer.

Content Links.   Embedded within the stories and biography are content links. Select medical terms, pharmacologic agents, and diagnostic tests are linked with brief content (definitions or descriptions) to provide real-time access to information enhancing students' understanding. Content links are accessed by clicking on the links within the stories.

Photographs and Video Vignettes.   Photographs and video vignettes are included throughout the Web site to enhance the stories. Approximately 640 photographs and 115 videos are associated with the stories. The photographs are embedded within the story, and video clips are accessed by clicking on links within the stories. Most video clips are one to two minutes long. In the printed version of the Faculty Navigation Guide, symbols embedded in each episode's stories (photograph [**P**]; video clip [**VC**]) alert faculty to supplements for that story.

Medical Records.   For many of the characters who experience health-related events that require health-care visits, a portion of a medical record is included with the story. A total of 15 medical records that detail inpatient or outpatient care are available; 4 of these medical records are updated over time to reflect follow-up visits (e.g., prenatal care, pediatric office visit, outpatient chemotherapy). On the Web site, an icon lets the user know when a medical record is embedded in the story; these records can be downloaded and printed, if desired. In the printed version of the Faculty Navigation Guide, a symbol (medical record [**MR**]) embedded in each episode's stories alerts instructors to medical record supplements for that story.

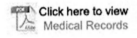

Click here to view Medical Records

Supporting Characters

Several characters are considered "supporting" characters, because their stories are not followed on a week-to-week basis. They are, however, important characters who appear frequently and have roles in the stories of several featured characters. Examples include Dr. Gordon in the emergency department; Dr. Rowe, a family practice physician; Dr. Jacobe, a psychiatrist; Carolyn Marquette, a pediatric nurse practitioner; and Terry Clark, a pregnant teenager.

Newspaper

A community newspaper features announcements and portions of health-related articles that correlate with events in *The Neighborhood* character stories. Like the character stories, the newspaper is updated in each episode. Common newspaper features include community events (e.g., a forest fire, a hospital strike), health promotion topics (e.g., nutrition,

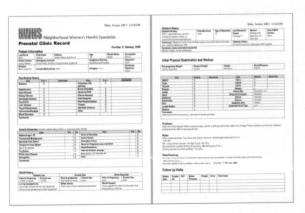

exercise, child safety seats, prenatal care), health concerns of older adults, issues involving substance abuse, domestic violence, and issues within the schools. The newspaper is enhanced by 55 photographs.

Community Facts

Like most real communities, *The Neighborhood* has a Community Facts link that acts as a community home page. Within this link, users will find a message from Neighborhood mayor Nathan Brice, along with links for population demographics, weather, income data (employment and average wages, unemployment and poverty rates, and cost-of-living data), and health-care information (inpatient and outpatient services, as well as health-care organizations).

VISUAL MAP OF *THE NEIGHBORHOOD* CHARACTERS

One of the unique characteristics of *The Neighborhood* is the interrelationships of characters. Not only are character stories within families interrelated, but the stories connect with those of other characters outside the family setting. This interrelatedness becomes more complex in each of the seasons as the stories unfold, and it is an essential feature in creating the feel of a community. The following diagrams show the various featured household and community characters in each of the three seasons. Arrows link character relationships outside the home setting.

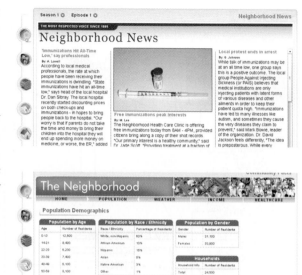

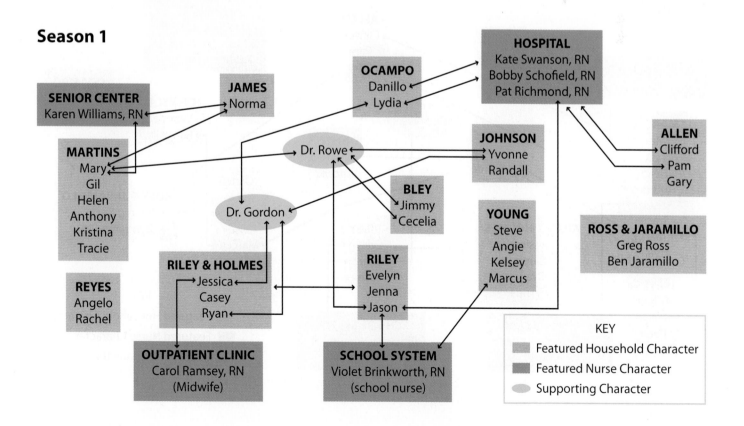

Season 1

SENIOR CENTER
Karen Williams, RN

MARTINS
Mary
Gil
Helen
Anthony
Kristina
Tracie

REYES
Angelo
Rachel

JAMES
Norma

Dr. Rowe

Dr. Gordon

RILEY & HOLMES
Jessica
Casey
Ryan

OUTPATIENT CLINIC
Carol Ramsey, RN
(Midwife)

OCAMPO
Danillo
Lydia

BLEY
Jimmy
Cecelia

RILEY
Evelyn
Jenna
Jason

SCHOOL SYSTEM
Violet Brinkworth, RN
(school nurse)

HOSPITAL
Kate Swanson, RN
Bobby Schofield, RN
Pat Richmond, RN

JOHNSON
Yvonne
Randall

YOUNG
Steve
Angie
Kelsey
Marcus

ALLEN
Clifford
Pam
Gary

ROSS & JARAMILLO
Greg Ross
Ben Jaramillo

KEY
Featured Household Character
Featured Nurse Character
Supporting Character

Season 2

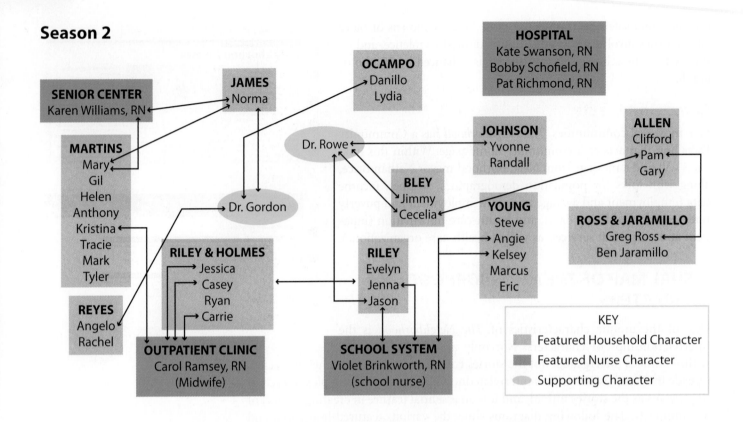

Season 3

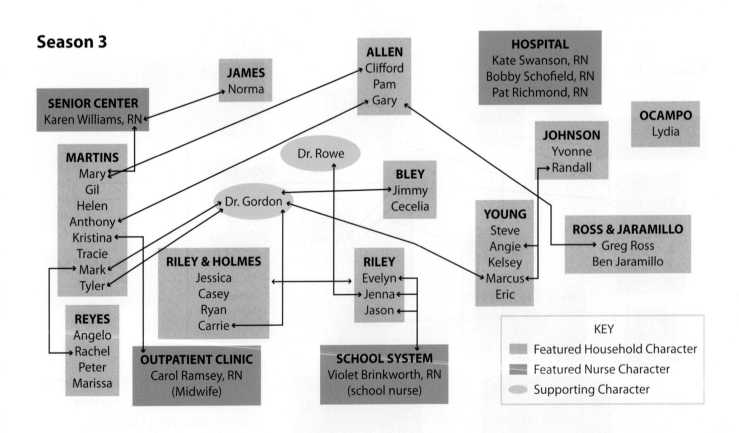

INSTRUCTIONAL TIPS AND TECHNIQUES

The stories in *The Neighborhood* represent many of the common health-related problems, social issues, and nursing practice issues that affect health care today; as such, they apply to most nursing courses, regardless of the curriculum. The instructor can determine how and to what extent the stories are applied in a course based on the course content and the placement (season) at which the course is offered in the curriculum. There are no embedded quizzes, questions, or specific learning activities in *The Neighborhood;* rather, it serves as a platform for the instructor to develop relevant and purposeful student-centered learning activities. *The Neighborhood* is not designed to replace classroom, online, or clinical instruction; it enhances student learning because it provides clinical and situational contexts to the content.

Faculty members who are new users may initially struggle with how to use *The Neighborhood* to enhance learning; this is not so much a reflection on the creativity or talent of faculty members as it is a reflection of current educational practice. Using *The Neighborhood* requires instructors to think differently about learning. One helpful suggestion is to think about teaching from the standpoint of what you want your students to be able to do. *The Neighborhood* provides a platform for practical application. For example, it is expected that students can write a care plan, prepare a teaching plan, prepare a health promotion activity, analyze risk factors, prepare discharge instructions, make a home visit, analyze effectiveness of care, and compare and contrast expected outcomes with actual outcomes. For the most part, these are practical applications only taught in clinical settings. However, *The Neighborhood* provides the opportunity for instructors to implement such activities in the classroom by linking to characters and events. Teaching in this way is an example of integrative teaching, which Benner and Sutphen (2007) describe as signature pedagogy of expert teachers.

The following tips will help you get started using *The Neighborhood* in your classroom:

- **Tip #1:** Become familiar with the characters, stories, and community events for the season/semester in which you teach so that you can identify the most appropriate links to the content in your class.
- **Tip #2:** Think broadly about applications. Although specific content covered in class might not be represented in a Neighborhood story, conceptual links between content and stories can almost always be made. For example, you might teach a class on rheumatoid arthritis (RA), but you will not find a character who has RA in *The Neighborhood*. However, one of the characters has lupus; both RA and lupus are autoimmune disorders, and they share many common clinical features. Making these connections will strengthen and deepen your students' understanding of the underlying concepts involved.
- **Tip #3:** Be sensitive to the timing of stories; stories unfold over time, and students are only able to see up to the current episode. It is important that learning activities are developed with consideration to this limitation. In other words, do not develop a learning activity related to a Neighborhood event that has not yet happened (from the perspective of the students). Although you can still make links to class content before an event happens, you might need to link the content differently. For example, while teaching about stroke in a Season 1 course, you may feel frustrated that one of the characters experiences

a stroke in Season 2, which the students in Season 1 cannot yet access. However, the character shows all the classic risk factors in Season 1, so you might plan a learning activity in which students conduct an analysis of risk factors for various characters to identify who is most at risk.

- **Tip #4:** Vary the learning activities and featured characters. No one likes to do the same thing over and over again, so it is important to modify the activities to keep learning interesting. Types of learning activities can range from those completed during class time to major course projects and assignments. It is most important that activities be purposeful. The beauty of *The Neighborhood* is that it is truly adaptable to almost any nursing course.
- **Tip #5.** Use *The Neighborhood* regularly. Student evaluations have shown that students become frustrated when they are asked to read *The Neighborhood* stories without application in class. Although it is not necessary to use the application in every class session to be successful, regular use is the perceived student benefit. Even during weeks when you do not have a specific class assignment, take a few minutes to reference *The Neighborhood* and give students a chance to share what is going on. This will help to keep them returning to *The Neighborhood* each week.

EXEMPLARY TEACHING STRATEGIES

Several instructional strategies can be used to teach using *The Neighborhood* characters and events, including the following learning activities: featured character case study, role-play, simulation, concept or topic analysis, games, comparing and contrasting, policy analysis, family history/genogram, concept map, small group discussion, and developing a care or teaching plan.

Featured Character Case Study

Perhaps the most obvious application of *The Neighborhood* is featuring the characters in a case study. This can be accomplished with any of the characters in any course; the possibilities for application of this type are endless. Case studies, particularly when done in small groups as an in-class assignment, provide a mechanism for dialog within the groups. Figure 1 (located at the end of this Section) illustrates an example of a featured case study. In addition, featured case studies are available at *The Neighborhood* Faculty User Forum; you can use these or create your own.

Role-Play

Role-play is a learning strategy in which learners assume the roles of other individuals and act out specific situations. The situation may be unstructured or semistructured. Other students watch the interactions during the role-playing session, offer feedback, and critique the students. *The Neighborhood* stories provide multiple opportunities for role-playing. Because students know the characters, it is simple for them to assume the role and act in a way that is consistent with the personality of the character.

There are three phases to a role-play learning activity:

1. An overview or prebriefing, so students understand the objectives of the role-playing activity
2. The actual role-playing, which should take between 5 and 15 minutes
3. A debriefing, which usually involves a discussion regarding what was learned

Figure 2 (located at the end of Section 1) is one example of a role-play learning activity, and there are additional examples at *The Neighborhood* Faculty User Forum; you can use these or create your own.

Simulation

Simulation involves the imitation of a clinical situation that a student might encounter. Over the past decade, human patient simulation has become a prominent teaching strategy used in nursing education programs. Multiple benefits of human simulation have been identified; the most important include the opportunity to provide a safe environment in which to learn and learner engagement.

Simulation is an ideal way to infuse *The Neighborhood* characters into learning activities, through either actual character events or what-if scenarios. Because of the breadth of situations within the stories, simulation activities can range from simple (e.g., focusing on communication and wound care in Season 1) to complex (e.g., management of life-threatening illnesses in Seasons 2 and 3). Figure 3 (located at the end of Section 1) shows one example of a simulation learning activity, and additional examples are available at *The Neighborhood* Faculty User Forum; you can use these or create your own.

Concept or Topic Analysis. A concept or topic analysis can be done in the form of a written assignment, a group project presentation, or an in-class assignment. In this activity, both a character and a problem are selected. Students are asked to analyze the character and the topic as they relate to the literature. Students gain a deep understanding of the topic as it presents in a clinical situation and how the character story is similar to and different from the presentation in the textbook or selected journal articles. Figure 4 (located at the end of Section 1) shows one example of a concept analysis learning activity, and additional examples are available at *The Neighborhood* Faculty User Forum; you can use these or create your own.

Games. The use of games to trigger active learning in the classroom and for independent learning is well described in the literature. There are multiple types of games that can be developed for instructional use; so many, in fact, that entire textbooks, sections of instructional textbooks, and Web sites are devoted to this topic alone. An important point about games is that they must be purposeful. A game that is fun but has no an obvious purpose adds little value to the learning experience and can be perceived as a waste of time by students. Figure 5 (located at the end of Section 1) shows one example of a Jeopardy game linked to *The Neighborhood*, and additional examples are available at *The Neighborhood* Faculty User Forum; you can use these or create your own.

Comparing and Contrasting. Another effective learning strategy is to compare and contrast a selected topic across multiple characters. This enables students to develop an enhanced understanding of similarities and differences in presentation, effects, and outcomes related to the topic. Several topics addressed in *The Neighborhood* link to this activity, including hypertension, diabetes, oxygenation, and substance abuse. Figure 6 (located at the end of Section 1) shows one example of a comparing and contrasting learning activity, and additional examples are available at *The Neighborhood* Faculty User Forum; you can use these or create your own.

Policy Analysis. *The Neighborhood* provides the ability to analyze policy initiatives as they relate to professional nursing practice and community events. Community events are included in the character stories and featured in *The Neighborhood* newspaper. A learning activity in which students study a specific policy or group of policies as they relate to characters or events in *The Neighborhood* helps students understand such initiatives as they apply to real-life situations. Figure 7 (located on the end of Section 1) features an example of a policy analysis learning activity involving injury prevention and protection; (also available on *The Neighborhood* Faculty User Forum); you can use this or create your own.

Family History/Genogram. An effective way to help students understand the benefits of taking a complete family history is by using information provided in *The Neighborhood*, specifically the biographical information of any of the characters. The complexity of the learning activity can be increased by enhancing existing content with additional information. With this additional information, students can draw a genogram for a given character or characters and use this information to identify risk factors for disease. Figure 8 (located on the end of Section 1) features an example of a genogram learning activity involving the Martin family; (also available on *The Neighborhood* Faculty User Forum); you can use this or create your own.

Concept Map. Concept maps have become popular as teaching strategies because they allow for the presentation of multiple primary concepts, interrelated concepts, and related linkages. They can be done as an independent learning assignment or as part of a group learning activity. There is significant variability with concept maps; therefore, there is no single correct way to use them. Learners identify the primary problems experienced by a *Neighborhood* character. Then, using a concept map, they show how the problems are interrelated. Figure 9 (located on the end of Section 1) features an example of a concept map activity (also available on *The Neighborhood* Faculty User Forum); you can use this or create your own.

Small Group Discussion. Small group discussion involves an exchange of ideas about a situation or a specified topic. This approach fosters active student engagement, particularly when learning groups are small. (Between four and six learners is ideal.) Small group discussion is most effective when questions are interesting and thought provoking. Small group discussion can be geared for very short periods (5–10 minutes) or longer periods, depending on the learning goals. This application is useful for traditional classroom and online learning environments. Figures 10 and 11 (located on the end of Section 1) feature examples of small group discussion activities featuring *Neighborhood* characters (also available on *The Neighborhood* Faculty User Forum); you can use these or create your own.

Developing a Care Plan or Teaching Plan. Learning to develop a care plan or a teaching plan can be challenging for students initially. Instructors can enhance this experience using the shared understanding of problems experienced by *Neighborhood* characters. Because data are already embedded in the stories, students and faculty have access to the same information, enabling instructors to provide more precise clarification and feedback to students. Figure 12 (located the end of Section 1) shows an example of a care plan learning activity featuring a *Neighborhood* character, and Figure 13 is an example of a teaching plan learning activity. These examples are also available on *The Neighborhood* Faculty User Forum; you can use these or create your own.

FIGURE 1 CASE STUDY PAM ALLEN

This case study follows Pam Allen and her family through the trajectory of her cancer diagnosis and eventual death. Refer to the Allen family stories in *The Neighborhood* (Seasons 1–3) and Pam Allen's medical records to complete this work.

- In Season 1, Pam is diagnosed with colorectal cancer (CA). Complete the following tables regarding an analysis of risk factors and recommended screenings in relationship to what we know about Pam.

Textbook Risk Factors for Colorectal CA	Screening Recommendations for Colorectal CA	Pam's Personal Risk Factors for Colorectal CA	Screenings Performed on Pam (if Any Known)

- What are the classic signs and symptoms of colorectal CA? What signs and symptoms does Pam have in Season 1?

Classic Signs and Symptoms According to Text	Pam's Signs and Symptoms

In episodes 13 and 14, Pam sees her physician. What assessment findings does the physician notice, and what diagnostic tests are done? What is the relationship of some of her symptoms to the findings?

- Assessment findings:

- Diagnostic tests performed and results:

- What is the relationship of Pam's symptoms to her clinical findings?

At the end of Season 1 and beginning of Season 2, Pam has surgery and begins adjuvant therapy.

- Which of the following best describes the goal of Pam's treatment plan at this point? (Circle one)   Cure   Control   Palliation

- What does adjuvant therapy mean, and what is it in Pam's case?

  _____

- What agents does Pam receive? _____

- Which agents are classified as chemotherapy, and which are considered biotherapy?

  _____

  _____

- What are the actions of the drugs?

  _____

  _____

  _____

- Describe the schedule for administration of her treatment. Explain the purpose of this schedule. Does this follow national recommendations? (Hint: Consult the National Comprehensive Cancer Network Web site at NCCN.org)

  _____

  _____

  _____

  _____

- What are the *major* side effects of these agents, and what would you include in your patient education?

  _____

  _____

  _____

  _____

- What is a PICC line, why is it inserted, and what would you need to teach Pam or Clifford about caring for it at home?

  _____

  _____

  _____

  _____

- In the following table, link Pam's experiences to concepts and nursing diagnoses. What do you consider the top six problems Pam experiences during this time? What concepts do these represent? If you were developing a care plan for Pam, what do you believe are the nursing diagnoses with highest priority?

Top Six Problems	Concepts Represented	Priority Nursing Diagnoses

- Up to this point, what impact has Pam's illness had on Clifford and Gary?

Clifford	Gary

At the beginning of Season 3, Pam suffers a setback. She experiences discomfort to the right upper quadrant of her abdomen, decreased appetite, yellowish tint to her sclera, and dark urine. She learns that the cancer has metastasized to her liver.

- Explain the physiologic causes of the symptoms.

Symptom	Physiologic Explanation
Discomfort in upper right abdomen	
Decrease in appetite	
Yellow sclera	
Dark urine	

- Pam has conflicting thoughts about beginning chemotherapy because of the side effects. Her physician and Clifford talk Pam into starting chemotherapy again. At this point, which of the following best describes the goal for Pam's treatment plan? (Circle one)   Cure   Control   Palliation

In Season 3, Episode 4, Pam's treatment is withheld. Refer to the story and Pam's medical record.

- What is her white blood cell count? _____

  - What problem does this represent? _____

- What is her platelet count? _____

  - What problem does this represent? _____

- What is the specific cause of these problems?
  _____

- If you were the nurse in the chemotherapy clinic, what nursing interventions and education would you provide to Pam and Clifford?
  _____
  _____
  _____

Tension exists between Clifford and Pam regarding her treatment wishes, representing concepts of family dynamics and ethics. Analyze the interactions between the nurse, Pam, and Clifford in Season 3, Episode 6.

- In what ways do you think this was handled well by the nurse? What could have been said or done differently?

- The goal of Pam's treatment shifts to palliation in Season 3, Episode 7. What are the specific goals and nursing interventions for Pam, Clifford, and Gary during this end-of-life care?

FIGURE 2 ROLE-PLAY JESSICA RILEY AND CAROL RAMSEY

Preparation and Briefing:

Divide students into groups of three to four individuals each. Select roles:

1. Jessica Riley
2. Carol Ramsey, CNM
3. Observer
4. Observer

Explain to students that the objective of the activity is to role-play an interview involving a nurse and patient who is possibly the victim of domestic violence. For five to ten minutes, students in the roles of Jessica and Carol should role-play the situation described next; observers should take notes about the nonverbal and verbal exchanges and provide feedback. (Consider videotaping the role-play if possible.)

Situation:

Jessica Riley from The Neighborhood *presents for a routine prenatal visit with Carol Ramsey, the Certified Nurse Midwife. Carol notices that Jessica has some bruises on her upper arms and an older bruise under her right eye. Jessica's boyfriend is waiting for her in the waiting room.*

Debriefing:

Following the five- to ten-minute role-play, lead the entire class in a discussion of the following questions:

1. What questions should Carol have asked, and how should they have been asked?

2. What information should be documented on Jessica's record?

3. What information should Carol share with Jessica before she leaves the clinic?

4. What is Carol's legal responsibility in this situation?

FIGURE 3 SIMULATION LEARNING ACTIVITY

Topic: Patient following outpatient colonoscopy with conscious sedation

Target Concepts: Assessment, oxygenation, medication management, communication, safety

Neighborhood Characters/Season Featured: Greg Ross and Benito Jaramillio—Season 1, Episode 14 (and after)

Learning Objectives:

1. Assess patient condition.
2. Recognize abnormal findings.
3. Implement appropriate interventions related to scenario.
4. Demonstrate appropriate therapeutic communication skills during scenario.
5. Reflect on scenario during debriefing; identify missed opportunities related to interventions and communication strategies.

Total Time Allotment for Simulation Activity:	**1 hour**
• briefing for all students	10 minutes
• data gathering	5 minutes
• exchange of report	5 minutes
• assessment of vital signs	5 minutes
• intervention related to vital signs	3 minutes
• response for help	2 minutes
• debriefing	30 minutes

Setting of Simulation Interaction:

• Outpatient procedures unit

Equipment and Props Needed:

• Hospital bed with bedside table and call light
• Blood pressure cuff
• Stethoscope
• Oxygen saturation probe
• Assortment of oxygen delivery devices, including Ambu bag.
• Medication cart (assortment of medications, including Narcan and Romazicon)
• Medical record from procedure
• Drug book
• IV fluid 0.9% NaCL to gravity, TKO rate

Active Participants Needed:

- Student Nurse #1 (to be played by student)
- Student Nurse #2 (to be played by student)
- Primary Nurse (to be played by instructor)
- Ben Jaramillio (to be played by student)

NEIGHBORHOOD LINK: GREG ROSS—SEASON 1, EPISODE 14

Actual Story: Greg continues to have pain and diarrhea and recognizes that he is having an acute exacerbation of colitis. He makes an appointment with the gastroenterologist, who gives Greg a prescription for oral prednisone and sulfasalazine and advises him to drink plenty of fluids. The physician also comments that Greg's blood pressure is 146/96 mm Hg. The gastroenterologist explains that his blood pressure is higher than it should be, and his abdominal pain might have something to do with it. Greg is told to have his blood pressure rechecked when he is feeling better.

What-If Scenario: *What if the gastroenterologist wanted to do a colonoscopy?* Greg's gastroenterologist recommends that he undergo a colonoscopy procedure. Greg goes to the outpatient gastrointestinal lab at Neighborhood Hospital. He has been NPO since breakfast and should tolerate conscious sedation for the procedure. Greg asks Ben to take a break from his intense training to pick him up at the hospital after the procedure. The primary focus of this scenario is communication and appropriate intervention.

Situation:

- Greg has just been transferred from the procedure room to the recovery area following a colonoscopy with conscious sedation.
- Two nursing students are assigned to care for Greg during the recovery period. A primary nurse is working with them. The students receive the report from the primary nurse, who tells them that during the procedure Greg received 10 mg Versed, and 4 mg morphine. The procedure occurred without incident, and Greg is in stable condition. The primary nurse instructs the students to assess Greg and provide post-procedure care.
- Ben is at Greg's bedside. It is expected that Greg will be discharged home within a few hours.

Roles:

Student Nurses: Receive assignment and the patient's chart with the patient history, conscious sedation medications given, and procedure that was completed. The student nurses are expected to get the report from the primary nurse before caring for the patient. The student nurses will have five minutes to review the chart and obtain the report from the primary nurse prior to starting the simulation (accepting care of the patient).

Primary Nurse: Give students their assignment and Greg's medical record to review. Ask students to review chart before getting report. The primary nurse will give report to the students before they begin caring for Greg.

Ben Jaramillio: When student nurses go in to assess Greg, Ben has pushed the call light on and tells the students he thinks something is wrong with Greg. However, he is unable to say what is wrong, other than that Greg just does not seem right. Ben becomes very loud and disruptive the longer it takes for the problem to be determined and action taken.

Scenario Data and Expected Student Behavior:

1. Assess and evaluate Greg's vital signs and level of sedation.
   - Respiratory: respiratory rate of 4 breaths/min, room air SP02 = 80%, decreased breath sounds at the bases; patient will continue to decompensate until reversal agent is given.
   - Neurological: patient is excessively sedated and will continue to become less responsive as time progresses until he receives reversal agent.

2. Assess Safety
   - Safety: side rails of bed will be down x4, and bed will be completely elevated.

3. Therapeutic Communication
   - Ben becomes concerned, overly anxious, and subsequently interferes with care.

4. Expected Student Actions
   - Raise side rails/lower bed.
   - Take a set of vitals.
   - Recognize sedation level and inadequate oxygen exchange.
   - Attempt to arouse patient.
   - Encourage deep breathing and administer proper oxygen delivery system.
   - Review medical record for medications given during procedure and critically think of reversal agent(s).
   - Obtain help from primary nurse if patient remains excessively sedated or there is no improvement in respiratory status.
   - Primary nurse may guide students to the use of a reversal agent for patient.
   - Calm Ben down and communicate they are getting help for Greg.

FIGURE 4 CONCEPT ANALYSIS PAPER

Choose one of the following *Neighborhood* characters—Anthony Martin, Jimmy Bley, or Ryan Riley—and identify three concepts best represented by that character. The following table contains a list of potential concepts.

Examples of Concepts

- Nutrition
- Fluid electrolyte balance
- Thermoregulation
- Oxygenation
- Inflammation
- Infection
- Tissue integrity
- Elimination
- Communication
- Coping
- Stress
- Acid–base balance
- Metabolism
- Perfusion
- Reproduction
- Motion
- Pain
- Fatigue
- Nausea and vomiting
- Family dynamics
- Mood and affect
- Anxiety
- Sleep
- Cellular regulation
- Intracranial regulation
- Clotting
- Sexuality
- Immunity
- Developmental delay
- Addiction
- Interpersonal violence
- Cognitive impairment
- Altered thought process

For each concept, describe the concept (based on the literature) and how the character exemplifies or exemplified the concept (currently or in the past). Comment on the interventions described in the stories, including whether they are consistent with recommended nursing and collaborative care in the literature.

Your paper should not exceed ten double-spaced pages (not including your title page or references). Follow APA style for your citations. You can use your textbooks as references, but you should also use nursing journals. Do not cite lecture notes, PowerPoint presentations, and so on; they are not a substitute for the nursing literature. The idea is that you read, reflect, and then write. Also, you do not need to cite *The Neighborhood* when you include specific examples from the stories.

This paper is worth _____% of your final course grade. Your project will be graded on the following criteria:

Character introduction (_____ points)

Concepts exemplified (_____ points)

Grammar, APA formatting, quality of presentation/references (_____ points)

This project can be done individually or in small groups (no more than four students per group). If you decide to work in a group, be aware that all group members will earn the same grade. Also be aware that after everyone contributes their sections, your group must read each other's work for clarity, use of references, and so on.

HEADINGS TO USE FOR YOUR PAPER

Introduction of Character

Provide a general overview of the character's story. (Pretend your reader does not know the character.) In this overview, you must mention the applicable featured concepts.

Featured Concepts Exemplified

Concept

Description of the concept

How character exemplifies/exemplified this concept

- *Risk factors*

- *Onset of problem*

- *Impact of problem on the character and family*

Interventions done for the character

Concept

Description of the concept

How character exemplifies/exemplified this concept

- *Risk factors*

- *Onset of problem*

- *Impact of problem on the character and family*

Interventions done for the character

Concept

Description of the concept

How character exemplifies/exemplified this concept

- *Risk factors*

- *Onset of problem*

- *Impact of problem on the character and family*

Interventions done for the character

Summary

24

FIGURE 5 NEIGHBORHOOD JEOPARDY

The basic game of Jeopardy requires that teams/players alternate in the selection of a category and points (e.g., "'Teach Me Something' for 400"). They are given an answer, and the team/player must state the question. Correct responses win the corresponding points, and the team/player with the most points at the end of the game wins. If a team/player is unable to answer a question, the opposite team/player gets the opportunity to answer the question and receive the points.

The five categories are linked to *Neighborhood* characters or stories. This can be done with multiple teams competing at the same time in one game or multiple simultaneous games in small groups. Categories can be changed depending on the specific course or class.

In the following example, the table illustrates categories that could be created for a game at any level. The instructor writes the questions/answers for each of the categories (total of 30); questions should get successively more difficult as the point values increase. The sample questions listed at the end of this section could be used as an early Level 1 game as a way to introduce the characters.

Who's Who	Teach Me Something	Name That Concept	Interventions	Drugs
100	100	100	100	100
200	200	200	200	200
300	300	300	300	300
400	400	400	400	400
500	500	500	500	500
600	600	600	600	600

SAMPLE QUESTIONS FOR DRUGS CATEGORY

Drugs 100	**Clue:** Clifford Allen takes this drug as conservative treatment for benign prostatic hyperplasia. **Answer:** What is Proscar?
Drugs 200	**Clue:** Gil Martin takes Atorvastin as a treatment measure for this condition. **Answer:** What is hyperlipidemia?
Drugs 300	**Clue:** Angelo Reyes anticipates long-acting glycemic control with this agent. **Answer:** What is NPH insulin?
Drugs 500	**Clue:** Failure to take this drug places Mrs. James at a very high risk for stroke. **Answer:** What is Coumadin?
Drugs 600	**Clue:** This drug, taken by Danilo Ocampo, is known to reduce mortality following acute myocardial infarction. **Answer:** What is metoprolol?

FIGURE 6 COMPARE AND CONTRAST: SUBSTANCE ABUSE (ALCOHOL) LEARNING ACTIVITY

With your learning group, compare and contrast the stories of *The Neighborhood* characters Casey Holmes, Mark Martin, and Bobby Schofield on several aspects of substance abuse.

	Casey Holmes	Mark Martin	Bobby Schofield
Risk factors for alcohol abuse			
Impact of alcohol on their lives			
Impact of alcohol on lives of others			
How is this typical or not typical of presentation in class or in textbooks?			
What interrelated concepts apply?			

Developed by Jean Giddens, PhD, Professor College of Nursing, University of New Mexico

FIGURE 7 LINKING POLICY TO CLINICAL APPLICATION

1. Go to the Healthy People 2010 Web site (www.healthypeople.gov), and review "Injury and Violence Protection." Which objectives link to preventing problems associated with head injury? For each of these, what supporting information and recommendations are made? (Organize your information using a table like the following example.)

Healthy People 2010 Objective	Information/Recommendations

2. Making links to *The Neighborhood*: Consider the stories of *The Neighborhood* characters and community events depicted in the Neighborhood News. List all examples of evidence in which head injury (from prevention to tertiary care) is represented in *The Neighborhood*. List the character or site, season and episode, and situation. (Organize your information using a table like the following examples.)

Character	Season and Episode	Situation

Neighborhood News	Season and Episode	Situation

Developed by Jean Giddens, PhD, RN, Professor College of Nursing, University of New Mexico

FIGURE 8 FAMILY HISTORY FOR ANTHONY AND KRISTINA MARTIN

Consider the Martin family in *The Neighborhood*. Using character information from *The Neighborhood*, along with the following supplemental information, draw a genogram for Anthony Martin and Kristina Martin. After drawing the genogram, list any risk factors that Anthony and Kristina have.

- Mary Martin (age 75) is the youngest of three children. She is in good health, with the exception of having glaucoma and cataracts. She was married for 52 years to Dominic Martin, who died last year at age 80 of prostate cancer. Mary and Dominic had three children: Gilbert (age 53), Isaac (died in a car accident—DUI at age 20), and Julia (age 49). Julia is a recovering alcoholic and has hypertension.

- Gilbert Martin married Jennifer Sanchez 25 years ago, and they had one son, Mark Martin (age 25). They divorced when Mark was 5 years old. Jennifer has severe asthma; she has not remarried or had other children. Gilbert married Helen Wilson Martin (age 48) 18 years ago. They had two children together: Anthony Martin (age 17) and Kristina Martin (age 16). Helen was previously married to Rick Ames and had one daughter, Tracie Ames (age 20). They divorced soon after Tracie was born.

- Helen has one older brother, Sean Wilson (age 52), who has schizophrenia. Her parents, Jerry and Ruth Wilson, are both deceased. Jerry was an alcoholic and died at age 57 from liver cancer. Ruth died from breast cancer when she was 66.

Adapted from an assignment developed by Mary Wright, RN, MSN College of Nursing, University of New Mexico

FIGURE 9 CONCEPT MAP: PAM ALLEN

Consider the story of Pam Allen from *The Neighborhood*. Pam has colorectal cancer and has undergone a colectomy with colostomy; she is also receiving chemotherapy and radiation therapy. Using the following table, identify what you consider the most significant problems Pam experiences as a result of each of these treatments.

Colectomy and Colostomy	Chemotherapy	Radiation Therapy

Next, draw a concept map that reflects the problems you identified previously. Following is the beginning of a concept map. Add to this map, using the information you identified in the preceding section. Be sure to show the interrelationship of concepts and problems to one another, as well as collaborative interventions that are described in the story or could be applied.

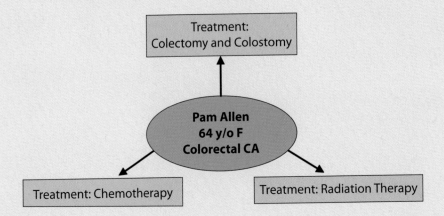

Developed by Jean Giddens, PhD, Professor College of Nursing, University of New Mexico

FIGURE 10 CARING IN *THE NEIGHBORHOOD*: GROUP DISCUSSION AND LEARNING ACTIVITY

Reading assignment as preparation for class:

1. Ocampo family story—Season 1
2. Brilowski, G. & Wendler, C. (2005). An evolutionary concept analysis of caring. *Journal of Advanced Nursing*, *50*(6), 641–650.

With your learning group, complete the following activities:

1. Discuss examples of caring behaviors that Danilo displays toward Lydia.
2. Categorize the caring behaviors by the attributes of caring (i.e., relationship, action, attitude, acceptance, and variability) that are identified in Brilowski and Wendler's article. Give the rationale for the categorization of each behavior.
3. Discuss the care Lydia experienced from Bobby (Lydia's primary nurse) when she was hospitalized in Episode 10. Does Bobby exhibit caring behavior? Why or why not?
4. Develop a plan of care that displays caring for Lydia using the attributes identified by Brilowski and Wendler.
5. Select one member of your learning group to present a summary of your work during the class wrap-up session.

Adopted from an assignment developed by Debra Brady, PhD, Associate Professor College of Nursing, University of New Mexico

FIGURE 11 GARY ALLEN AND COGNITIVE IMPAIRMENT:
SMALL GROUP DISCUSSION

Gary Allen (from *The Neighborhood*) has Down syndrome. In your learning groups, engage in a discussion related to Gary and how he exemplifies impaired cognition.

1. Gary Allen has innate cognitive impairment. What does this term mean?

2. Based on Gary's story, how would you characterize his level of intellectual disability? Base your answer on specific examples from Gary's story.

3. *Gary presents to the emergency department of Neighborhood Hospital after work and tells you it hurts to pee.*

   What questions would you typically ask a male who presented with these symptoms? How would you elicit the same information from Gary?

4. *Gary is diagnosed with a urinary tract infection. The physician prescribes Bactrim for five days.*

   What specific discharge instructions would you write, and how would you explain to Gary how to take his medicine?

Developed by Jean Giddens, PhD, RN, Professor College of Nursing, University of New Mexico

FIGURE 12 CARE PLAN ASSIGNMENT

Develop a care plan for Mrs. James of *The Neighborhood*, focusing on her visit to Karen Williams at the Senior Center in Season 1, Episode 3.

Start by completing the database on the first two pages. This information can be found in her weekly stories and the biographical information.

Biographical Data

Name:	Gender: M F	Age:	Race/Ethnicity:
LMP: Marital Status:		Occupation:	Source/Reliability:

History

Presenting Problem/Chief Complaint:

History of Presenting Problem (Symptom Analysis):

Past Medical and Surgical History (from Biographical Information):

Current Medications (include dose and frequency from Biographical Information):

Allergies:

Family History:

Social History:

Examination Findings

Vital Signs: T   BP   HR   RR

General Survey (overall appearance, gait, level of orientation, etc):

Lower Extremities:

Problem List (Nursing Diagnoses)

NURSING CARE PLAN

CLIENT ID (INITIALS): _____   SETTING: _____   STUDENT: _____   DATE: _____

Assessment Data	Nursing Diagnosis	Expected Client Outcome(s) or Client Goals	Nursing Interventions and Activities	Evaluation

FIGURE 13 DEVELOPING A TEACHING PLAN: GROUP PROJECT

This is a two-part assignment that involves developing a teaching plan and presenting it to the class. You should complete this assignment with your learning group. Your final grade for this assignment will be the average of points for Parts 1 and 2.

Part 1: Developing a Teaching Plan

With your learning group, design a teaching plan for one of the following *Neighborhood* characters. Base all of your work on the character as he or she appears during any point of time during Episodes 1–7, focusing on the identified stage of change.

- Jimmy Bley (preparation stage of change)
- Norma James (precontemplation stage of change)
- Casey Holmes (precontemplation stage of change)
- Jenna Riley (precontemplation stage of change)

For the teaching plan, include all of the following:

1. What data do you need to formulate a comprehensive teaching plan for a client? List the data needed and why. Cite your references.
2. What assessment data do you have that might affect your teaching plan for this individual?
3. Develop five objectives that may be appropriate for your teaching plan.
4. Identify four subjects that you will teach and the methods you will use. State your rationale for the chosen methods and include your references.
5. How would you determine that your teaching plan was effective? What methods would you use to evaluate your teaching?

Part 1 will be graded on the following criteria:

• Assessment data needed with rationale	15 points
• Assessment data you have for your client	15 points
• Objectives and planning	20 points
• Interventions with rationale	20 points
• Evaluation	20 points
• Grammar, spelling, sentence structure, APA format	10 points
Total Points Possible	100 points

Part 2: Student Presentations

After developing the teaching plan, present it to the class, as if you are teaching *The Neighborhood* character. The group may provide a lecture, demonstration, group discussion, gaming application, video, CD, or any other method appropriate to the material being taught to the selected *Neighborhood* character. Each group will have 20 minutes for the presentation.

Part 2 will be graded on the following criteria:

• Presentation is well organized, clear, and effectively structured. Information is presented in a logical, interesting sequence that the audience can follow.	8 points
• Presentation begins with a clear purpose. Objectives are reviewed at the beginning of the presentation and met by the end.	10 points
• Learning objectives, content, and teaching strategies are consistent.	15 points
• The content presented is comprehensive, accurate, and believable.	10 points
• Approach is creative.	10 points
• Conclusion is clear.	5 points
• Class is included in the learning process.	10 points
• There is evidence of balanced group participation in the presentation.	9 points
• Class evaluation of the teaching effectiveness*	15 points
• Self and group analysis*	8 points
Total Points Possible	100 points

Note: Each student will complete an evaluation of teaching effectiveness and evaluate each group member using forms provided by the instructor.

SPECIALTY COURSE USE AND SUGGESTED CHARACTERS

COURSE USE OVERVIEW

This section of the Faculty Navigation Guide links *The Neighborhood* character stories to content typically found in nursing courses. It is important to recognize that this section does not identify *all* possible linkages, because the extension of "what if" applications are not captured here. In addition, note that all of the teaching strategies described in Section I can be applied to most of these links. So, for example, an instructor who is interested in identifying different ways to teach the concept of elimination will find six characters who specifically experience problems related to elimination (see "Nursing Fundamentals—Basic Nursing Skills"). For each of these characters, the instructor could develop multiple types of classroom learning activities. In fact, 50 different character-linked activities could be generated from this concept alone—and this does not include the "what if" scenarios. In addition, a notation (**MR**) is included to indicate that a corresponding medical record is available for the episode and characters. A newspaper link table is provided for each of the courses to lead nursing faculty to additional story enhancements for learning.

The potential applications of *The Neighborhood* stories to learning activities in nursing courses are truly endless, and to list all possible links would be impossible. However, this section is a helpful place to start. *The Neighborhood* Faculty User Forum is envisioned to be a repository of teaching strategies developed by faculty who are willing to share their work with others. Make sure to check this site periodically for newly added learning activities, and consider posting some of your own.

NURSING FUNDAMENTALS—BASIC NURSING SKILLS

Basic nursing principles and skills are featured throughout the stories in all three seasons of *The Neighborhood*. However, because these courses are typically taught in the first semester or term of most nursing programs, the most likely focus is on Season 1 stories. The following tables outline links to fundamental nursing concepts and basic nursing skills.

FUNDAMENTAL CONCEPTS

Concept Focus	Character Season/Episode	Comments
Anorexia	Pam Allen Season 2	As a consequence of chemotherapy and radiation therapy (**MR**)
Communication	Norma James Season 2, Episodes 6–10	Aphasia after stroke (**MR**)
Elimination	Pam Allen, Season 1, Episodes 9–13	Oddly colored and shaped stools; constipation ends up being colorectal cancer; new colostomy and Foley catheter in postoperative period (**MR**)
	Clifford Allen Season 1, Episodes 1–11	Urinary retention associated with benign prostatic hyperplasia (BPH); transurethral prostatectomy (TURP) Season 1, Episode 9: Foley catheter insertion and bladder irrigation (**MR**)

FUNDAMENTAL CONCEPTS *continued*

Concept Focus	Character Season/Episode	Comments
	Greg Ross Season 1, Episode 14 Season 2, Episode 4	Diarrhea associated with acute exacerbation of colitis (**MR**)
	Jessica Riley Season 2, Episode 4	Constipation associated with pregnancy
	Norma James Season 2, Episodes 6, 7	Problems with fecal and urinary incontinence after stroke; Foley catheter insertion (**MR**)
	Eric Young Season 3, Episode 3	Infant diarrhea
End of life	Pam Allen Season 3, Episodes 6–9	End stages of cancer; hospice nurse is involved
Fatigue	Pam Allen Season 1, Episodes 12–15 Seasons 2, 3	Fatigue associated with cancer and cancer treatment (**MR**)
	Danilo Ocampo Seasons 1, 2	Fatigue and activity intolerance associated with chronic condition of heart failure and associated with stress of caregiver role
	Yvonne Johnson All Seasons	Fatigue as a symptoms of systemic lupus erythematosus (SLE)
	Jimmy Bley All Seasons	Fatigue and activity intolerance associated with chronic obstructive pulmonary disease (COPD)
Infection	Norma James Season 1, Episodes 1–4 Season 2, Episode 7	Wound infection (diabetic ulcer); links with Karen Williams at the Senior Center Urinary tract infection from indwelling catheter
	Lydia Ocampo Season 1, Episodes 10–12	Incision infection after open reduction with internal fixation (ORIF); links with nurses at Neighborhood Hospital
	Pam Allen Season 1, Episode 14 Seasons 2, 3	Infection risk postoperatively in Season 1, Episode 14; infection risk in Seasons 2 and 3 associated with chemotherapy
	Ryan Riley Season 1, Episodes 14, 15	Respiratory syncytial virus (RSV) (**MR**)
	Carrie Holmes Season 3, Episode 8	Seen in emergency department for otitis media
	Marcus Young Season 1, Episode 9	Conjunctivitis—acute, one-time event
Mobility	Lydia Ocampo Season 1, Episodes 10–15	Mobility problems after hip fracture; issues continue in other seasons; links with nurses at Neighborhood Hospital (**MR**)
	Norma James Season 2, Episodes 6–10	Mobility issues associated with stroke; rehabilitation

continued

FUNDAMENTAL CONCEPTS *continued*

Concept Focus	Character Season/Episode	Comments
	Mark Martin Season 3, Episodes 4–15	Mobility issues associated with paraplegia after motor vehicle crash
	Marcus Young Season 3, Episodes 5–11	Bicycle accident, multiple fractures; acute care through home care/rehabilitation; links to Neighborhood Newspaper in Season 3, Episode 5
Nausea/Vomiting	Jessica Riley Season 1, Episodes 10, 11	Nausea associated with pregnancy
	Pam Allen All Seasons	Nausea in Season 1 related to postoperative nausea after colectomy; in Seasons 2 and 3, related to chemotherapy and radiation (**MR**)
	Helen Martin Seasons 1, 2	Nausea in Season 1 related to cholelithiasis; Season 2 nausea/vomiting are associated with postoperative status
Nutrition	Ryan Riley Season 1	Failure to thrive evolves over Season 1 (**MR**)
	Jenna Riley Seasons 1, 3	Adolescent obesity; ongoing story
	Helen Martin Season 1	Adult obesity; cholelithiasis; attempts to manage condition through dietary modification
	Norma James Season 2, Episodes 7–10	Swallowing difficulties after stroke lead to need for tube feeding (**MR**)
	Pam Allen Seasons 2, 3	Anorexia, nausea, and vomiting as side effects of chemotherapy and radiation lead to nutritional deficits (**MR**)
	Lydia Ocampo Season 1, Episode 10 Season 3	Dementia and nutrition problems begin after hip fracture and hospitalization; problems accelerate when placed in a nursing home in Season 3
Oxygenation	Jimmy Bley All Seasons	Advanced nursing skills in Season 3, Episodes 7–11 (respiratory failure, use of ventilator, sepsis)
	Ryan Riley Season 1, Episode 14	RSV (**MR**)
	Kelsey Young Seasons 1, 2	Asthma (**MR**)
Pain	Ryan Riley Season 1, Episode 1	Infant pain from colic
	Clifford Allen Season 1, Episode 9	Postoperative pain (bladder spasms) (**MR**)
	Cecelia Bley All Seasons	Chronic pain from osteoarthritis
	Helen Martin Seasons 1, 2	Intermittent pain associated with cholelithiasis
	Gil Martin All Seasons	Chronic back pain in all seasons

FUNDAMENTAL CONCEPTS *continued*

Concept Focus	Character Season/Episode	Comments
	Greg Ross Season 1, Episode 14 Season 2, Episode 4	Pain associated with acute exacerbations of colitis
	Pam Allen Season 1, Episode 14	Postoperative pain (abdominal surgery)
	Carrie Holmes Season 3, Episode 8	Infant pain from diarrhea
Safety	Lydia Ocampo All Seasons	Risk for injury in home; risk for injury while hospitalized due to exacerbated confusion; use of restraints in Season 1, Episode 10 due to combativeness in postoperative period (**MR**); links with nurses at Neighborhood Hospital
Self-care	Lydia Ocampo All Seasons	Dementia; functional limitations
	Danilo Ocampo All Seasons	Limitations due to caregiver issues
Sensory-perceptual	Jimmy Bley Seasons 1–3	Hearing deficits
	Mary Martin Seasons 1–3	Visual deficits; links with Karen Williams at Senior Center
	Angelo Reyes Season 1, Episodes 12–14	Diabetic retinopathy; undergoes surgery for vitreous hemorrhage
Skin integrity	Norma James Season 1, Episodes 1–4	Diabetic foot ulcer on leg; links with Karen Williams at Senior Center
	Lydia Ocampo Season 3, Episodes 2–10	Decubitus ulcer as a consequence of Alzheimer's disease, poor nutritional intake, and nursing home care
	Mark Martin Season 3, Episodes 5–10	Develops a decubitus ulcer as complication of paraplegia
Sleep	Danilo Ocampo Seasons 1, 2	Problems sleeping due to poorly controlled heart failure; caregiver stress—particularly after Season 1, Episode 10
	Lydia Ocampo Season 2, Episodes 8, 9	Dementia; tends to wander at night in Season 2
	Jessica Riley All Seasons	Sleep deprivation associated with multiple roles
Spirituality	Pam Allen Season 1, Episode 7 Season 2, Episodes 5, 6, 9 Season 3, Episodes 8, 9	Active member of church; receives support from members of church; anointing of sick; calls on parish priest (Father John) for spiritual comfort
	Mary Martin Season 3, Episodes 3, 5, 13	Prays for injured grandson

BASIC NURSING SKILLS

Featured Skill/Equipment	Character Season/Episode	Comments
Blood transfusion	Lydia Ocampo Season 1, Episode 11	Transfusion to treat anemia (postoperative complication after ORIF)
Documentation	Kate Swanson Season 1, Episode 1	Describes difficulty finding time to chart; point-of-care charting
	Carol Ramsey Season 1, Episode 2	Describes medical record transfer into a new system and the need to write office notes on a yellow pad
Feeding tube	Norma James Season 2, Episodes 7, 8	After stroke
Foley catheter	Clifford Allen Season 1, Episode 9	Postoperative after TURP—has continuous bladder irrigation (CBI) (**MR**)
	Pamela Allen Season 1, Episode 14	Postoperative after colectomy (**MR**)
	Lydia Ocampo Season 1, Episodes 10–12	Postoperative after ORIF (**MR**); links with nurses at Neighborhood Hospital
	Norma James Season 2, Episodes 6–10	After stroke (**MR**)
Injections (immunizations)	Karen Williams (Senior Center Nurse) Season 1, Episode 11	Supervises nursing students at immunization clinic
Intravenous (IV) therapy	Clifford Allen Season 1, Episode 9	Postoperative after TURP—has CBI (**MR**)
	Pamela Allen Season 1, Episode 14 Seasons 2, 3	Postoperative after colostomy (**MR**) PICC line for chemotherapy (**MR**)
	Lydia Ocampo Season 1, Episodes 10–12	Postoperative after ORIF (**MR**)
	Norma James Season 2, Episodes 6–10	After stroke (**MR**)
	Helen Martin Season 2, Episode 4	After cholecystectomy—IV therapy, including patient-controlled analgesia (PCA)
	Angelo Reyes Season 2, Episode 8	IV therapy associated with Emergency Departmnet (ED) visit for diabetic ketoacidosis (**MR**)
	Danilo Ocampo Season 2, Episode 10	IV therapy associated with ED visit for acute myocardial infarction (AMI)/cardiac arrest (**MR**)
	Jimmy Bley Season 3, Episodes 7–9	IV therapy associated with respiratory failure and sepsis
Nasogastric (NG) tube	Pam Allen Season 1, Episode 14	Postoperative care after colectomy (**MR**)

BASIC NURSING SKILLS *continued*

Featured Skill/Equipment	Character Season/Episode	Comments
Oxygen therapy	Jimmy Bley Season 3, Episodes 7–15	Intubation and subsequent oxygen therapy including oxygen therapy in home
Positioning, transfers, body mechanics	Lydia Ocampo Season 1, Episodes 10–15 Seasons 2, 3	After ORIF (**MR**) Long-term care facility
	Norma James Season 2, Episodes 6–10	Mobility issues associated with stroke; rehabilitation (**MR**)
	Mark Martin Season 3, Episodes 4–15	Mobility issues associated with paraplegia after motor vehicle crash
Postoperative care	Clifford Allen Season 1, Episode 9	After TURP (**MR**)
	Lydia Ocampo Season 1, Episode 10	After ORIF (**MR**); link to nurses at Neighborhood Hospital
	Pamela Allen Season 1, Episode 14	After colectomy (**MR**)
	Helen Martin Season 2, Episode 4	After cholecystectomy
Restraints	Lydia Ocampo Season 1, Episode 10	Use of restraints due to combativeness in postoperative period (**MR**); link to Bobby Schofield in Neighborhood Hospital
	Anthony Martin Season 2, Episode 13	Psychosis, combative, restrained in ED and on unit to ensure safety
Wound care	Lydia Ocampo Season 1, Episodes 10–12 Season 3	Surgical incision decubitus ulcer
	Mark Martin Season 3, Episodes 4–11	Decubitus ulcer

NEWSPAPER LINKS TO FUNDAMENTAL CONCEPTS AND BASIC SKILLS

Topic	Season/Episode
Immunizations (injections)	Season 1, Episode 1
End of life	Season 1, Episode 11
Medication management	Season 3, Episode 5
Nutrition	Season 1, Episode 13 Season 2, Episode 4 Season 2, Episodes 14, 15 (link to Violet Brinkworth) Season 3, Episode 2

continued

NEWSPAPER LINKS TO FUNDAMENTAL CONCEPTS AND BASIC SKILLS *continued*

Topic	Season/Episode
Oxygenation	
Forest fire	Season 2, Episode 5
Smoking ban	Season 2, Episode 12
Sensory-Perceptual	
Hearing loss prevention	Season 2, Episode 8
Macular degeneration	Season 3, Episode 8
Sleep	Season 2, Episode 11

ADULT HEALTH NURSING

Several character stories link closely to topics found in medical–surgical nursing courses. Stories are found in all three seasons; therefore, it is important to remember that, depending on where your course falls in the curriculum, you can use stories from previous seasons. For example, if your course is a Season 2 course, you can use Season 1 and Season 2 stories.

Multiple household characters link directly to medical–surgical concepts. Because the stories are all told from the perspective of the character, it is important to consider the stories of other household members to gain a perspective of the effects of an individual's health-related problem on other members of the household. In addition to the household characters, there are three featured characters in the Neighborhood Hospital and stories in the Neighborhood Newspaper that link to adult health course topics. The following tables present links to topics commonly addressed in adult health/medical–surgical nursing courses.

RESPIRATORY SYSTEM

Problem	Character Season/Episode	Comments
Emphysema	Jimmy Bley All Seasons	Progression of disease from Season 1 to Season 3
Pneumonia	Jimmy Bley Season 3, Episodes 4–7	Evolution of a cough and upper respiratory infection to pneumonia
Respiratory failure Acute phase through transition to home	Jimmy Bley Season 3, Episodes 7–11	Acute exacerbation of emphysema triggered by pneumonia; includes issues associated with transitioning to home and the rehabilitation process due to a deconditioned state after discharge

CARDIOVASCULAR SYSTEM

Problem	Character Season/Episode	Comments
Acute myocardial infarction (AMI)	Danilo Ocampo Season 2, Episode 10	As a complication of poorly managed heart failure (**MR**)
Anemia	Lydia Ocampo Season 1, Episode 11	Links as a complication of ORIF

CARDIOVASCULAR SYSTEM *continued*

Problem	Character Season/Episode	Comments
	Pam Allen Season 1, Episode 14	Rectal bleeding from colorectal cancer
	Yvonne Johnson Season 3, Episode 10	Links as a complication of renal failure
Atrial fibrillation	Norma James All Seasons	Links as a contributory factor to stroke
Heart failure	Danilo Ocampo Seasons 1, 2	Presents typical symptoms and home management; acute exacerbation of symptoms in Season 1, Episodes 11, 14, 15 and in Season 2, Episodes 6–10
Hypertension	Norma James All Seasons	As a comorbid condition
	Danilo Ocampo Seasons 1, 2	As a comorbid condition
	Greg Ross All Seasons	New diagnosis in Season 1, Episode 7; focus is on side effects from antihypertensive medication
Septic shock	Jimmy Bley Season 3, Episode 9	As a complication of pneumonia and respiratory failure

NEUROLOGIC SYSTEM

Problem	Character Season/Episode	Comments

Spinal cord injury
  Acute phase and
    rehabilitation hospital
  Transition and home care
	Mark Martin
	Season 3, Episodes 5–10
	
	Season 3, Episodes 11–15
		Includes issues associated with common complications (depression, decubitus ulcer, autonomic dysreflexia) and impact on family; links to Neighborhood Newspaper in Season 3, Episode 4

Stroke
  Acute phase and
    rehabilitation hospital
  Home care
	Norma James
	Season 2, Episodes 6–14
	
	Season 3, ongoing
		Includes issues with nonadherence to treatment plans in Season 1; multiple complications after stroke (speech, swallowing, incontinence, depression) and caregiving issues with transition home (**MR**); links to Karen Williams at Senior Center

MUSCULOSKELETAL SYSTEM

Problem	Character Season/Episode	Comments
Chronic back pain	Gil Martin Season 1, Episodes 3, 6, 7, 9 Season 2, Episodes 3, 9	Coping mechanisms associated with ongoing chronic pain

Hip fracture
  acute phase
  rehabilitation after ORIF
	Lydia Ocampo
	Season 1, Episodes 10–12
	Season 1, Episodes 13–15
	Season 2, Episodes 1, 2
		Multiple related postoperative complications include delirium, anemia, mobility, and infection (**MR**); multiple issues with rehabilitation and transition home

continued

MUSCULOSKELETAL SYSTEM *continued*

Problem	Character Season/Episode	Comments
Osteoarthritis	Cecelia Bley All Seasons	Story focus for Season 1, Episodes 2 and 6–10; in Season 2, concern regarding addiction to pain medication
Osteoporosis	Mary Martin Season 1, Episodes 7-10	Screening, diagnosis, and treatment

GASTROINTESTINAL SYSTEM

Problem	Character Season/Episode	Comments
Cholelithiasis	Helen Martin Seasons 1– through Season 2, Episode 4	Follows initial symptoms and diagnosis through surgery; postoperative pain and nausea
Colorectal cancer	Pam Allen Season 1, Episode 14 through Season 3	Initial signs occur in Season 1, Episodes 12–14; issues associated with surgical procedure, body image, coping, nausea, vomiting, fatigue, nutrition, and neutropenia; end-of-life issues in Season 3 (**MR**)
Crohn's disease	Greg Ross All Seasons	Exacerbations in Season 1, Episodes 13–15 and in Season 3, Episodes 4, 5. (**MR**)

UROLOGIC SYSTEM

Problem	Character Season/Episode	Comments
Renal insufficiency and failure	Yvonne Johnson Season 3	As a complication of SLE; progression of renal insufficiency to renal failure
Benign prostatic hyperplasia	Clifford Allen Season 1, Episodes 3, 6, 7, 9	Pharmacotherapy ineffective; symptoms progress to need for TURP (**MR**)
Urinary tract infection	Norma James Season 2, Episode 7	Associated with indwelling catheter

METABOLIC AND NUTRITION

Problem	Character Season/Episode	Comments
Obesity	Helen Martin All Seasons	Ongoing issue with weight; linked to gallbladder disease in Seasons 1 and 2
Protein calorie malnutrition	Lydia Ocampo Season 3	Poor nutrition in nursing home
Type 1 diabetes	Angelo Reyes All Seasons	Excellent adherence, well-controlled; complications featured: ketoacidosis and retinopathy
Type 2 diabetes	Norma James All Seasons	Poor adherence and control; complications featured: foot ulcer, hypertension, and stroke

IMMUNE SYSTEM

Problem	Character Season/Episode	Comments
Systemic lupus erythematosus (SLE)	Yvonne Johnson All Seasons	Follows progression of disease from subtle to overt symptoms

ACID BASE/FLUID ELECTROLYTE DISTURBANCES

Problem	Character Season/Episode	Comments
Dehydration/hypernatremia	Angelo Reyes Season 2, Episode 8	Associated with ketoacidosis (**MR**)
Hyperkalemia	Angelo Reyes Season 2, Episode 8	Associated with ketoacidosis (**MR**)
Ketoacidosis	Angelo Reyes Season 2, Episode 8	Also has dehydration and hyperkalemia (**MR**)
Respiratory acidosis	Jimmy Bley Season 3, Episode 7	Associated with emphysema and respiratory failure

VISUAL AND AUDITORY SYSTEMS

Problem	Character Season/Episode	Comments
Cataracts	Mary Martin All Seasons	Undergoes cataract surgery in Seasons 1 and 2
Diabetic retinopathy	Angelo Reyes All Seasons	Experiences vitreous hemorrhage and undergoes vitrectomy in Season 1, Episode 12
Glaucoma	Mary Martin All Seasons	Not the major focus of story, but part of health history
Hearing loss	Jimmy Bley All Seasons	Contributes to communication issues with wife

NEIGHBORHOOD HOSPITAL LINKS

Topic	Season/Episode	Comments
Colon cancer	Bobby Schofield Season 1, Episode 14	Links to Pamela Allen
Hip fracture care	Bobby Schofield Kate Swanson Episodes 10–13	Links to Lydia Ocampo

NEWSPAPER LINKS TO ADULT HEALTH NURSING

Topic	Season/Episode
Blood supply	Season 1, Episode 2
Cancer	
Cancer awareness	Season 2, Episode 3
Skin cancer	Season 2, Episode 8
Breast cancer	Season 3, Episode 13

continued

NEWSPAPER LINKS TO ADULT HEALTH NURSING *continued*

Topic	Season/Episode
Hearing loss prevention	Season 2, Episode 7
Hospital visitation	Season 1, Episode 14
Nutrition	Season 2, Episode 4 Season 2, Episodes 14, 15; links to Violet Brinkworth, school nurse Season 3, Episode 2

Respiratory
  Smoking cessation
  Influenza
  Forest fire
  Smoking ban
	
	Season 1, Episode 9
	Season 1, Episode 11
	Season 2, Episode 5; links to Jimmy Bley
	Season 2, Episode 12

Trauma
  Spinal cord injury
  Pelvic fracture
	
	Season 3, Episode 4; links to Mark Martin
	Season 3, Episode 5; links to Marcus Young

Vision (macular degeneration)	Season 3, Episode 8

MATERNITY AND WOMEN'S HEALTH

Several featured characters in *The Neighborhood* represent women's health issues. The pregnancies of three characters (Jessica Riley, Angie Young, and Rachel Reyes) are followed from conception to birth, detailing prenatal and postpartum care. In all cases, a prenatal medical record is included. The stories of the nurse midwife (Carol Ramsey) provide further examples of pregnancy care and related practice issues. Other women's issues are reflected in the stories of Violet Brinkworth, Helen Martin, and Kristina Martin, and in the Neighborhood Newspaper. Because the stories are told from the perspective of the character, it is important to consider the impact on family members as well. The following tables present links to topics commonly found in maternity and women's health nursing courses.

PREGNANCY

Characteristic	Character Season/Episode	Comments
High-risk pregnancy Cesarean section	Rachel Reyes Seasons 2, 3	Prenatal care; complications include preeclampsia in Season 3, Episode 4; hemolysis, elevated liver enzymes and low platelet count (HELLP) syndrome and premature delivery of twins in Season 3, Episode 5 (**MR**)
Unplanned teen pregnancy	Jessica Riley Seasons 1, 2	Prenatal care; links to domestic violence; abdominal trauma resulting in placental abruption; full-term, healthy infant (**MR**); links to Carol Ramsey, nurse midwife

PREGNANCY *continued*

Characteristic	Character Season/Episode	Comments
Patient care provider—prenatal care, delivery, and postpartum care	Carol Ramsey Seasons 1–3	Nurse midwife; story reflects multiple patient and provider issues
Planned pregnancy	Angie Young Seasons 1, 2	Prenatal care; full-term, healthy infant; no complications (**MR**)

WOMEN'S HEALTH ISSUES

Issue / Condition	Character Season/Episode	Comments
Contraception	Carol Ramsey Season 1, Episodes 6, 7	Nurse midwife patient care provider
	Jessica Riley Season 2, Episode 15	Contraception patch; postpartum anemia; links to Carol Ramsey, nurse midwife.
	Kristina Martin Season 2, Episode 7	Oral contraceptives; links to Carol Ramsey, nurse midwife
Infertility	Rachel Reyes Season 1 Season 2, Episodes 1–6	Infertility workup and treatment; becomes pregnant in Season 2
Menopause	Helen Martin All Seasons	Reference to menopause primarily in Season 1, Episodes 1–3 and Season 2, Episode 8
Sexuality, sexually transmitted infection (STI), and contraception in schools	Violet Brinkworth Season 3, Episodes 4–8	Attempting to provide adequate sex education and contraception in middle and high schools; principal in opposition
Sexually transmitted infection	Kristina Martin Season 3, Episode 5	Chlamydia; links to Carol Ramsey, nurse midwife

NEWSPAPER LINKS TO MATERNITY AND WOMEN'S HEALTH

Topic	Season/Episode
Domestic violence hotline	Season 1, Episode 12
Childbirth classes	Season 2, Episode 1
Domestic violence toward pregnant women	Season 2, Episode 1
Teen pregnancy	Season 2, Episode 7
Gay/lesbian parenting	Season 2, Episode 8
Mother kills newborn infant	Season 3, Episode 8
Gay/lesbian awareness	Season 3, Episode 14

PEDIATRIC AND FAMILY NURSING

There are 13 featured infant, child, and adolescent characters in *The Neighborhood* stories. Infant through toddler-aged characters include Ryan Riley, Carrie Holmes, Eric Young, Peter and Marissa Reyes, and Tyler Martin. School-aged characters include Marcus and Kelsey Young and Jason Riley. Adolescent characters include Jenna Riley, Kristina and Anthony Martin, and Randall Johnson. Some of these characters (Eric Young, Carrie Holmes, Tyler Martin, and the Reyes twins) do not appear in *The Neighborhood* until Seasons 2 or 3. Most of these characters are healthy; their stories reflect well-child visits, typical episodic problems seen among children, or the effect of other situations occurring in the home. When possible, the stories of the younger children reflect their growth and development milestones.

In addition to these stories, stories involving the school nurse character (Violet Brinkworth) can be incorporated because of her interactions with children and adolescents. Finally, several links to pediatric and family nursing content are found in the Neighborhood Newspaper. Because the stories are told from the perspective of the character, it is important to consider the effects on other family members as well. The following tables present links to topics commonly found in pediatric and family nursing courses.

HEALTH PROMOTION AND WELLNESS

Featured Health Topic	Character Season/Episode	Comments
Newborn care	Carrie Holmes Season 2, Episode 13	Full-term infant; describes after-birth care
	Eric Young Season 2, Episode 9	Full-term infant; describes after-birth care
Well child visit and immunizations	Tyler Martin Season 2, Episodes 10, 14 Season 3, Episode 9	Information regarding height/weight, growth charts, vital signs, and immunizations are included
	Ryan Riley Season 1, Episode 3 Season 2, Episode 1 Season 3, Episodes 1, 14	Information regarding height/weight, growth charts, vital signs, and immunizations are included
	Carrie Holmes Season 3, Episode 14	Information regarding height/weight, growth charts, vital signs, and immunizations are included
	Eric Young Season 2, Episodes 9–11 Season 3, Episodes 2, 8, 15	Information regarding height/weight, growth charts, vital signs, and immunizations are included
	Peter and Marissa Reyes Season 3, Episodes 3–13	Information regarding height/weight, growth charts, vital signs, and immunizations are included
	Randall Johnson Season 1, Episode 7	Sports physical examination; does not want mother in room during examination; nurse practitioner gets mother to agree to wait in the waiting room
Screenings in school	Violet Brinkworth Season 1, Episode 4	Hearing and vision screening

HEALTH-RELATED PROBLEMS

Problem	Character Season/Episode	Comments
Allergic reaction	Tyler Martin Season 3, Episode 1	Allergy to peanuts
Asthma	Kelsey Young All Seasons	Ongoing story; has acute exacerbation in Season 2, Episodes 5, 6 (**MR**); links to Violet Brinkworth

HEALTH-RELATED PROBLEMS *continued*

Problem	Character Season/Episode	Comments
Attention deficit hyperactivity disorder	Jason Riley Seasons 1–3	Focus of story is problems in school and issues obtaining diagnostic workup and diagnosis; links to Violet Brinkworth
Colic	Ryan Riley Season 1, Episode 1	ED visit; parent coping
Conjunctivitis	Marcus Young Season 1, Episode 9	Acute, one-time event
Dehydration	Ryan Riley Season 1, Episode 14	RSV and dehydration
	Eric Young Season 3, Episode 3	Dehydration associated with diarrhea
Dental caries	Tyler Martin Season 2, Episodes 8–14	As a result of poor hygiene and bottle mouth
Diabetes mellitus type 2	Jenna Riley Seasons 2, 3	Risk factors present in Season 1; early symptoms in Season 2; formally diagnosed in Season 3, Episodes 3–5
Diarrhea	Eric Young Season 3, Episode 3	Infant diarrhea
Hyperbilirubinemia	Peter and Marissa Reyes Season 3, Episode 5	As a complication of prematurity
Infant respiratory distress syndrome	Peter Reyes Season 3, Episode 5	As a complication of prematurity
Nutrition	Ryan Riley Season 1, Episodes 7, 10, 15	Failure to thrive; poor infant weight gain
	Kristina Martin All Seasons	Obsessed about being thin; excessive intentional weight loss
	Jenna Riley All Seasons	Obesity
Otitis media	Carrie Holmes Season 3, Episode 8	Seen in ED for otitis media
Prematurity	Peter and Marissa Reyes Season 3, Episodes 5–15	As a complication of maternal preeclampsia
Sexually transmitted infection	Kristina Martin Season 3, Episode 5	Chlamydia; links to Carol Ramsey
Trauma	Marcus Young Season 3, Episodes 5–11	Bicycle accident, multiple fractures; story depicts acute care through home care/rehabilitation; links to Neighborhood Newspaper in Season 3, Episode 5
Type 2 diabetes	Jenna Riley Seasons 2, 3	Risk factors present in Season 1; early symptoms in Season 2; formally diagnosed in Season 3, Episodes 3–5

continued

HEALTH-RELATED PROBLEMS *continued*

Problem	Character Season/Episode	Comments
Upper respiratory infection	Eric Young Season 3, Episode 10	Mild case in infant
Upper respiratory infection/RSV	Ryan Riley Season 1, Episode 14 Season 2, Episode 11	Required hospitalization in Season 1 (**MR**)

FAMILY AND SOCIAL ISSUES

Problem	Character Season/Episode	Comments
Domestic violence	Ryan Riley and Carrie Holmes All Seasons	Infant neglect in Season 1; mother is victim of domestic violence; social services follows well-being of children
Chronically ill parent	Randall Johnson All Seasons	Story addresses effect of mother's progressive illness on Randall
	Tyler Martin Season 3	Story addresses effect of traumatic injury on Tyler's father
Family in crisis	Martin family All Seasons	Story addresses effect on family in constant chaos
Parenting stress	Evelyn Riley All Seasons	Extreme stressors dealing with significant issues affecting welfare of all three children and grandchildren
Potential Internet pedophile	Jenna Riley Season 3, Episodes 4–7	Story addresses Internet "boyfriend" and potential risks; links to Neighborhood Newspaper Season 2, Episode 10 and Season 3, Episode 10
Poverty and financial stress	Ryan Riley and Carrie Holmes All Seasons	Mother is single, works at restaurant and receives Medicare and WIC; boyfriend assists with finances at times
	Johnson Family All Seasons	Yvonne loses job and benefits due to chronic illness; effect of change in socioeconomic status on teen

SCHOOL NURSE TOPICS

Problem	Character Season/Episode	Comments
Asthma	Violet Brinkworth Season 2, Episode 5	Kelsey Young has asthmatic attack; school nurse management
Conjunctivitis outbreak management	Violet Brinkworth Season 1, Episode 9	Links to Marcus Young
Drug overdose	Violet Brinkworth Season 3, Episodes 13, 14	Student experiences overdose; principal criticizes school nurse for how she handles situation
Hearing and vision screening	Violet Brinkworth Season 1, Episode 4	Links to Jason Riley
Immunizations	Violet Brinkworth Season 3, Episode 10	Recordkeeping for children in Neighborhood Schools

SCHOOL NURSE TOPICS *continued*

Problem	Character Season/Episode	Comments
Learning problems	Violet Brinkworth Season 1, Episodes 2, 10 Season 2, Episodes 2, 3	Links to Jason Riley
Nutrition in schools	Violet Brinkworth Season 1, Episodes 6, 12 Season 2, Episodes 8, 10, 15 Season 3, Episode 1	Attempts to implement improved nutrition choices in schools and vending machines; encounters resistance from students and parents
Sexuality, STIs, and contraception in schools	Violet Brinkworth Season 3, Episodes 4–8	Attempts to provide adequate sex education and contraception in middle and high schools; principal opposes

NEWSPAPER LINKS TO PEDIATRIC AND FAMILY NURSING

Topic	Season/Episode	Topic	Season/Episode
Immunizations/fears	Season 1, Episode 1	Internet teen site	Season 2, Episode 10
Pertussis death	Season 1, Episode 1	Music benefits, children	Season 2, Episode 11
Extracurricular activity	Season 1, Episode 2	Bicycle safety	Season 2, Episode 14
Poison hotline established	Season 1, Episode 4	Vending machines in schools	Season 2, Episode 15
Traumatic infant death	Season 1, Episode 5	Steroid use, adolescents	Season 3, Episode 1
Health fair	Season 1, Episode 7	Teen cooking class	Season 3, Episode 2
Oral health, children	Season 1, Episode 7	Abduction, rape of child	Season 3, Episode 2
School violence	Season 1, Episode 8	Substance abuse	Season 3, Episode 3
Pit bull attack on child; pit bull ban proposed	Season 1, Episode 10 Season 1, Episode 12	Child trauma	Season 3, Episode 5; link to Marcus Young
Childhood obesity	Season 1, Episode 13	Teen smoking	Season 3, Episode 7
Infant/child car seats	Season 2, Episode 1	Teen mother kills infant	Season 3, Episode 8
Middle school science fair	Season 2, Episode 5	Youth swimming lessons	Season 3, Episode 10
Hearing loss prevention	Season 2, Episode 7	Internet sexual predator	Season 3, Episode 10
Teen pregnancy	Season 2, Episode 7	Boy Scout food drive	Season 3, Episode 12

MENTAL HEALTH NURSING

Several mental health issues are featured in character stories and in the Neighborhood Newspaper. The primary characters who experience mental health challenges include members of the Martin family (Anthony, Helen, Gilbert, Mark, and Kristina), Lydia Ocampo, Clifford Allen, Jimmy Bley, and Bobby Schofield. Because the stories are told from the perspective of the character, it is important to consider the effects their problems have on those around them as well. For the Martin family, this is especially evident. The following tables present links to topics commonly found in mental health nursing courses.

PSYCHOTIC DISORDERS

Problem	Character Season/Episode	Comments
Delirium	Lydia Ocampo Season 1, Episodes 10, 11	Delirium superimposed on dementia triggered by surgical procedure **(MR)**
Schizophrenia	Anthony Martin Seasons 1–3	Early symptoms in Season 1; psychotic break in Season 2, Episode 6

COGNITIVE DISORDERS

Problem	Character Season/Episode	Comments
Attention deficit hyperactivity disorder	Jason Riley All Seasons	Links to teasing, problems with social relationships, and behavioral issues
Dementia	Lydia Ocampo All Seasons	Progressive dementia from Alzheimer's disease and caregiver issues

MOOD DISORDERS

Problem	Character Season/Episode	Comments
Depression	Clifford Allen All Seasons	Primary diagnosis, exacerbated by death of spouse
	Mark Martin Season 3	Situational depression triggered by traumatic injury resulting in paraplegia
	Norma James Season 2, Episodes 6–15	Situational depression triggered by stroke resulting in hemiparesis
	Anthony Martin Season 3, Episode 8	Dual diagnosis with schizophrenia

OTHER MENTAL HEALTH ISSUES

Problem	Character Season/Episode	Comments
Anxiety	Helen Martin All Seasons	Overt symptoms begin Season 1, Episode 9
Domestic violence	Jessica Riley and Casey Holmes All Seasons	Subtle initial indicators of domestic violence that escalates over time, especially with Jessica's pregnancy; links to Carol Ramsey
Eating disorder	Kristina Martin All Seasons	Obsession with thinness; begins excessive dieting in Season 1, Episode 11
Substance abuse	Bobby Schofield All Seasons	Multiple substances; substance abuse as it affects professional nursing practice; diversion program
	Casey Holmes All Seasons	Multiple substances; links to domestic violence
	Mark Martin All Seasons	Alcohol; links to driving while intoxicated and traumatic injury

OTHER MENTAL HEALTH ISSUES *continued*

Problem	Character Season/Episode	Comments
	Clifford Allen Seasons 2, 3	Alcohol; featured as ineffective coping
	Gil Martin All Seasons	Alcohol; featured as ineffective coping

NEWSPAPER LINKS TO MENTAL HEALTH NURSING

Topic	Season/Episode	Topic	Season/Episode
Domestic violence murder story	Season 1, Ongoing story from Episodes 1–14	Rape and homicide	Season 3, Episodes 2–4
		Substance abuse	Season 3, Episode 3
Gun violence	Season 1, Episode 8	Drunk driving	Season 1, Episode 5 Season 3, Episodes 4, 6
Drug use	Season 1, Episode 9 Season 3, Episode 7		
Homeless man's death	Season 1, Episode 11	Maternal-infant homicide	Season 3, Episode 8
Domestic violence hotline	Season 1, Episode 12	Meditation	Season 3, Episode 9
		Sexual predator	Season 3, Episode 10
Domestic violence risks in pregnancy	Season 2, Episode 1	Drug use fatality	Season 3, Episode 11; links to Casey Holmes
Support groups forming	Season 2, Episode 9		
Man exposes self	Season 2, Episode 13; links to Anthony Martin		

GERIATRIC NURSING

There are six featured geriatric household characters in *The Neighborhood*: Danilo and Lydia Ocampo, Jimmy and Cecelia Bley, Norma James, and Mary Martin. In addition, Karen Williams (the geriatric nurse specialist at the Neighborhood Senior Center) is a featured character whose episodely story reflects multiple issues of concern among older adults. The Neighborhood Newspaper also includes multiple references to health-care concerns of older adults. Because the stories are told from the perspective of the character, it is important to consider the effects on other family members as well. The following tables present links to topics commonly found in geriatric nursing courses.

HEALTH-RELATED CONDITIONS

Problem	Character Season/Episode	Comments
Acute myocardial infarction	Danilo Ocampo Season 2, Episode 10	As a complication of poorly managed heart failure **(MR)**
Anemia	Lydia Ocampo Season 1, Episode 11	Links as a complication of ORIF

continued

HEALTH-RELATED CONDITIONS

Problem	Character Season/Episode	Comments
Atrial fibrillation	Norma James All Seasons	Links as a contributory factor to stroke
Cataracts	Mary Martin All Seasons	Undergoes cataract surgery in Seasons 1, 2
Delirium	Lydia Ocampo Season 1, Episodes 10, 11	Delirium superimposed on dementia triggered by surgical procedure
Dementia	Lydia Ocampo All Seasons	Progressive dementia from Alzheimer's disease; caregiver issues
Depression	Norma James Season 2, Episodes 6–15	Situational depression triggered by stroke resulting in hemiparesis
	Clifford Allen All Seasons	Depressive disorder exacerbated by wife's illness and death
Diabetes mellitus type 2	Norma James All Seasons	Poor adherence, poor control; complications featured: foot ulcer, hypertension, and stroke
Emphysema	Jimmy Bley All Seasons	Progression of disease from Seasons 1 to 3
Glaucoma	Mary Martin All Seasons	Glaucoma is part of health history, but not major emphasis of stories; increased intraocular pressure as a result of nonadherence to eye drop regimen
Hearing loss	Jimmy Bley All Seasons	Story focus is the effect of hearing loss on relationship and communication (particularly with his wife)
Heart failure	Danilo Ocampo Seasons 1, 2	Presents typical symptoms and home management; acute exacerbation of symptoms in Season 1, Episodes 11, 14, 15 and in Season 2, Episodes 6–10
Hip fracture Acute phase through rehabilitation	Lydia Ocampo Season 1, Episode 10 Season 2, Episode 2	Multiple related postoperative complications, including delirium, anemia, mobility, and infection; story describes issues with rehabilitation, transitional care, and caregiving **(MR)**
Hypertension	Norma James All Seasons	As a comorbid condition
	Danilo Ocampo Seasons 1, 2	As a comorbid condition
Osteoarthritis	Cecelia Bley All Seasons	Story focus for Season 1, Episodes 2 and 6–10; in Season 2, she has ongoing concern regarding addiction to pain medication
Osteoporosis	Mary Martin Season 1	Screening in Season 1, Episode 7; diagnosis and treatment begin in Season 1, Episode 10
Protein calorie malnutrition	Lydia Ocampo Season 3	As a consequence of progressive dementia and living in nursing home

HEALTH-RELATED CONDITIONS

Problem	Character Season/Episode	Comments
Pneumonia	Jimmy Bley Season 3, Episodes 4–7	Follows the evolution of a "cough" and simple upper respiratory infection to pneumonia
Respiratory acidosis	Jimmy Bley Season 3, Episode 6	Associated with emphysema and respiratory failure
Respiratory failure Acute phase, hospitalization, and transition home	Jimmy Bley Season 3, Episodes 7–11	Acute exacerbation of emphysema triggered by pneumonia; includes issues associated with transitioning to home and the rehabilitation process due to a deconditioned state after discharge
Septic shock	Jimmy Bley Season 3, Episode 9	As a complication of pneumonia and respiratory failure
Stroke Acute phase through rehabilitation	Norma James Season 2, Episodes 6–14 Season 3, Ongoing	Includes issues with noncompliance with treatment plans in Season 1; multiple complications after stroke (speech, swallowing, incontinence, depression) and caregiving issues as she transitions to home **(MR)**

FAMILY AND SOCIAL ISSUES

Problem	Character Season/Episode	Comments
Caregiving	Norma James Season 2, Episodes 11–14 Season 3, Episodes 1–4	Son moves in to be mother's caregiver
	Danilo Ocampo Seasons 1, 2	Managing care of wife with Alzheimer's disease and after hospital discharge; receives assistance from family member for a few episodes; after family member leaves, Danilo Ocampo is overwhelmed
	Cecelia Bley Season 3, Episodes 11–15	Managing care of husband after hospital discharge; receives assistance from family members
	Mary Martin Season 3, Episodes 10–15	Mary becomes Mark's primary caregiver after discharge from spinal cord injury rehabilitation
Financial concerns	Norma James All Seasons	Limited income; payment for medications a concern
	Mary Martin Season 1, Episodes 3, 14	Widow with limited income; moves in with son; cuts corners with glaucoma medication to make it last longer
Functional status	Karen Williams Season 1, Episode 1 Season 3, Episode 7	Assessment of functional status in elderly clients

continued

FAMILY AND SOCIAL ISSUES *continued*

Problem	Character Season/Episode	Comments
Health promotion (elder)	Mary Martin Season 1, Episodes 7, 9, 10	Interest in participation at health fair; compliant with medication and walking to minimize osteoporosis
	Cecelia Bley Season 1, Episode 7 Season 3, Episode 1	Interest in participation at health fair and receiving flu shot; encourages Jimmy to receive flu shots and quit smoking
Power of attorney	Danilo Ocampo Season 1, Episode 6	Initial planning for wife's care in the event that he dies before she does
	Lydia Ocampo Beginning Season 2, Episode 10	No plans were finalized by husband before his death; family attorney has power of attorney over her care
Transitional care	Lydia Ocampo Season 1, Episodes 12–15 Season 2, Episodes 1–3	Issues surrounding discharge coordination and care issues after arriving at home
	Norma James Season 2, Episodes 8–14	Issues surrounding discharge coordination and care issues after arriving at home
	Jimmy and Cecelia Bley Season 3, Episodes 11–15	Issues surrounding discharge coordination and care issues after arriving at home

SENIOR CENTER NURSE TOPICS

Topic	Character Season/Episode	Comments
Elder abuse	Karen Williams Season 1, Episode 12	Recognizes possible elder abuse; contacts social services; links to Neighborhood Newspaper in Season 2, Episode 9
Independent living	Karen Williams Season 1, Episode 1	Family attempting to "force" man into moving to assisted living
Health-care access	Karen Williams Season 1, Episodes 3, 10 Season 2, Episode 14	Facilitates and encourages seniors to obtain appointments for various conditions
Health promotion	Karen Williams All Seasons	Smoking Awareness Episode, Season 1, Episode 9 Flu Vaccinations, Season 1, Episode 11 Senior Center Outing, Season 2, Episode 2 Fitness for Elders, Season 3, Episode 13 (links to Neighborhood Newspaper)
Health teaching	Karen Williams All Seasons	Osteoporosis—Mary Martin, Season 1, Episode 14 Forest fire—Season 2, Episode 5 Cataract surgery—Season 2, Episode 15 Medication management—Season 3, Episodes 3, 5
Professional boundaries	Karen Williams Season 2, Episode 1	Sets limits with seniors who request special assistance and favors
Social isolation	Karen Williams Season 1, Episode 10 Season 3, Episodes 1, 7	Recognizes social isolation among some residents

NEWSPAPER LINKS TO GERIATRIC NURSING

Topic/Concept	Season/Episode	Topic/Concept	Season/Episode
Retirement community planned	Season 3, Episode 6	Caregiver issues	Season 2, Episode 9
Flu shots at senior center	Season 1, Episode 11	Elder abuse in nursing home	Season 2, Episode 9
Flu deaths rising	Season 1, Episode 11	Retirement financial concerns	Season 2, Episode 13
Senior center outing	Season 2, Episode 2; links to Karen Williams	Medication management	Season 3, Episode 5; links to Karen Williams
Senior center visits rising	Season 2, Episode 2; links to Karen Williams	Macular degeneration	Season 3, Episode 8
Pet therapy	Season 2, Episode 2	Elder exercise	Season 3, Episode 13

COMMUNITY HEALTH

There are multiple opportunities to use and apply *The Neighborhood* stories in community health courses. Topics found in the character stories and the Neighborhood Newspaper span all types of community events. In the following table, various community topics that are commonly addressed in community health courses are described, along with the character or characters.

COMMON COMMUNITY HEALTH TOPICS

Topic	Character Season/Episode	Comments
Battered women's shelter	Jessica Riley Season 3, Episodes 9–11	Seeks protection from Casey with her two children
Community assessment	Not applicable	Go to Community Facts link on home page for listing of community health-care resources, demographics, jobs, income, and so on
Community health department	Kristina Martin Season 2, Episode 7 Season 3, Episode 5	Utilizes the community health department for oral contraceptives and for sexually transmitted infection workup
	Mark and Tyler Martin Season 2, Episode 14 Season 3, Episodes 2, 9	Free immunizations and dental care
Forest fire	Community event Season 2, Episode 5	Mentioned in several stories, most significant effect on Jimmy Bley and staff at Neighborhood Hospital
Health fair	Mary Martin and the Bley and Young Families Season 1, Episode 7	Events and screening described within stories; links to Neighborhood Newspaper, Season 1, Episode 7
Immunizations	See Pediatric and Family Nursing	
Public safety	Angie Young Season 3, Episodes 9–13	Attempts to lobby city to install speed bumps; links to Neighborhood Newspaper, Season 3, Episodes 11 and 13
Smoking ban	Bobby Schofield Season 1, Episode 9	Links to Neighborhood Newspaper, Season 1, Episode 9

NEWSPAPER LINKS TO COMMUNITY HEALTH

Topic/Concept	Season/Episode
Blood supplies	Season 1, Episode 2 (×2)
Citizen deaths	
Domestic homicide	Season 1, Episodes 4–14
Homeless man	Season 1, Episode 11
Infant murder	Season 3, Episode 8
Child abduction, rape	Season 3, Episodes 2, 3
Community activities	
Senior center trip	Season 2, Episode 2 (links to Karen Williams)
Science fair	Season 2, Episode 5
Cardiopulmonary resuscitation (CPR) class	Season 2, Episode 10
Music event	Season 2, Episode 11
Special Olympics	Season 2, Episodes 13-14 (links to Gary Allen)
Running club	Season 3, Episode 4
Medication management lecture	Season 3, Episode 5 (links to Karen Williams)
Macular degeneration lecture	Season 3, Episode 8
Swimming lessons	Season 3, Episode 10
Gay/lesbian awareness	Season 3, Episode 14
Community health policy	
Workplace smoking ban	Season 1, Episode 9
Pit bull ban	Season 1, Episode 12
MP3 player ban	Season 2, Episode 7
Junk food ban	Season 2, Episodes 14, 15 (links to Violet Brinkworth)
Citywide smoking ban	Season 2, Episode 12
Substance abuse	Season 3, Episodes 3, 6
Trash burning ban	Season 3, Episode 11
Speed bumps	Season 3, Episodes 11, 13
Community services	
Poison control hotline	Season 1, Episode 4
Domestic violence	Season 1, Episodes 6, 12 Season 3, Episode 7
Homeless shelter	Season 3, Episode 12
Senior center	Season 2, Episode 2 (links to Karen Williams)
Support group	Season 2, Episode 9
Dental screenings	Season 2, Episode 8 (links to Tyler Martin)
Grief and bereavement	Season 3, Episode 1
Meditation group	Season 3, Episode 9

Topic/Concept	Season/Episode
Epidemics/outbreaks	
Influenza outbreak	Season 1, Episode 11
Childhood obesity	Season 1, Episode 13
Teen smoking increasing	Season 3, Episode 7
Spider bites	Season 3, Episode 12
Cancer mortality rising	Season 3, Episode 13
Environmental health	
Water pollution	Season 1, Episode 3 (×2)
Smoking ban	Season 1, Episode 9 Season 2, Episode 12
Forest fire	Season 2, Episode 5
Noise control	Season 2, Episode 11
Water supply	Season 3, Episode 6
Trash burning	Season 3, Episode 11
Health-care issues	
Caregiver issues	Season 2, Episode 9 (links to Danilo Ocampo)
Teen pregnancies	Season 2, Episode 7
Sleep deprivation	Season 2, Episode 11
Health care facilities	
Cancer center	Season 1, Episode 15 Season 2, Episodes 3, 12
Retirement community	Season 3, Episode 6
Immunizations	Season 1, Episode 1 (×4) Season 1, Episode 11
Injury prevention	
Child safety seats	Season 2, Episode 1
Bicycle safety	Season 2, Episode 14 (links to Young family)
Occupational health	Season 1, Episodes 2, 9
Occupational injury	Season 3, Episode 1
Public safety issues	
Terrorism	Season 1, Episode 4
Substance abuse	Season 1, Episodes 5, 9 Season 3, Episodes 3, 4 (links to Mark Martin) Season 3, Episode 11 (links to Casey Holmes)
Gun scare at school	Season 1, Episode 8
Pit bull attack	Season 1, Episode 10
Domestic violence	Season 2, Episode 1
Internet predators	Season 2, Episode 10 Season 3, Episode 10 (links to Jenna Riley)
Bicycle injury	Season 3, Episode 5 (links to Marcus Young)

NURSING LEADERSHIP AND PROFESSIONAL CONCEPTS COURSE

The nurse character stories provide the basis for most of the links made to content that is typically taught in a leadership or professional nursing roles course. Concepts are divided between typical practice issues and roles of professional nurses. The Neighborhood Newspaper also presents stories that provide the basis for many learning activities. The following tables summarize the content, concepts, character stories, and newspaper linkages that can be made.

PROFESSIONAL PRACTICE ISSUES

Topic/Issue	Character Season/Episode	Comments
Bed control	Kate Swanson Pat Richman Season 2, Episode 5	Bed control due to excessive hospital admissions and ED need associated with forest fire; links to Neighborhood Newspaper, Season 2, Episode 5
Budget	Karen Williams Season 2, Episode 2 Season 3, Episode 6	Budget restraints in clinic; must justify service for funding; writes letter to request additional funding
Ethics	Lydia Ocampo Season 1, Episode 10	Placed in restraints; links to Bobby Schofield, who medicated her to keep her quiet
	Violet Brinkworth Season 2, Episode 6 Season 3, Episode 1	Medical privacy issues; links to Health Insurance Portability and Accountability Act (HIPAA)
	Kate Swanson Pat Richman Season 3, Episodes 3, 4	Accused rapist and murderer on inpatient unit reporting poor care; links to Neighborhood Newspaper, Season 3, Episodes 2–4
Impaired nurse	Bobby Schofield All Seasons	Closely links to stories of Kate Swanson and Pat Richman; story progresses from initial behavior to diversion program with the Board of Nursing
Insurance and payment systems	Jessica Riley Biography page	WIC assistance and Medicaid
	Mary Martin Season 1, Episode 14	Prescription assistance program
	Gil Martin Season 2, Episode 15 Anthony Martin Season 3, Episode 8	Maxes out insurance coverage for mental health
	Yvonne Johnson Season 3, Episodes 8, 12–14	Loses job and insurance; COBRA insurance coverage, attempting to obtain social security disability
Legal—power of attorney	Danilo Ocampo Season 1, Episode 6 Lydia Ocampo Season 2, Episodes 11, 12	When Danilo dies, Lydia has no family to care for her

continued

PROFESSIONAL PRACTICE ISSUES *continued*

Topic/Issue	Character Season/Episode	Comments
Mandatory reporting	Karen Williams Season 1, Episode 12	Suspects elder abuse, notifies social services
	Kate Swanson Pat Richman Season 2, Episodes 5, 6	Suspects drug impairment of staff nurse; links to Bobby Schofield
Medical records	Carol Ramsey Season 1, Episode 2	Describes difficulty associated with transferring old medical records into a new computerized system.
	Violet Brinkworth Season 1, Episode 13 Season 3, Episode 10	Maintaining and updating medical records of students in Neighborhood Schools
Nursing shortages and workload	Pat Richman All Seasons	Ongoing theme in story
	Kate Swanson Season 1, Episodes 1–3, 6, 15 Season 2, Episode 3	Increased patient loads in context of hospital inpatient unit
	Bobby Schofield Season 1, Episode 2	Staffing shortages in context of hospital inpatient unit
	Violet Brinkworth Season 1, Episode 5	Shortage of help; issues associated with covering three schools
	Karen Williams Season 2, Episode 2	Increasing number of senior visits to clinic despite reduced nursing hours
	Carol Ramsey Season 1, Episodes 1, 14 Season 3, Episodes 1, 13	Increasing patient loads in context of advance practice nurse in group practice
Nursing strike	Kate Swanson Pat Richman Season 3, Episodes 5–10	Links to Neighborhood Newspaper, Season 3, Episodes 5, 8–10
Policy	Neighborhood Hospital nurses Season 2, Episodes 5, 6	Mandatory overtime policy announced; eventually leads to strike
	Pat Richman Season 2, Episodes 13, 14	Employee policy for drug testing
	Violet Brinkworth Season 3, Episodes 13, 14	School principal disciplines Violet for not following after-school policy regarding notification for health-care emergencies
	Karen Williams Season 3, Episode 6	Letter writing for clinical financing
Recruitment	Karen Williams Season 2, Episode 10 Violet Brinkworth Season 3, Episode 9	Calls from nurse recruiter with job offer at Neighborhood Hospital
	Pat Richman Season 1, Episodes 1, 7 Season 3, Episode 10	Recruitment and hiring of hospital nurses

PROFESSIONAL PRACTICE ISSUES *continued*

Topic/Issue	Character Season/Episode	Comments
Referral/collaboration of care	Violet Brinkworth Season 1, Episode 9 Season 2, Episode 5 Season 3, Episodes 2, 13	Several examples of referral to another health-care provider based on assessment and clinical judgment
	Carol Ramsey Season 1, Episode 9 Season 2, Episodes 3, 12	Examples of referral to another health-care provider based on assessment and clinical judgment
	Karen Williams Season 1, Episode 3 Season 3, Episode 12	Examples of referral to another health-care provider based on assessment and clinical judgment
Social services	Jessica Riley Season 1, Episode 15 Season 2, Episodes 13, 14	Social services involved due to concern for child safety; links to Carrie Holmes and Ryan Riley, Season 3, Episodes 2, 6
Workplace morale	Pat Richman All Seasons	Story from perspective of nurse manager
	Kate Swanson Season 2, Episodes 5-6	Story from perspective of staff nurse

ROLES OF THE PROFESSIONAL NURSE

Role/Behavior	Character Season/Episode	Comments
Advocate	Karen Williams Season 1, Episodes 3, 10–12 Season 2, Episodes 8, 14 Season 3, Episodes 7,11	Examples of patient advocacy in her practice
	Carol Ramsey Season 2, Episodes 11, 12 Season 3, Episodes 2, 3	Examples of patient advocacy in her practice
	Kate Swanson Season 2, Episode 4	See Bobby Schofield, Season 1, Episode 10 for example of lack of advocacy
Boundary setting	Karen Williams Season 2, Episode 1	Role-modeling
Care provider	Kate Swanson All Seasons	Context of acute care in hospital, new graduate
	Bobby Schofield All Seasons	Context of acute care in hospital
	Karen Williams All Seasons	Context of community care in senior center

continued

ROLES OF THE PROFESSIONAL NURSE *continued*

Role/Behavior	Character Season/Episode	Comments
	Violet Brinkworth All Seasons	Context of community-based care in schools
	Carol Ramsey All Seasons	Context of advanced nursing practice
Community service	Kate Swanson Season 1, Episodes 1, 11 Season 2, Episode 3	Volunteer at immunization clinic Volunteer at senior center for flu shots Volunteer at Walk for Life event
	Carol Ramsey Season 2, Episode 1	Teaches childbirth classes as community service
Educator	Karen Williams Season 1, Episodes 9–11, 14 Season 2, Episodes 5, 15 Season 3, Episodes 3, 5, 10, 11	Multiple examples of teaching as a component of nursing practice
	Carol Ramsey Season 1, Episode 6 Season 2, Episodes 1, 7, 15 Season 3, Episodes 5, 7	Multiple examples of teaching as a component of nursing practice; teaches childbirth classes as community service
	Violet Brinkworth Season 3, Episodes 4–8	Sex education classes in the middle school
Empathy	Kate Swanson Season 1, Episodes 10–13 Season 2, Episode 10	Empathy, attachment, and grief related to Mr. and Mrs. Ocampo; see Bobby Schofield, Season 1, Episodes 8, 14 for examples of lack of empathy

Linking to community resources	Karen Williams
	
	Season 1, Episode 3
	
	Season 1, Episode 10
	Season 3, Episodes 1, 7
		Mrs. James—transportation to
		   physician office
		Mrs. James—properly
		   fitting shoes
		Brian James—transitional care
		Senior Center Ride Service

Manager/leader	Pat Richman All Seasons	Nurse manager at Neighborhood Hospital
Orientation/mentor	Carol Ramsey Season 3, Episode 7	Begins process of orienting and mentoring a new midwife who has joined the practice
	Violet Brinkworth Season 2, Episode 11	Begins process of orienting two new health aides to work at schools
Professional behavior	Kate Swanson, Karen Williams All Seasons	These two characters are positive role models of professionalism (with a few exceptions on Kate's part)

NEWSPAPER LINKS TO NURSING LEADERSHIP AND PROFESSIONAL CONCEPTS

Topic/Concept	Season/Episode	Topic/Concept	Season/Episode
Accreditation (hospital)	Season 3, Episode 14	**Policy**	
Bed control (inpatient)	Season 1, Episode 7	Workplace smoking	Season 1, Episode 9
	Season 2, Episode 5	Citywide smoking ban	Season 2, Episode 12
		Pit bull ban	Season 1, Episode 12
Ethics/legal issues		Visitation policy	Season 1, Episode 14
Gay/lesbian rights	Season 2, Episode 8	Advance directive	Season 1, Episode 14
Nursing home abuse	Season 2, Episode 9	Mandatory overtime	Season 2, Episode 6
Withholding treatment	Season 3, Episode 4	MP3 player ban	Season 2, Episode 7
Negligence incident	Season 3, Episode 7	Junk food ban	Season 2, Episodes 14, 15
		Trash burning ban	Season 3, Episode 11
Health care financing	Season 2, Episode 13	Speed bumps	Season 3, Episodes 11, 13
Nursing shortage			
Nurses quitting jobs	Season 1, Episode 8		
Health-care career fair	Season 1, Episode 8		
Unfilled positions	Season 2, Episode 3		
Nursing schools	Season 2, Episode 6		
Nursing shortage	Season 2, Episode 6		
task force	Season 3, Episode 14		
Nursing strike	Season 3, Episodes 5, 8–10		

HEALTH PROMOTION

Health promotion concepts are represented throughout the character stories and the Neighborhood Newspaper. For this reason, health promotion courses link well to *The Neighborhood* regardless of the placement of the course within the curriculum. Several characters make ongoing efforts to improve or enhance health, whereas others do not seem to give much thought to health promotion behaviors. The following tables summarize the links that can be made in character stories and the Neighborhood Newspaper.

CHARACTER STORIES

Topic	Character Season/Episode	Comments
Childbirth classes	Carol Ramsey Season 2, Episode 1 Angie and Steve Young Season 2, Episode 1 Rachel and Angelo Reyes Season 2, Episode 15	Describes plans to attend classes or teach classes; links to Neighborhood Newspaper, Season 2, Episode 1
Dental screening and community-based dental care	Mark Martin, Tyler Martin , Tracie Ames Season 2, Episodes 8, 14 Season 3, Episode 2	Aunt Tracie takes Tyler to screening; follow-up dental work needed

continued

CHARACTER STORIES *continued*

Topic	Character Season/Episode	Comments
Exercise and fitness	Ben Jaramillo All Seasons	Exercise as a way of life
	Kate Swanson Season 1, Episode 3 Season 2, Episode 3 Season 3, Episode 13	Run for the Fish participant; having trouble finding time for exercise; Walk for Life organizer; aerobics class
	Karen Williams Season 3, Episode 13	Geriatric exercise
Health fair	Mary Martin, Bley and Young Familes, Carol Ramsey Season 1, Episode 7	Events and screening described within stories; links to Neighborhood Newspaper, Season 1, Episode 7
Hearing and vision screening	Violet Brinkworth Season 1, Episode 4	Screening at Neighborhood School; links to Jason Riley
Hearing protection	Casey Holmes Season 1, Episode 4	Context of on-the-job ear protection
Immunizations	See Pediatric and Family Nursing	
Medication management (elders)	Karen Williams Season 3, Episode 5	Links to Neighborhood Newspaper
	Norma James Season 1, Episode 13 Season 2, Episodes 2, 11	Refilling prescription Hoarding medications
Nutrition	Violet Brinkworth Seasons 1–3, ongoing	Efforts to improve nutrition at school
Safe sex/sex education	Carol Ramsey Season 1, Episodes 6, 7 Season 2, Episode 7 Season 3, Episode 5	At health fair and with clients; links to Kristina Martin
	Violet Brinkworth Season 3, Episodes 4, 6, 7	School-based education and resistance from principal
Smoking cessation	Steve Young Season 1, Episodes 4–6 Season 2, Episode 12 through Season 3	Depicts one unsuccessful attempt to stop smoking, followed by success
	Jimmy Bley Season 1, Episodes 8–12 Season 2, Episodes 3–6 Season 2, Episodes 10–14	Depicts three unsuccessful attempts to stop smoking
Prenatal care	See Maternity and Women's Health	
Well infant and child care	See Pediatric and Family Nursing	

NEWSPAPER LINKS TO HEALTH PROMOTION

Topic/Concept	Season/Episode
Immunizations	Season 1, Episode 1 (×4)
	Season 1, Episode 11
Cancer prevention	
Walk for Life	Season 2, Episode 3
Skin cancer	Season 2, Episode 8
Community health fair	Season 1, Episode 7
Diet and nutrition	Season 2, Episode 4
	Season 3, Episode 2
Exercise and fitness	
Community exercise initiative	Season 1, Episode 13
Running club	Season 3, Episode 4
Elder exercise	Season 3, Episode 13
Swimming lessons	Season 3, Episode 10
Hearing loss prevention	Season 2, Episode 7

Topic/Concept	Season/Episode
Health promotion classes	
Smoking cessation	Season 1, Episode 9
Childbirth classes	Season 2, Episode 1
Elder exercise class	Season 3, Episode 13
Healthy cooking class	Season 3, Episode 2
Medication management	Season 3, Episode 5
Injury prevention	
Child safety seats	Season 2, Episode 1
Bicycle safety	Season 2, Episode 14
Sports injuries	Season 2, Episode 3
Occupational health	Season 1, Episode 2
Oral health	
Cavity prevention	Season 1, Episode 7
Dental screenings	Season 2, Episode 8

FEATURED CHARACTER OVERVIEWS AND STORIES

HOUSEHOLD CHARACTERS

Key: **[P]** = photograph   **[VC]** = video clip   **[MR]** = medical record

ALLEN HOUSEHOLD

ALLEN FAMILY STORY OVERVIEW

Character	Season 1	Season 2	Season 3
CLIFFORD ALLEN	Clifford is generally well and has plans to retire in the next couple of years. During this season he is diagnosed with BPH and has a TURP after trying unsuccessful medical treatment. Shortly after this, his wife is diagnosed with colorectal cancer. When Pam has surgery, Clifford takes off work to care for Pam and Gary.	During this season, Clifford is overwhelmed as he takes care of Pam (while she undergoes chemotherapy and radiation) and Gary. He experiences insomnia and weight loss, and begins drinking alcohol in the evenings as a coping measure.	Pam has a recurrence of cancer. When she elects to stop treatment, Clifford becomes very depressed. After Pam dies, he struggles with grief, loss and depression. He makes a decision to retire and care for Gary on a full-time basis.
PAM ALLEN	Pam is a middle-aged woman who presumes to be in perfect health. She spends most of her time managing the home and caring for Gary. After experiencing rectal fullness and blood in her stool, Pam is diagnosed with advanced stage colorectal cancer. She has surgery and prepares for chemotherapy and radiation treatment.	Pam undergoes chemotherapy and radiation on an outpatient basis. She experiences stomatitis, nausea, diarrhea, and fatigue. She finds it difficult to keep up with home management and caring for Gary. Following chemotherapy, Pam feels pretty good for a while and begins to believe she has beaten the cancer.	At the beginning of Season 3, Pam learns that the cancer has metastasized to her liver and pancreas. She initially agrees to undergo chemotherapy again, but shortly after decides to stop treatment. The focus of story is around end-of-life care issues and family coping responses. Pam dies during this Season.
GARY ALLEN	Gary is a generally health adult male with Down syndrome. He lives at home and works at a grocery store. He is involved in many activities and depends on his parents for transportation and most daily activities	Gary knows that his mother is sick, but does not really comprehend what is going on. He continues to work, but recognizes the stress within the home.	Gary is greatly impacted by his mother's illness and has a loss of consistency in his routine. In an attempt to protect him, Clifford sends Gary to live with friends for the last few weeks of his mother's life.

CONCEPTS   *Body Image, Coping, Cognitive Grief, Impairment, Elimination, End of Life, Family Dynamics, Immunity, Interpersonal Relationships, Mood and Affect, Nutrition, Pain, Role Performance, Sexuality, Sleep, Spirituality*

CLIFFORD ALLEN
Season 1

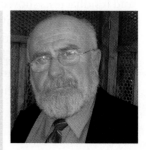

Biographical Information

Clifford is a 64-year-old male who has been married to his wife Pam for 40 years. Their only child, 24-year-old Gary, has Down syndrome and lives with them. Clifford is a middle manager for a small manufacturing company, where he has worked for the past 20 years.

Overall, Clifford is in good health, although he has recently been undergoing conservative treatment for benign prostatic hypertrophy. He has a history of depression and his brother committed suicide as a teenager. Clifford had a brief episode during college, for which he did not seek treatment. He had another episode shortly after Gary was born. At that time, with encouragement from his wife, Clifford sought treatment, which consisted of counseling and antidepressant agents. He quit taking the medications after about 6 months and decided he would just learn to deal with depression on his own. Although he has had mild episodes of depression over the years since that time, Clifford has been unwilling to seek treatment because he fears the social stigma associated with being labeled as medically depressed. He is also concerned that his employer will find out about it through his use of the medical benefits. It is Clifford's opinion that his employer would perceive depression as a sign of weakness. Overall, he has done well without the medications.

Clifford has been thinking about retiring within the next few years. He and his wife have always planned to do some traveling, but mostly he looks forward to being able to escape the busy and stressful work environment. Clifford and Gary are involved with activities at their church; they also enjoy a walk each evening after supper. Clifford belongs to a bowling league and is at the bowling alley a few evenings each week.

Episode 1
No news this week.

Episode 2
After dinner, Clifford and Gary go for a walk. Then they go to the bowling alley for the evening. Clifford notices that his bladder feels somewhat full while bowling. **[P]**

Episode 3
Clifford calls to make an appointment to see his urologist for a follow-up examination for his benign prostatic hypertrophy (BPH) treatment. He has been taking finasteride (Proscar) for the past 6 months, but he doesn't feel that it's been particularly effective. He still has problems urinating and, in fact, believes his symptoms are worse than they were before he started taking the medication. Although Clifford reported the lack of improvement of his symptoms to his physician several months ago, he was asked to "stick with" the medication regimen for 6 months and then return for a reevaluation of his condition. When he calls the office, Clifford learns that the physician is booked through the end of the week and out of town the following week. **[P]**

Episode 4
No news this week.

Episode 5
No news this week.

Episode 6
Clifford sees the urologist this week. He shares with the physician that he often feels as if his bladder is full after voiding, he has a hard time starting his stream, and, when he does void, the urinary stream is weak. He also reports that he gets up frequently at night to void. His score on the American Urological Association Symptom Index is 28. Six months ago, his score was 18. Based on the current symptoms and findings from the digital rectal exam, the urologist confirms with Clifford that the medication has not been effective. He schedules Clifford for further tests, including an outpatient uroflometry test, a post-void residual test, a prostate-specific antigen (PSA) blood test, and a urinalysis. **[VC]**

Episode 7
This week, Clifford undergoes the uroflometry test, the post-void residual test, and a PSA test at the outpatient

diagnostics clinic. Results from the uroflometry and post-void residual tests show a significant obstruction of urinary flow. The PSA is negative, and the urinalysis is consistent with bladder inflammation. In a follow-up phone call, the urologist shares with Clifford the results of the tests and recommends a transurethral resection of the prostate (TURP) procedure in the upcoming weeks. **[P]**

Episode 8
No news this week.

Episode 9
This week, Clifford is admitted to Neighborhood Hospital for a TURP procedure. He has been very anxious about having the procedure performed because of the potential complication of impotence.

Clifford's surgery goes smoothly, and he experiences no complications. In the immediate postoperative period, he has a three-way Foley catheter with continuous bladder irrigation. He experiences pain and has occasional bladder spasms due to blood clots. Two days after surgery, the catheter is removed, and Clifford is discharged home. He is somewhat distressed on the day he goes home because he experiences some uncontrolled dribbling. He performs Kegel exercises, as instructed by the discharge nurse. **[MR] [VC]**

Episode 10
Clifford remains off work, recovering from the TURP procedure. He is having fewer problems with dribbling and is relieved that he does not have a problem with impotence. Clifford is anxious to go back to work. **[P]**

Episode 11
Clifford is feeling much better and enjoys the newfound ease of urinating. The dribbling has also subsided. He wishes he had been more assertive with the physician and had the surgery earlier. He goes back to work, but is still feeling very tired at the end of the day. He realizes that the surgery took more out of him than he had expected. **[P]**

Episode 12
No news this week.

Episode 13
Pam shares with Clifford that she is having routine follow-up tests at the physician's office this week. He does not think too much about this news and is focused on catching back up with work. **[P]**

Episode 14
Clifford is shocked when he gets a phone call from Pam informing him that she is being admitted to the hospital and needs surgery. He immediately worries about the possibility of cancer. He leaves work at once to be with Pam.

The following day, Clifford and Gary stay at the hospital most of the day. Immediately after surgery, the physician talks with Clifford at length to explain Pam's condition. As soon as the physician says "colon cancer," Clifford is in such a state of shock that he does not hear anything else that is said. He has a hard time interpreting just what is going on. **[P]**

Episode 15
Clifford takes the entire week off work to take care of Pamela and Gary. He finds the colostomy bag on Pam's abdomen disgusting and avoids looking at it unless he must. Clifford refuses to believe that the prognosis is poor; he knows Pam was cured of cancer last time, and he is sure she can do it again. He is angry with her when she tells him that she is not sure she wants to go through with chemotherapy and radiation.

Clifford feels overwhelmed with the job of managing the home, taking care of Gary, and helping Pam. He is accustomed to Pam taking care of most things and has a hard time getting organized; in fact, he often finds himself sitting in a chair in the living room, staring at the walls, unable to get anything done. Clifford takes Gary to and from work all week and, although he shares with Gary that his mother is sick and had to have surgery, he does not elaborate on Pam's condition. **[VC]**

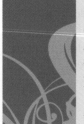

CLIFFORD ALLEN
Season 2

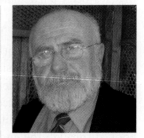

Biographical Information

Clifford is a 64-year-old male who has been married to his wife Pam for 40 years. Their only child, 24-year-old Gary, has Down syndrome and lives with them. Clifford is a middle manager for a small manufacturing company, where he has worked for the past 20 years.

Clifford's wife has recently been diagnosed with colon cancer, which has turned his world upside down. She is beginning chemotherapy and radiation

Continued

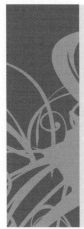

therapy, and he finds this very stressful. He is trying to work, take care of his son, and support his wife. He does not have strong coping skills, and his history of depression further complicates matters. He has not been treated for depression for a number of years, partly because he fears the social stigma associated with being labeled as medically depressed and partly because he is concerned that his employer would find out through the use of the medical benefits. It is Clifford's opinion that depression would be perceived as a sign of weakness by his employer.

Before his wife became sick, Clifford was thinking about retiring within the next few years, but now he is concerned about medical bills and does not believe he can afford to retire anytime soon. Clifford and his son Gary are involved with church. Since Pam became ill, Clifford has not regularly gone for a walk with Gary, and he has also stopped bowling in his league.

Episode 1

Clifford has been trying to keep himself occupied so that he does not constantly think about Pam. Although he has been told that her prognosis is poor, he wants her to undergo the radiation and chemotherapy treatments. He accompanies Pam to the outpatient clinic to have a peripherally inserted central catheter, or PICC line, placed. **[P]**

Episode 2

Clifford takes Pam to her chemotherapy treatments this week and drops Gary off at work. He is able to go into the office by late morning and still get part of a day of work in, but he has a hard time focusing on his work. **[P]**

Episode 3

Clifford is glad to see Pam feeling better this week. He decides that the oncology nurse was probably exaggerating the treatment side effects, because Pam is obviously doing fine. He continues to be very preoccupied and is having a hard time focusing on his work.

Episode 4

No news this week.

Episode 5

Clifford is feeling overwhelmed. Pam is feeling very sick, and he has to work and take care of Gary. Pam is too weak to do anything. He feels sick to his stomach when he needs to help her empty her colostomy bag. He does not want to look at it, let alone smell it. He appreciates the help from people from church, but he still feels helpless. He is having a hard time sleeping at night and has lost his appetite. He has a couple of drinks of scotch each evening to help him relax. **[VC]**

Episode 6

Clifford is feeling very down. He wants to believe that Pam is going to get better, but by the way she is acting, he thinks she is giving up. He thinks she should be more optimistic and just believe things will be okay. He has begun to lose weight and continues to drink alcohol in the evenings. He has a hard time being productive at work and has avoided social interactions with friends. He is angry when Pam suggests that he might need to get some help for depression. **[VC]**

Episode 7

No news this week.

Episode 8

Clifford is glad that Pam has completed the chemotherapy regimen. He is hopeful that everything will get back to normal. He loves Pam, but this illness has changed things. Although he does not mean it, he does not like to touch her, he does not like the way she smells, and he does not like the colostomy bag. He feels very tired from the ordeal.

Episode 9

Clifford is glad to see Pam begin to feel better—this makes him feel better as well. He realizes he has lost 15 pounds over the past several months. **[P]**

Episode 10

No news this week.

Episode 11

Clifford has been sleeping much better lately. He has also stopped drinking alcohol in the evening. He actually feels like he has a little energy and has been looking forward to going to work. Clifford realizes he has not really spent much time with Gary over the past few months. He feels as if he has been in a fog—existing without really living. He takes his son fishing, which is the first activity they have done together in a very long time. **[P]**

Episode 12

Clifford takes Pam and Gary on a weekend vacation and has a wonderful time. After getting home he talks to Pam about taking a Caribbean cruise next year. He is disappointed that

Pam is not enthusiastic about the idea and wishes she would think more positively. He decides to start looking at some travel plans anyway. **[VC]**

Episode 13
No news this week.

Episode 14
Clifford goes bowling this week and joins his friends for a card game. He is feeling rested and energetic; his friends tell him he looks better now than he has in months. He tells his friends he is so thankful that Pam has beaten the cancer again.

Episode 15
Clifford and Gary have resumed their nightly walks after dinner. Clifford realizes how hard the past year has been on him and vows to never let family issues get in the way of meeting his own needs. Clifford goes online to research his company's retirement requirements and evaluate his options. **[P]**

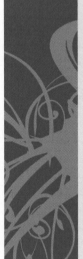

CLIFFORD ALLEN
Season 3

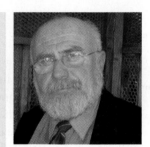

Biographical Information
Clifford is a 65-year-old male who has been married to his wife Pam for 41 years. Their only child, 25-year-old Gary, has Down syndrome and lives with them. Clifford is a middle manager for a small manufacturing company, where he has worked for over the past 21 years.

During the past year, Pam was diagnosed with colorectal cancer, had a colectomy and colostomy, and underwent chemotherapy and radiation therapy. Following her treatments, the oncologist was optimistic, and Pam began feeling good again. However, a few weeks ago, Pam became ill again. They were told that her cancer had metastasized to her liver and pancreas, and her prognosis was very poor.

Clifford has a history of depression, although he has not undergone treatment for several years. While Pam was going through chemotherapy and radiation several months ago, he became depressed, but did not seek treatment. He has been feeling very angry since learning of Pam's metastatic cancer.

Episode 1
A few weeks ago, Pam began feeling ill again and learned that her colon cancer had metastasized to her liver and pancreas. Her prognosis is poor. Clifford is angry with everyone. He is angry with Pam for getting sick again, he is angry with the physicians for not telling him how sick she was, and he is angry with God for doing this to her. He does not understand why Pam has been ambivalent about further chemotherapy treatment, but is pleased when she elects to begin treatment. In spite of the prognosis, he still believes everything will be okay. **[VC]**

Episode 2
Clifford takes Pam to have a PICC line reinserted for chemotherapy. He tells his employer that things might be rough for a while and he might need to take some time off. His boss at work is very understanding of the situation and lets him know he can take the time as he needs it. However, Clifford knows he has used up his family leave benefits.

Episode 3
This has been a bad week for Clifford. He tries to take care of Pam while she is nauseated, but he feels helpless. He cannot sleep and loses his appetite. Again, he feels as if he is in a fog and is almost nonfunctional. He makes arrangements for Gary to stay with some people from church for the next few weeks, because he knows he cannot cope with his son right now. He begins to drink alcohol heavily in the evenings again. He goes to work, but just sits in his office and stares at the walls. He has quit going to church on Sundays because he does not see any point in going at this time. **[P]**

Episode 4
No news this week.

Episode 5

Pam continues her chemotherapy. Clifford has become almost nonfunctional. The people caring for Gary become very concerned about Clifford and suggest that Gary continue to stay with them until things improve at home. Clifford becomes very angry with them and says he feels as though he is losing his son and wife at the same time. Because of Clifford's actions, they notify the parish priest about what is going on.

Father John visits with Clifford and asks him how things are going. Clifford shares with him that he does not understand why God is doing this to them. He also confides that he is afraid that Pam might not make it. Father John recommends that he get counseling or come back and talk with him again so that Clifford can better support his wife. Clifford tells Father John he needs to think about it, but that he is not really interested in talking to anybody. He does not think he has time for therapy, even if he wanted to go.

Episode 6

Clifford has an angry outburst at the clinic this week when Pam refuses to have her chemotherapy treatment. The nurse at the clinic gradually calms him down and talks with him about changing the focus of care. When he gets home, he sobs uncontrollably, and he gets drunk later that evening. He has not slept well in a week and has eaten very little. He also has no energy and has been suffering from frequent headaches. Many people have come to the home to help out, but it is obvious to everyone that Clifford is not managing things well at all.

Episode 7

Clifford meets the hospice nurse and decides he likes her and believes that hospice will be helpful. However, he continues to be angry with Pam for stopping treatment and "giving up." He feels powerless and as if everything is out of his control. He continues to drink heavily. He refuses to talk to Pam about caring for Gary when she dies; he wants to talk with her about getting better.

Father John, the parish priest, makes a visit to their home. Clifford shares with him that he doesn't think he can go on without Pam. Father John reminds him that he must go on—not only for himself, but also for Gary. He also reminds Clifford that he needs to put Pam's mind at ease. Clifford tells Father John there really is not much to look forward to. Father John recognizes the situation to be serious and convinces Clifford to get counseling immediately. **[VC]**

Episode 8

Clifford sees the psychiatrist, Dr. Jacobe, twice this week. On the first visit, he shared his previous history of depression some 20 years ago and the fact that his brother committed suicide when they were teenagers. He also shared his ongoing feelings about not wanting to go on without Pam, that he has been a worthless husband, and that he has nothing to look forward to. The psychiatrist recognizes that Clifford is depressed and prescribes bupropion (Wellbutrin). Clifford actually felt better after his first session and decided to get the prescription filled. On the second visit this week, Clifford is able to talk more about the possibility of his wife's death and feelings of anger, abandonment, and hopelessness. Dr. Jacobe talks with Clifford about how to deal with those feelings and, most importantly how to keep from taking them out on his wife and son. Because Clifford reports ongoing insomnia, the physician gives him a prescription for zolpidem (Ambien) to facilitate sleep.

Clifford also has benefited from the social worker who has been working with the family, specifically regarding how to talk to Gary about what is happening with Pam and prepare him for her death. Although Clifford struggles with these conversations, he has accepted the fact that Pam is dying and that he needs to talk with Gary. **[VC]**

Episode 9

Clifford can see that Pam is declining fast. She has had nothing to eat or drink for the past 5 days, and she is putting out very little urine. With the help of the hospice nurse, Clifford knows the medications well and has been able to take charge of managing her pain.

Clifford notices that Pam's respiratory rate has become more irregular and calls the hospice nurse for advice. He is told that it is likely that she will die soon and to continue to manage her pain the way he has been. Clifford asks that she come to see Pam herself. When the hospice nurse arrives, she finds Pam resting comfortably and confirms the change in her breathing pattern. She reassures Clifford. Clifford is finally able to fully accept that Pam is dying. He tells her that he will be okay and that he will take good care of Gary. He calls Father John and asks him to come. Clifford is at Pam's side when she dies peacefully early the following morning. Clifford has never experienced such pain.

Two days after she dies, Clifford keeps his appointment with Dr. Jacobe, the psychiatrist. It is a much-needed appointment, and he talks about his overwhelming sense of loss and grief. Fortunately, Clifford has tremendous support from his church and friends. **[P]**

Episode 10

Clifford keeps his weekly appointments with Dr. Jacobe, the psychiatrist, and continues to take the Wellbutrin. The dose has been slowly increased, and Clifford thinks it has been helpful. He talks about his loss and grief, and the overwhelming support from members of the church. Dr. Jacobe asks Clifford to start thinking about his plans for taking care of Gary and ongoing self-management.

Episode 11

No news this week.

Episode 12

Clifford is now seeing Dr. Jacobe just twice a month and has been making progress. He has attempted to establish a regular routine for Gary. Clifford knows how important it is that he stays mentally and physically well for Gary's benefit, and he makes a commitment to see himself through this challenging period of his life. **[P]**

Episode 13

It would have been Pam's birthday this week. Clifford cries off and on all day. In spite of his sadness and sense of loneliness, Clifford and Gary decide to make a birthday cake to honor her. This week, Clifford also officially announces his retirement, which will become effective at the end of the month. He tells his colleagues that he realizes he has an opportunity to do something positive with the remainder of his life—to give his full attention to Gary.

Episode 14

No news this week.

Episode 15

On Clifford's last day of work, his company gives him a retirement party and several nice gifts. During the party, he shares plenty of laughs and tears with his coworkers and feels grateful for their sincerity. As he leaves the office for the last time and gets into his car to drive home, Clifford experiences the emotion of multiple losses—the end of a career and the loss of his wife. He is profoundly sad and lonely. Within this experience of grief and loss, Clifford remains hopeful and is receptive to the ongoing support of friends and church members. He looks forward to meeting with the psychiatrist the next morning.

PAMELA ALLEN
Season 1

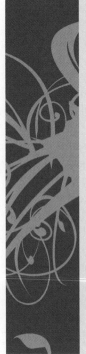

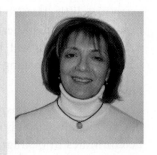

Biographical Information

Pamela is a 65-year-old female who has been married to Clifford for 40 years. Their only child, 24-year-old Gary, has Down syndrome and lives with them. In the past, Pamela worked as an administrative assistant in a law firm. After Gary was born, Pam gave up her career to care for Gary.

Pam describes her health as excellent. She has no current medical conditions or problems for which she seeks treatment. She frequently experiences constipation, which she treats with over-the-counter agents. She considers the constipation more of an annoyance than anything else. The only medical condition she has ever had requiring treatment was endometrial cancer at age 50. The cancer was diagnosed at a very early stage, and she underwent a total hysterectomy and bilateral salpingo-oophorectomy. Because there was no evidence of lymph node involvement, Pam was considered cured and has been cancer-free ever since. Her last examination was 14 months ago.

Pam is very close and devoted to her son Gary. Her goal is to optimize his potential, despite his limitations. She provides almost everything he needs, including transportation to and from his part-time job and to various activities. Her favorite hobby is quilting, and she belongs to a quilting group. Pamela regularly wins awards for her quilts, which are highly sought after; she sells a few each year for additional income.

Episode 1

No news this week.

Episode 2

Pam enjoys an afternoon with her quilt club this week. She talks with the other women about the travel plans she and Clifford have after he retires. **[P]**

Episode 3

No news this week.

Episode 4

No news this week.

Episode 5

No news this week.

Episode 6

Pam knows that Clifford is often uncomfortable when he is unable to urinate completely. She knows he tends to downplay his symptoms, not wanting to look like a complainer. She is glad that he has decided to go for some tests. **[P]**

Episode 7

Pam learns from Clifford that he is going to have surgery on his prostate; she is relieved to know he does not have prostate cancer. She hopes he does not get too stressed out from the entire process. Pam and Gary participate in a church-cleaning activity one evening this week.

Episode 8

No news this week.

Episode 9

Pam continues to keep Gary's routine as uninterrupted as possible, while managing to be at the hospital with Clifford. She is relieved that there were no complications from the surgery. She is having problems with constipation this week and takes laxatives to relieve herself. The following day she experiences diarrhea with an odd reddish-brown color and odor. **[P]**

Episode 10

Pam spends most of her time this week helping Clifford recover from surgery and taking care of Gary. She experiences little relief from the constipation that has recently plagued her; she has been straining to have bowel movements and notices that her stools are thinner than usual. **[P]**

Episode 11

No news this week.

Episode 12

Pam continues to experience constipation and odd-shaped stools, and now she senses fullness in her rectum and pelvic areas, even after defecating. The appearance of reddish-brown in her stools has been more regular. She has also felt tired lately. On Friday afternoon, Pam finally decides to call for an appointment with her physician to discuss the symptoms. She is told to come to the office on the following Monday morning. Given her past history of cancer, she has a feeling of dread and becomes worried that something serious may be wrong. Pam begins to worry about her son and wonders if Clifford could manage if she were to get sick and die. She decides it might be best to just wait and see what the physician has to say before sharing any of this with Clifford. **[P]**

Episode 13

Pam sees the physician Monday morning. He immediately notices that she looks pale. After eliciting a history, the physician conducts an examination, including a digital rectal examination. The physician tells Pam that he is able to palpate a mass and that her stool tested positive for occult blood. He would like to conduct further tests, including blood work and a computed tomography (CT) scan of the abdomen. These tests are performed on an outpatient basis over the next few days. Pam is very worried at this point. She tells Clifford that she is having some tests done, but does not elaborate or show that she is concerned. **[P]**

Episode 14

Pam follows up with her physician regarding her test results. The physician tells Pam that she has a mass in her upper rectum and lower colon that extends into surrounding structures. A CBC confirms that she is anemic. He tells her that she needs to be admitted to the hospital for surgery. Pam calls Clifford to inform him that she is being scheduled for surgery the following day. Pam is sent to the preadmission clinic for a preoperative work-up and teaching.

The following morning, Pam is admitted to the hospital and taken to surgery for a colectomy and possible colostomy. When she wakes up in recovery, she is nauseated and experiences a tremendous amount of pain. She has tubes in her arms, bladder, and nose. She feels a bandage and a strange object on her stomach. After she is transferred to the surgical unit, she sees her surgeon, who confirms her worst nightmare. Pam is told she had a large cancerous tumor in her lower colon and upper rectum. The surgeon was unable to remove all of it because the tumor had adhered to the side walls of her lower abdominal cavity. The physician also biopsied lymph nodes in her groin, which were thought to contain cancerous cells. **[MR]**

Episode 15

Pam is discharged from the hospital this week. She is told that her condition is serious, and further treatment with chemotherapy and radiation therapy is recommended. These treatments would start in about one month, after she has healed from surgery. Pam tells her physician and Clifford that she is not sure she wants chemotherapy and radiation treatment.

At home, Pam is slowly learning to care for the colostomy. A home-care nurse makes a few visits to help her adjust to her colostomy and provide other aspects of support; Pam is grateful for the help. She is very aware that Clifford is disgusted with her colostomy. **[P]**

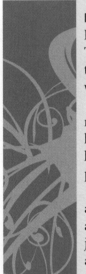

PAMELA ALLEN
Season 2

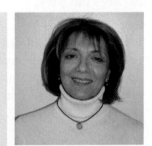

Biographical Information

Pamela is a 65-year-old female who has been married to Clifford for 40 years. Their only child, 24-year-old Gary, has Down syndrome and lives with them. In the past, Pamela worked as an administrative assistant in a law firm. After Gary was born, Pam gave up her career to care for Gary.

Pam has recently been diagnosed with advanced colorectal cancer. Last month, she had surgery (colectomy and colostomy), and she is still adjusting to having the colostomy. Because the tumor extended into the perineum and lymph nodes, she has been advised to start radiation and chemotherapy. She previously underwent treatment for endometrial cancer at age 50.

Pam has always been very close and devoted to her son Gary. Her goal has always been to optimize his potential, despite his limitations. She provides almost everything he needs, including transportation to and from his part-time job and to various activities. At this time, she is very concerned about not being able to take care of Gary. She also is worried about Clifford and his ability to cope with these changes.

Episode 1

Pam has begun to regain the strength she had before surgery and has resumed many of her regular routines with Gary. Although she was initially reluctant to begin chemotherapy, after talking to Clifford she decided to go ahead and begin treatment. Her first chemotherapy is scheduled to begin early next week. She goes to the outpatient clinic to have a peripherally inserted central catheter, or PICC line, placed. This will prevent frequent needle sticks and allow the infusion of medications and blood samples to be drawn through the line when needed. She thinks this will be an advantage, but is a bit anxious about having one more thing to care for. She is feeling optimistic that the treatment will cure her cancer. Pam receives the Sacrament of Anointing of the Sick at her church and hopes that this will help her through her treatment. **[P]**

Episode 2

Pam begins her chemotherapy treatment this week. Her treatment regimen includes leucovorin followed by 5-fluorouracil (5-FU) daily for 5 days every month for the next 4 to 5 months. The oncology nurse explains the common side effects of treatment, which could include mild to moderate nausea or changes in her interest in food. To prevent nausea, she is given ondansetron (Zofran) before chemotherapy. In addition, she is told to watch for changes in her stool consistency, because 5-FU can cause loose stools. Pam experiences nausea, slight changes in her appetite, and a slight loosening of her stools, which is controlled with Lomotil. She tries to drink plenty of fluids. **[MR] [P]**

Episode 3

Pam is feeling physically better this week. The nausea has subsided, and she has a good appetite. This week she started external lymph node radiation therapy to her right groin. The radiation treatment schedule is Monday through Friday for 6 weeks. She takes Gary to and from work, just as she had before her surgery, and still takes care of most household chores. Caring for her colostomy and PICC line are daily reminders of her situation, which bring with them emotions and fears about the cancer. She is self-conscious of the colostomy bag and its contents, knowing that it is difficult for Clifford to deal with, and it has interfered with their intimacy. She has not told Gary how sick she is, but she knows he is aware that she is not feeling well. Pam worries about Gary's long-term care if she dies; she is not sure Clifford can handle it. Pam decides to start working on a special quilt for Gary. **[P]**

Episode 4
No news this week.

Episode 5
Pam recently completed another round of chemotherapy and is still undergoing radiation. This week, she feels as if she hit a wall. She is extremely fatigued and nauseated, has diarrhea, and has developed sores in her mouth. The diarrhea makes managing the colostomy bag a challenge. Her hair has thinned, and she has redness and irritation of the skin in her right groin area from the radiation treatment. She doesn't feel like she has the energy to do anything—even Gary's routine care has become a huge task.

Fortunately, people from her church have come to help. Every day, somebody comes into the home to do housework and either brings or prepares meals. They have also made arrangements to transport Gary to and from work and other activities. Pam feels relieved to have the help, but hates feeling so tired and helpless. It is difficult to explain to others just how tired she is. The one bit of good news she had from her doctor is that her white blood cell (WBC) count has remained above $3,000/mm^3$, and her platelets have remained above $100,000/mm^3$ during therapy. She is mildly anemic, which explains part of her fatigue. **[MR] [VC]**

Episode 6
Pam continues to feel completely exhausted. She had no idea she could ever feel so tired; she feels worse the longer she has the treatments. She continues to feel nauseated and never feels like eating. Pam continues to have sores in her mouth and diarrhea. She is beginning to wonder if she will even survive the treatments. She feels so tired, for example, that reaching for a glass of water on the coffee table while lying on the couch is a huge effort. She receives a blood transfusion this week because she has become progressively anemic.

Pam feels badly about not being able to be a mother to her son or a wife to Clifford, but frankly she has little interest in doing anything right now. Although she has completed the radiation therapy, she is still getting the chemotherapy. Friends from the church continue to come in daily to help. She knows Clifford is not coping well with her illness, and she suggests that he get counseling for depression. She also is aware of his new pattern of drinking alcohol in the evening, which worries her.

Episode 7
No news this week.

Episode 8
Pam has finally completed the chemotherapy and is looking forward to feeling better. She was happy to have the PICC line removed. She knows she will continue to feel tired for a while, but the sores in her mouth, diarrhea, and her appetite have all improved. She has lost weight through this ordeal, and when she looks at herself in the mirror, she hates what she sees. She sees a skinny woman with draping skin, a bag of stool on her abdomen, and thinning hair. She feels as if she has lost all that she was; she does not look the least bit feminine or attractive and understands why Clifford seems to physically avoid her. Pam is soothed through her ongoing relationship with Gary, who continues to seek comfort from her. **[MR] [P]**

Episode 9
Pam continues to feel a little better and is slowly able to take care of more household tasks—although she still gets tired easily. She has started to go back to church services with Gary and Clifford and also has decided to start working on Gary's quilt again. **[P]**

Episode 10
No news this week.

Episode 11
Pam goes to her quilting group for the first time since becoming sick. She is worried about what the women in her group will think when they see her, but is very glad to get out and see some of her friends again. She goes with Clifford and Gary to a volunteer service meeting at the church. **[P]**

Episode 12
Pam actually feels good enough now to go with Clifford and Gary on an out-of-town trip for a weekend. It has been so long since she has felt well enough to enjoy herself and her family. Although she still tires easily, the fatigue is becoming less of an obstacle. Her appetite has returned, and she is gaining some of her weight back.

Pam is relieved that Clifford seems to be back to his "old self" again and has stopped drinking in the evening. He suggests to Pam that they go on a cruise next year; she tells him she is not sure how things will be next year, and they should just take life one day at a time. Pam continues to work on Gary's quilt.

Episode 13
No news this week.

Episode 14
Pam is really regaining her energy and agrees to lead a volunteer group at the church. She is almost finished with Gary's quilt and is thinking about entering it in a quilting contest at the annual Neighborhood Arts and Crafts Fair.

Episode 15
Pam wins the grand prize for her quilt and is awarded $1,500 for it. She has never been offered so much money for a quilt, but also realizes she has never made a more beautiful quilt. She decides to sell it, aware that her family could use the extra money and that she can always make Gary another quilt. Pam feels guilty about it afterward—the quilt was part of her cancer therapy, and she made that quilt especially for Gary. **[P]**

PAMELA ALLEN
Season 3

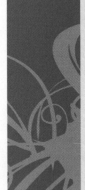

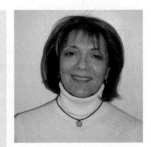

Biographical Information
Pamela is a 66-year-old female who has been married to his Clifford for 41 years. Their only child, 25-year-old Gary, has Down syndrome and lives with them. In the past, Pamela worked as an administrative assistant in a law firm. After Gary was born, Pam gave up her career to care for Gary.

During the past year, Pam was diagnosed with colorectal cancer, had a colectomy and colostomy, and underwent chemotherapy and radiation therapy. Following completion of her treatments, the oncologist was optimistic, and Pam began feeling good again. However, a few weeks ago, Pam became ill again. They were told that her cancer had metastasized to her liver and pancreas, and her prognosis was very poor.

Episode 1
A few weeks ago, Pam began experiencing intermittent right upper quadrant discomfort and a decline in her appetite again. More recently, she noticed a hint of yellow coloration to the sclera of her eyes and a dark color to her urine. She called her oncologist and was seen immediately. After a series of diagnostic tests, Pam is given very grave news: the cancer has metastasized to her liver and pancreas. The oncologist outlined two treatment options: another course of chemotherapy with bevacizumab (Avastin) or palliative treatment.

Pam hates to even think about more chemotherapy, but she also knows that if she does not undergo chemotherapy, she will surely die. Part of her reluctance to get treatment is based on her understanding of the severity of side effects. Clifford is angry with her for considering any option other than chemotherapy, and the physician also strongly encourages Pam to undergo the chemotherapy. Pam has had time to think about everything. Deep down, she knows she will die—she just doesn't know if living longer while enduring the adverse effects of treatment outweighs avoiding the adverse effects at the expense of a shorter life. After talking with her priest, Father John, and despite the fact that she really does not want to go through chemotherapy again, Pam agrees to this treatment.

Episode 2
Pam has another PICC line inserted and begins the chemotherapy. She will be receiving bevacizumab, 5 mg/m^2 every 2 weeks, at the outpatient chemotherapy unit. On her way to the first chemotherapy treatment, Pam experiences a high degree of nausea. **[MR] [P]**

Episode 3
Mouth sores, diarrhea, and vomiting have returned with the new chemotherapy agent. Pam can't get relief from the nausea and vomiting, even after trying several different

anti-nausea medications. Her platelet count has also dropped due to the chemotherapy.

Episode 4

Despite various anti-nausea medications, Pam continues to have constant nausea and diarrhea. She has lost 15 pounds. Her muscles and joints ache, and she has persistent headaches. Lab results prior to her next treatment show her total white blood cell (WBC) count is 2,300/mm^3. Treatment is delayed due to her symptoms and her WBC count. **[MR]**

Episode 5

Pam feels worse than ever—in fact, she feels much worse than the last time she went through chemotherapy. She has decided this is not worth it, and she tries to tell Clifford she does not want to continue treatments. **[VC]**

Episode 6

Pam continues to feel terrible this week. When it is time for her next appointment, she tells Clifford—in no uncertain terms—that she does not want to continue with the chemotherapy treatments. However, he picks her up, carries her out to the car, and takes her to the clinic. She is too weak to refuse. At the clinic, Pam tells the nurse that she does not want any more treatments, but her husband made her come. The nurse talks with Clifford and tells him Pam has the right to stop treatment. Pam is embarrassed by his reaction in the clinic and wishes he would just let it go. Once Clifford has calmed down, the nurse engages in a discussion about changing the focus of care and introduces the concept of hospice care to the couple. **[VC]**

Episode 7

Pam and Clifford have elected to interview a hospice nurse and hear what the program has to offer them. During the home visit, the hospice nurse learns that Pam has not been eating well, has continued to lose weight, and that she has been experiencing a great deal of pain. Pam tells the hospice nurse she wants pain medication to make her comfortable. Later in the week, Pam tells Clifford she is ready to die and wants to talk with him about Gary. She is frustrated that Clifford will not talk with her.

Episode 8

Pam and Clifford experience a good relationship with the hospice nurse and other team members. The agency has supplied them with a hospital bed, bedside commode, and a medication box to help organize her pills. Clifford is fond of the social worker who has begun working with them, specifically regarding how to talk to Gary about what is happening with Pam and to prepare him for her death. Although Clifford struggles with these conversations, he has accepted the fact that Pam is declining and they need to talk to Gary. **[P]**

Pam has had very little to eat or drink this week and is rarely urinating. The hospice nurse notices that she has abdominal fullness (ascites) due to the accumulation of fluid in the peritoneal cavity and appears more jaundiced. Her pain continues, but the nurse establishes a pain management plan that works for Pam. The hospice nurse is in phone contact nearly every day to assess Pam's pain and make adjustments to the medication.

Pam sleeps most of the day, but when she is awake, she is alert and able to engage in conversation. During one of those moments, she tells Clifford that she regrets selling the quilt. Friends from the church continue to visit, bring food for Clifford and Gary, and offer support in whatever ways they can. **[P]**

Episode 9

Pam has had nothing to eat or drink for the past 5 days. There has been no stool in the colostomy bag for several days. She now has a Foley catheter because she is too weak to get up to use the bedside commode; it only has small amounts of dark, concentrated urine. She is more alert in the mornings and talks to those around her. The hospice aide comes in every other day to bathe her and provide comfort care. The hospice nurse has implemented a good pain management regimen, and Pam is more comfortable this week.

When Pam's respiratory rate becomes irregular, Clifford calls the hospice nurse and asks her to come to the home. The hospice nurse finds Pam resting comfortably. When she approaches her, Pam slowly wakes, but is quite weak and unable to talk. She offers a smile when she recognizes the nurse. Her breathing pattern has changed, and the nurse reassures Clifford. He is finally able to truly accept that Pam is dying. Clifford tells her that he will be okay and that he will take good care of Gary. Father John comes by the house to give Pam the Sacrament of Anointing of the Sick. Pam drifts off to sleep and does not wake again. She dies early in the morning the next day, peacefully, with her family at her side.

GARY ALLEN
Season 1

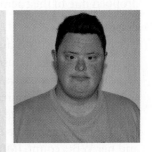

Biographical Information

Gary is a 24-year-old male with Down syndrome. He lives with his parents, Clifford and Pamela. He is very close to his parents and has not been interested in living elsewhere. Gary has a part-time job as a courtesy clerk at a grocery store near their home. He is also given other duties as assigned, such as collecting baskets from the parking lot and helping customers with carrying groceries out. He works every afternoon from 1 pm to 5 pm. He has been doing this type of work for about 5 years now, and he loves having a job.

Gary has had only a few health-related problems during his life, including hypothyroidism since infancy and, more recently, keratoconus in both eyes, which affects his vision. Gary is unable to drive and relies on his parents for transportation. When they are unavailable to provide transportation, Gary rides the bus.

Gary helps his parents with many things around the house. He has learned to do laundry and help with the dishes and cleaning. Gary is able to make his own breakfast and lunch now (e.g., heat soup in a pan, make a sandwich, heat something in a microwave), but he is unable to interpret cooking directions or recipes. Gary does best when in controlled settings or in a routine setting with which he is familiar.

Gary enjoys a very active life. He is involved in various Special Olympics programs, including golf, swimming, and bowling; an Explorer Scout troop comprised of individuals with cognitive disabilities; and his church. Gary also rides his bike a couple miles three times a week, and he enjoys daily walks with his father. These various activities have afforded him multiple social connections and allowed him to enjoy friendships with a number of individuals.

Episode 1
No news this week.

Episode 2
Each day this week, Gary goes to work in the afternoon, comes home, and watches television until dinner time. After dinner, he takes a walk with his father around the neighborhood. [P]

Episode 3
No news this week.

Episode 4
No news this week.

Episode 5
Gary works each day this week. He bruises his fingers when he gets them caught in a grocery cart. He is instructed to stay in the store and greet customers for the rest of the week. [P]

Episode 6
No news this week.

Episode 7
Gary and his mother go to church to participate in a church-cleaning activity. Gary loves to go to these activities because he likes to help with projects. He has many friends at the church, and he likes the fact that they talk to him. Later in the day, he takes a bike ride. [P]

Episode 8
No news this week.

Episode 9
Gary's mother shares with him that his father must stay at the hospital to fix a problem with his bladder. Gary understands that you go to the hospital when you are sick or for tests or procedures, but he does not grasp what she means by "bladder problems." He is worried about his father and relieved when Pam tells him that his father is fine. [P]

Episode 10

Gary enjoys having his father at home during the week. Gary helps his mother take care of him. He also spends time in the afternoons at the swimming pool with his Special Olympics team. **[P]**

Episode 11

No news this week.

Episode 12

Gary goes on a bus trip with the youth group at church to a one-day church retreat. He has a great time with the members of the youth group. He gets home shortly after dinner time and is so excited that he has a hard time telling his mother and father what he did that day. He also has a hard time falling asleep that night.

Episode 13

No news this week.

Episode 14

Gary is aware that his mother is at the hospital because she is sick. His father makes arrangements for friends from church to spend time with him in the evenings. Although Gary doesn't like the fact that his parents are not home, he is happy to talk with the people from church. He spends time making models and shows his car collection to his church friends. **[P]**

Episode 15

When Pam arrives home from the hospital, Gary is sensitive to the fact that she does not feel well. He notices that she spends a lot of time lying around. He helps his father with chores around the house and wonders why his father spends so much time sitting in the living room chair and why they don't take their walk after dinner. On Sunday morning, he reminds his father that it's time for church, but is told they will not go this week.

GARY ALLEN
Season 2

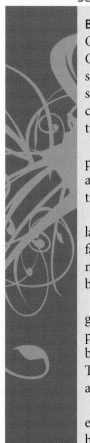
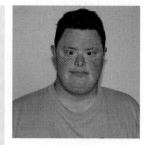

Biographical Information

Gary is a 24-year-old male with Down syndrome. He lives with his parents Clifford and Pamela. Gary has a part-time job as a courtesy clerk at a grocery store near their home. He is also given other duties as assigned, such as collecting shopping baskets from the parking lot and helping customers with carrying groceries out. He works every afternoon from 1 pm to 5 pm. He has been doing this type of work for about 5 years now, and he loves having a job.

Gary has had only a few health-related problems during his life, including hypothyroidism since infancy and, more recently, keratoconus in both eyes, which affects his vision. Gary is unable to drive and relies on his parents for transportation. When they are unavailable to provide transportation, Gary rides the bus.

Gary helps his parents with many things around the house. He has learned to do laundry and help with the dishes and cleaning. Gary is able to make his own breakfast and lunch now (e.g., heat soup in a pan, make a sandwich, heat something in a microwave), but he is unable to interpret cooking directions or recipes. Gary does best when in controlled settings or in a routine setting with which he is familiar.

Gary enjoys a very active life. He is involved in various Special Olympics programs, including golf, swimming, and bowling; an Explorer Scout troop comprised of individuals with cognitive disabilities; and his church. Gary also rides his bike a couple miles three times a week, and he enjoys daily walks with his father. These various activities have afforded him multiple social connections and have allowed him to enjoy friendships with a number of individuals.

Gary has always relied on his mother for help with living skills. His mother, however, has recently been ill, and she has been unable to help him in the ways in which he is accustomed. His father has been helping him more, but his father seems so sad. Gary is aware of the changes going on around him, but does not understand them.

Episode 1

Gary sees the PICC line in his mother's arm and asks her about it. Pam tells him that she will be getting medicine in the tube to help her get well. Gary cannot quite picture medicine going in the tube. He goes to Poly Hockey with his Special Olympics group. **[P]**

Episode 2

Gary can tell that his mother does not feel well this week and asks her if she is taking the medicine to get better. He goes on a camping trip with the Explorer Scout troop this week. **[P]**

Episode 3

Gary's Mom takes him to and from work this week. He can tell she is feeling tired. He still wonders about the tube in her arm and when she will take the medicine. He spends time in his room working on Word Search puzzles and coloring. **[P]**

Episode 4

No news this week.

Episode 5

Many people at Gary's church have been giving him rides to and from work and have been spending time at the house helping his mother. He is always happy to have them there because they talk to him and they are always very nice. They often stay long enough to cook dinner. He is glad to have dinner, but he likes the food his mother makes even better. When he gets tired of the extra people in the house, he retreats to his room to watch television.

Episode 6

Gary notices that his mother spends all of her time lying on the couch. He does not think his mother looks the same, and she smells different. He knows she is sick and he asks her when she is going to take her medicine. Pam tells him she is taking the medicine, but it just makes her feel tired. Gary does not understand any of this. The ladies from the church continue to come over, but his father has not taken him to church lately and has not been able to get him to all of his Special Olympics activities. He misses spending time with his friends.

Episode 7

No news this week.

Episode 8

Gary learns from his mother that she has finished taking all of her medicine. She tells him that she hopes to be able to start doing more things with him again. Gary loves his mother and has never complained about her lack of attention while she has been sick. He spends time in the garage crushing cans to earn money for his scout troop. **[P]**

Episode 9

Gary goes back to church this week for the first time in a long time. He is so happy to see his friends there. He tells his mother they should not miss church any more.

Episode 10

No news this week.

Episode 11

Gary and his Dad go fishing. Gary loves to fish. He fails to catch anything, but he doesn't care, because he enjoys sitting with his Dad and throwing rocks in the water. **[P]**

Episode 12

Gary goes with his parents on a short vacation. He loves to take trips and see new places and things. One of the visits they make is to the Museum of Natural History. Gary enjoys looking at the dinosaur bones and the mammal section.

Episode 13

No news this week.

Episode 14

Gary plays in a Special Olympics golf tournament this week. He does not win the gold medal, but he has a lot of fun. **[P]**

Episode 15

Gary accompanies his mother to the arts and crafts fair. His mother wins a prize. Later in the afternoon, a nice man named Greg spends time talking to Gary and his mother. Greg tells Gary that his name starts with the letter "G," just like Gary's name does. The man buys a quilt from his mother. Gary is happy to see his mother smile. Gary is also very happy that his Dad has been asking him to take walks in the evenings. While on a walk, he tells his Dad about his new girlfriend at work.

GARY ALLEN
Season 3

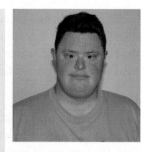

Biographical Information

Gary is a 25-year-old male with Down syndrome. He lives with his parents Clifford and Pamela. Gary has a part-time job as a courtesy clerk at a grocery store near their home. He is also given other duties as assigned, such as collecting shopping baskets from the parking lot and helping customers with carrying groceries out. He works every afternoon from 1 pm to 5 pm. He has been doing this type of work for about 6 years now.

Gary has had only a few health-related problems during his life, including hypothyroidism since infancy and, more recently, keratoconus in both eyes, which affects his vision. Gary is unable to drive and relies on his parents for transportation. When they are unavailable to provide transportation, Gary rides the bus.

Gary helps his parents with many things around the house. He has learned to do laundry and help with the dishes and cleaning. Gary is able to make his own breakfast and lunch now (e.g., heat soup in a pan, make a sandwich, heat something in a microwave), but he is unable to interpret cooking directions or recipes. Gary does best when in controlled settings or in a routine setting with which he is familiar.

Gary enjoys a very active life. He is involved in various Special Olympics programs, including golf, swimming, and bowling; an Explorer Scout troop comprised of individuals with cognitive disabilities; and his church. Gary also rides his bike a couple miles three times a week, and he enjoys daily walks with his father. These various activities have afforded him multiple social connections and have allowed him to enjoy friendships with a number of individuals.

Gary has been told that his mother is sick again. This makes him feel very sad.

Episode 1
Gary's mother tells him she is very sick again—even sicker than last time. Gary is very worried about this and asks his mother if she is going to get more medicine. **[P]**

Episode 2
When Gary sees the PICC line in his mother's arm, he tells her she is going to get medicine. Gary's mother confirms his understanding. Gary goes bowling with his Special Olympics friends this week.

Episode 3
Gary sees his mother and is worried about how sick she is. She keeps throwing up, and she tells his Dad that she just can't eat anything. He gets upset when he sees his Dad get angry. His Dad tells Gary that he is going to stay with the Marshall family, their friends from church, for a little while until his mother is feeling better. He likes the Marshalls and willingly goes to stay with them, but is worried about his mother. He takes Word Search puzzles to keep him busy.

Episode 4
No news this week.

Episode 5
Gary has been at the Marshall's house for several weeks now and, although he likes being with them, he misses his mother. He hears his Dad yelling at the Marshalls and wonders why he is so upset. Gary visits his mother frequently and is worried about how sick she looks. He spends a lot of time in his room making models. The Marshalls take Gary to work and to as many of his activities as they can manage.

Episode 6
Gary remains with the Marshalls. They take Gary over to his house and find Clifford sitting in the living room crying and Pam in the bedroom crying. Gary is very sad and starts to cry, but he does not know what's wrong. He hugs his mother for a very long time, and she tells him she is very, very sick and might die soon. Gary knows what this means because his grandparents died a few years ago. He is very upset and unable to go to work. **[P]**

Episode 7
No news this week.

Episode 8

Gary goes to work every day this week and continues to stay with the Marshalls. He has come to feel very comfortable in their home and is actually pretty happy. He gets sad every time he sees his mother and father, and wonders why the medicine his mother is taking is not helping her get well. **[P]**

Episode 9

The Marshalls learn that Pam will soon die. They talk to Gary and ask him if he wants to be with his mother and father. He says yes. When Gary gets to the house, he notices the house smells bad. Clifford holds him in his arms and tells him he is so sorry that he could not make his Mom well. Gary is shocked at how his mother looks. Her skin is yellow, and her face is hollow. She is breathing very fast, and her eyes are closed. Gary is comforted by Father John's presence. He talks to his Mom about going to heaven, but Gary is unsure if she hears him. After his mother dies, Gary goes back to the Marshalls home, where they sit with him and let him talk about how he is feeling. **[P]**

Episode 10

After his mother's funeral, Gary goes back to live at home with his Dad. He is glad the bad smells are gone. He checks all the rooms to be sure his mother is not there. Clifford tells Gary that they are on their own now, and they need to stick together.

Episode 11

No news this week.

Episode 12

Gary learns from his Dad that he is going to retire and stay home with him every day. Gary is very happy to hear this and asks him when they can go fishing again. While some friends from the church are over at the house, Gary proudly shows off the medals he has won over the years in Special Olympics. **[P]**

Episode 13

Gary helps his Dad bake a cake in honor of his mother's birthday. It makes him happy to do this because he likes cooking with his dad—and because he loves birthdays. **[P]**

Episode 14

No news this week.

Episode 15

Gary receives a package in the mail this week. In the package is the quilt his mother had sold several months ago at the art fair. There is a note attached to the quilt, and it reads: **[P]**

> Dear Gary,
>
>   I was saddened to learn that your mother recently passed away. Your mother made this beautiful quilt. I would like you to have it to keep you warm at night.
>
>   Your friend,
>   Greg Ross

BLEY HOUSEHOLD

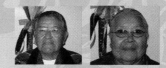

BLEY FAMILY STORY OVERVIEW

Character	Season 1	Season 2	Season 3
JIMMY BLEY	Jimmy has emphysema and hearing loss. He is able to do most things needed around the house, but he needs to pace himself. He does not perceive that his breathing problems are all that bad. He is still a smoker, and he uses an inhaler when absolutely necessary, but he is not oxygen-dependent. He makes an unsuccessful attempt to quit smoking during this season.	Story continues with a description of daily activities and another unsuccessful attempt to quit smoking.	During this season, Jimmy gets the flu, which leads to respiratory failure and sepsis. He is admitted to the ICU, requiring intubation and mechanical ventilation. He suffers from delirium during the acute illness. Following discharge, he has less oxygen capacity is oxygen-dependent at home. He becomes depressed and is given a prescription for Wellbutrin.
CECELIA BLEY	Cecelia is a very mentally sharp woman in excellent health. She has osteoarthritis that causes pain in the morning, but feels better as the day progresses. She takes care of most of the routine home activities. She often is frustrated trying to communicate with her husband Jimmy.	Story continues with a description of daily life with joint pain. When her pain increases, Cecilia sees a physician and is formally diagnosed with osteoarthritis.	When Jimmy becomes ill, Cecelia is very concerned for him; she stays with him at the hospital and has strong support from her family members.

CONCEPTS   *Acid Base, Addiction, Cognitive Impairment, Communication, Coping, Culture, Family Dynamics, Mobility, Moods and Affect, Oxygenation, Pain, Role Performance, Sensory/Perceptual*

JIMMY BLEY
Season 1

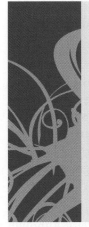

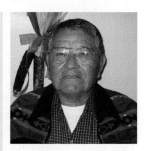

Biographical Information

Jimmy is a 78-year-old Native American male with moderate emphysema and hearing loss. He is a retired veteran who served as an electronics technician in the Army for his entire career. In his retirement, Jimmy has taken an interest in computers. He spends most of his time surfing the Internet or playing games on the computer; he also likes to build computers. Jimmy has been married for 56 years to his wife Cecelia. They argue a lot, but they would not know what to do without one another just the same. They have several grown children, grand-children, and great-grandchildren who live within the community. Jimmy often goes with his wife to the Neighborhood Senior Center for bingo night.

Jimmy considers himself healthy. He describes his hearing loss as mild. He has a hearing aid, but does not like to wear it and thus does not make changing

Continued

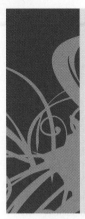

the batteries a priority. He does not perceive his hearing loss to be much of a problem. Likewise, Jimmy describes his emphysema as "not that bad." However, he becomes short of breath with most activities; thus, it takes time for him to complete tasks. He compensates by taking his time to do most things. Over time, he learned that he must pace himself; if he does not, he becomes exhausted, and it takes several days to recover. Jimmy is very aware of his limits—yet, at the same time, he does not generally consider his illness to be very bad. Although he would not admit it, he recognizes that his breathing has become more of a problem during the past couple of years. He continues to smoke and knows he should quit, but he just can't seem to get interested in quitting because he enjoys it.

Episode 1

Jimmy goes shopping with Cecelia. He knows that she has more energy than he does when it comes to shopping, and he has a tendency to become tired rather quickly. When she asks him if he's tired, Jimmy tells her that it's not that he is tired, but he gets bored with the shopping trips. He doesn't even consider staying home, because their outings have been part of their routine for years. Jimmy gets annoyed with Cecelia when she yells at him while driving, claiming he does not hear an ambulance. He has been driving all of his life, and he thinks he can hear well enough; besides that, he doesn't drive with his ears.

Episode 2

The bathroom sink faucet breaks this week. Cecelia suggests that they ask one of the boys to fix it, but Jimmy wants to do it himself. It takes him three days to complete the repair. On the first day, he takes the faucet apart to see what is wrong with it. On the second day, he makes a trip to the hardware store for supplies, and on the third day, he replaces the faucet with the new supplies. Cecelia is annoyed that it takes him so long, but at the same time, she is used to it.

Episode 3

No news this week.

Episode 4

Each week, Jimmy mows the lawn at their home. It usually takes him 3 to 4 days to do it, because he does just a little at a time. He refuses to have someone do it for him. This week, Jimmy becomes very short of breath while mowing and needs to stop and rest. Because his shortness of breath does not subside, he goes ahead and uses his albuterol inhaler. Jimmy uses this only when absolutely necessary, and his current inhaler is 2 years old. He is aware that it is past the expiration date, but he doesn't want to get a new one, because that would be a waste of money. **[P]**

Episode 5

No news this week.

Episode 6

Cecelia tells Jimmy that the kids and grandchildren are going to be coming over during the weekend to celebrate a birthday. Jimmy does not hear her say this. Over the weekend, when the kids show up, he asks Cecelia why nobody told him they were all coming over.

The family stays at their home most of the day. During their visit, Jimmy enjoys himself with two of his grandsons by playing computer games with them. After the family leaves, he feels very tired and short of breath, and needs to use his inhaler. Cecelia suggests to Jimmy that he quit smoking and get more exercise instead of sitting at the computer all day. **[P]**

Episode 7

Cecelia asks Jimmy to come with her to the community health fair. Jimmy declines, telling her that he is too busy. He actually doesn't go because he knows it would just make him tired. Cecelia brings a smoking cessation flyer home for him to look at. He reminds her that the last time he tried to quit smoking it nearly killed him. **[P]**

Episode 8

Jimmy's daughter and Cecelia accompany Jimmy to his family physician, Dr. Rowe, for a routine visit for his emphysema. Dr. Rowe tells Jimmy that his lung capacity continues to decline and that he really needs to stop smoking. Jimmy agrees to try to quit. Dr. Rowe refers him to the Neighborhood Patient Education Center. He is told that success is highest with group classes. He agrees to give a smoking cessation class a try. **[P]**

Episode 9

Jimmy attends his first smoking cessation class. Although he likes the nurse who leads the class, he is not sure what to think or do; he feels out of place when asked to share with the group his experiences related to smoking and what smoking means to him. He finds one lady to be particularly annoying; she wears heavy perfume, laughs loudly, and always wants to dominate the discussion. After the class is over, he is not so sure about the class, but decides it's worth going to for a while. In the meantime, he decides to cut back his smoking to about one-half his normal amount. **[P]**

Episode 10
Jimmy and his son accompany Cecelia to her x-ray tests and blood test at the diagnostic lab. Jimmy is uncomfortable because he has a serious craving for a cigarette. Later in the day, they go to play bingo at the Neighborhood Senior Center. Jimmy has a hard time concentrating on the game because he keeps thinking about smoking. He goes to the smoking cessation class again this week; the annoying lady is there, and once again she gets on his nerves.

Episode 11
No news this week.

Episode 12
Jimmy is not successful with his smoking reduction plan. Although he intended to cut back the amount he smoked by about one-half, over the past few weeks, he has crept back up to almost the same number of cigarettes that he smoked before. He finds that he actually feels as though he can breathe better when he smokes. This week, he decides to stop going to the smoking cessation classes because he can't stand the lady with the perfume. He does not talk to the nurse who leads the class because he doesn't want to disappoint her.

Episode 13
No news this week.

Episode 14
The nurse who leads the smoking cessation class calls Jimmy in response to his absence. Jimmy tells her that he couldn't come last week because of car trouble, but he might make it to the next class. Jimmy wins $20 playing bingo this week. **[P]**

Episode 15
Jimmy and Cecelia go to a school band concert to listen to their grandson play. Jimmy does not wear his hearing aid and is glad he didn't—he thinks the music is awful, but, of course, would never admit that he doesn't like it.

JIMMY BLEY
Season 2

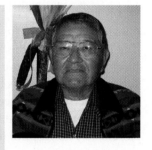

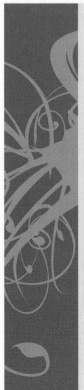

Biographical Information
Jimmy is a 78-year-old Native American male with moderate emphysema and hearing loss. He is a retired veteran who served as an electronics technician in the Army for his entire career. In his retirement, Jimmy has taken an interest in computers. He spends most of his time surfing the Internet or playing games on the computer; he also likes to build computers. Jimmy has been married for 56 years to his wife Cecelia. They argue a lot, but they would not know what to do without one another just the same. They have several grown children, grandchildren, and great-grandchildren who live within the community. Jimmy often goes with his wife to the Neighborhood Senior Center for bingo night.

Jimmy considers himself healthy. He describes his hearing loss as mild. He has a hearing aid, but does not like to wear it and thus does not make changing the batteries a priority. He does not perceive his hearing loss to be much of a problem. Likewise, Jimmy describes his emphysema as "not that bad." However, he becomes short of breath with most activities; thus, it takes time for him to complete tasks. He compensates by taking his time to do most things. Over time, he learned that he must pace himself; if he does not, he becomes exhausted, and it takes several days to recover. Jimmy is very aware of his limits—yet, at the same time, he does not generally consider his illness to be very bad. Although he would not admit it, he recognizes that his breathing has become more of a problem during the past couple of years. He continues to smoke and knows he should quit, but he just can't seem to get interested in quitting because he enjoys it.

Episode 1

Jimmy and his wife attend a granddaughter's soccer game. It is very cold outside, and Jimmy feels more short of breath than usual when walking back to the car. He never returned to the smoking cessation classes, because he just didn't believe it was worth it. He finds that he is okay just using his inhaler when needed, but realizes he should quit smoking. He uses his inhaler while walking to the car.

Episode 2

Jimmy has been cleaning out the garage for the past few days and notices that it takes him quite awhile to catch his breath. He feels especially short of breath and uses his inhaler again. He also notices that the past several times he's mowed the grass, it's been more exhausting than usual. Cecelia has also noticed these changes and has been nagging him about how much better he would feel if he quit smoking. Jimmy and his daughter accompany Cecelia to the clinic. **[P]**

Episode 3

Jimmy makes a decision this week to quit smoking but decides *not* to tell anyone, just in case things don't work out. He picks up some brochures with smoking cessation tips and reads them to get motivated.

Episode 4

Jimmy smokes his last cigarette today. He has selected one tip he thinks might help: Every time he thinks about or really craves a cigarette, he will take one and place it in a jar he has hidden in his bedroom closet. **[P]**

Episode 5

The local forest fire has kept Jimmy indoors. He knows if he goes out, he will have problems breathing. Cecelia tells Jimmy that the dryer is broken "AGAIN!" Jimmy looks at it and determines he needs to go to the store for parts to fix it. Cecelia also wants to go out, but he tells her they should stay home until the air clears.

Episode 6

The air is clear enough for Jimmy to venture out with Cecelia again. They go to the Neighborhood Senior Center to play bingo and to the hardware store to buy parts for the dryer. Jimmy is glad that he didn't tell anyone about his quitting, because he is smoking again; still, he feels better since he's "cut down" on the number of cigarettes per day. Over the weekend, Jimmy enjoys having his family at the house. He spends most of his time playing computer games with his grandchildren.

Episode 7

Jimmy accompanies Cecelia and his daughter to the nurse practitioner to see about Cecelia's arthritis pain. While sitting in the waiting room, he notices another man come in with portable oxygen. The man appears to be short of breath from the walk in to the office from the parking lot. Jimmy is glad he does not have to tote an oxygen tank around with him.

Episode 8

No news this week.

Episode 9

Jimmy goes to his son's home to help him fix a computer. They have to move furniture in order to pull the computer out. In shifting the furniture, Jimmy becomes very short of breath and is without his inhaler. He panics and struggles to get air. He sits down for about 30 minutes to rest and catch his breath. His son is concerned and inquires about the last time his Dad has talked to a doctor about his breathing. Jimmy tells his son his breathing is fine; he is just a little out of shape. **[P]**

Episode 10

Jimmy sees Dr. Rowe for routine follow-up care. He has a routine chest x-ray taken to evaluate his condition. Jimmy tells Dr. Rowe that he's been feeling fine; he just gets short of breath on occasion. The physician talks with Jimmy about the progression of his disease and reinforces the need to stop smoking. She inquires about his attempts at doing so. Jimmy tells Dr. Rowe about "white smoke," but Dr. Rowe isn't sure what he is talking about. Thinking about his experience last week and the words of his physician, Jimmy again thinks about ways to stop smoking. On the Internet, he reads about nicotine gum and places an order online. **[VC]**

Episode 11

Jimmy received the nicotine gum and has been following the directions. He is down to chewing one piece every few hours and is proud of his progress. Again, he enjoys watching the stash of cigarettes grow as he puts one in the jar every time he craves one. This really helps motivate Jimmy.

Cecelia is down with the flu this week; one of Jimmy's daughters and a granddaughter spend a lot of time at the house taking care of things for them. **[P]**

Episode 12

No news this week.

Episode 13

While outside doing a little yard work, Jimmy sees the dogs fighting with a cat that has gotten in the yard. Jimmy scurries across the yard to break it up. The cat runs off, but one of his dogs has a big scratch across its nose. Jimmy becomes very upset and short of breath, and wants a cigarette. To calm himself down, he reaches into his shirt pocket and takes three pieces of nicotine gum, thinking more is better. It burns his tongue, and he feels dizzy and becomes sweaty. **[P]**

Episode 14
Jimmy decides Cecelia is probably right about the nicotine gum, concluding that it is just too dangerous. He decides it is probably safer to smoke just a few cigarettes a day and use his inhaler when needed. He is glad Cecelia does not nag him when she sees him smoking. He coughs nearly every morning for a few minutes when he wakes up; he attributes this to his body readjusting to the cigarettes.

Episode 15
Cecelia "drags" Jimmy to the Neighborhood Arts and Crafts fair. He really does not want to go, but it is an activity they go to each year. Jimmy gets tired and finds a bench to sit on while his wife and daughters walk around to each exhibit. A couple of other men who are also waiting for their wives begin to talk with Jimmy, but he has a hard time hearing them because of all of the extraneous noise in the exhibit hall. **[P]**

JIMMY BLEY
Season 3

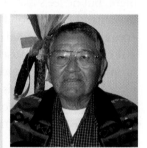

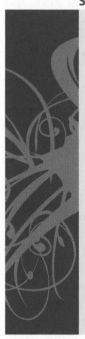

Biographical Information
Jimmy is a 79-year-old Native American male with moderate emphysema and hearing loss. He is a retired veteran who served as an electronics technician in the Army for his entire career. In his retirement, Jimmy has taken an interest in computers. He spends most of his time surfing the Internet or playing games on the computer; he also likes to build computers. Jimmy has been married for 57 years to his wife Cecelia. They argue a lot, but they would not know what to do without one another just the same. They have several grown children, grandchildren, and great-grandchildren who live within the community. Jimmy occasionally goes with his wife to the Neighborhood Senior Center for bingo night.

Jimmy considers himself healthy. He describes his hearing loss as mild. He has a hearing aid, but does not like to wear it and thus does not make changing the batteries a priority. He does not perceive his hearing loss to be much of a problem. Likewise, Jimmy describes his emphysema as "not that bad." Recently, his episodes of shortness of breath have interfered with activities more than usual, and he has made efforts on two occasions to stop smoking. Both times, Jimmy was not successful. He is privately very aware of the fact that his breathing has worsened and is using his inhaler much more frequently.

Episode 1
Jimmy's daughter hears an announcement on the radio that free flu shots are being offered at a local health clinic. She tells both of her parents, but Jimmy is sure it will just make him sick. He is already not feeling great and does not want to take the vaccine. His daughter tells him that both of them are considered at high risk for getting the flu. Jimmy feels that he is basically fairly healthy and never gets sick anyway, so he will just take his chances.

Episode 2
Although Jimmy has had less energy and a cough, he enthusiastically agrees to help his 13-year-old granddaughter navigate the Internet to help her find what she needs for a school science project. Feeling very tired, he takes a nap after she leaves. **[P]**

Episode 3
No news this week.

Episode 4
Jimmy continues to feel very tired and has a nagging cough. He gets short of breath very easily while doing chores outside. Over the weekend, he has so much difficulty mowing the lawn that he lets his son-in-law finish the job for him. He goes in the house, lies on the couch to watch TV, and naps off and on for the rest of the afternoon. His son and daughter suggest that he go to his doctor. Jimmy tells them his appointment is in another month or so, and he can wait to see his doctor then. Jimmy's cough at night has become more frequent, although he tends to sleep through it.

Episode 5

Jimmy has begun waking in the middle of the night with a persistent, productive cough. He finds himself needing his inhaler as soon as he is awake. Jimmy believes he has just caught a bad cold. To help him sleep, Jimmy props himself up on several pillows. Cecelia sets up a humidifier in the room at night, which seems to help. He spends most of the day resting and taking over-the-counter cold medicine in an effort to treat this "cold." Jimmy is resistant to Cecelia's suggestion to see a doctor. "It is just a cold," he tells her. **[VC]**

Episode 6

Jimmy feels a bit better this week. He still has a cough at night, but he feels like he has more energy and is sleeping a bit better. He feels good enough to accompany Cecelia on errands, but is very tired by the time they get home. Jimmy's son comes by the house and takes care of the yard work; Jimmy does not object to this, believing that he should conserve his strength—he is sure that by next week he will feel up to doing the yard work. He has intermittent "coughing fits," and Cecelia tells Jimmy to quit the cigarettes.

Episode 7

This week, Jimmy feels worse than before. He is surprised at how long the symptoms have persisted. He continues to have a persistent, productive cough. He finds that he becomes short of breath much more easily than he normally does, and it takes him twice as long to shower and get dressed in the morning. His appetite has dropped off, and he has not been drinking as many fluids as he needs—partly because of the effort involved in eating and drinking.

Jimmy wakes up suddenly in the middle of the night and is unable to catch his breath. He tries to use his inhaler, but this doesn't seem to help. He can't move air well enough to take a deep breath and get any medication into his lungs. He feels like he is suffocating and becomes very anxious. Cecelia wants to call for an ambulance, but Jimmy insists on going to the hospital in their car. Cecelia calls her daughter, and they take him to the emergency department. Walking from the house to the car is very difficult and compromises Jimmy further. Jimmy is seen and treated in the emergency department by Dr. Gordon and is admitted to the intensive care unit (ICU) with a diagnosis of pneumonia and acute respiratory failure. **[P]**

Episode 8

Jimmy has spent the past week intubated on a ventilator and is receiving antibiotics. He is very scared and anxious. Although he is unable to talk, he is comforted by having his family with him; when they are present, Jimmy is much calmer. A family member stays with him as long as the nursing staff allows a visitor. Although the pneumonia is resolving, the nurses in the ICU have not yet been successful in weaning Jimmy from the ventilator. **[P]**

Episode 9

Jimmy has taken a turn for the worse. He has become septic, and his blood pressure has dropped significantly. He remains on a ventilator, is receiving medications to maintain his blood pressure, and is on multiple antibiotics. He is confused and disoriented. The nurses keep him heavily sedated to manage his anxiety and control patient-ventilation asynchrony. **[P]**

Episode 10

Jimmy's condition stabilized at the end of last week, and he is now quickly improving. Jimmy is not confused, but feels like he's just awakened from a bad dream. He cannot recall much of anything. The experience has left him very weak and frightened.

The ICU nurses successfully wean Jimmy off the ventilator, and he is moved to the step-down unit. He is on oxygen, and his oxygen saturation is monitored carefully. A nurse brings in a fan to help relieve Jimmy's sense of shortness of breath. It really makes him feel better.

Episode 11

Jimmy's condition has improved. Because he is deconditioned, respiratory, physical, and occupational therapists have been working with him to help him regain mobility and the ability to perform activities of daily living (ADLs). Case management is involved with assessing his discharge needs. Because his oxygen saturation falls below 90% when he is off oxygen doing any kind of activity, it is determined that he will need supplemental oxygen at home. He also will need to continue with outpatient physical and occupational therapy after discharge. He is unable to ambulate without the use of a walker. A dietitian meets with Jimmy and Cecelia to talk about ways to improve Jimmy's nutritional status.

Because of this ordeal, Jimmy has become very depressed. He does not interact much with his family or the staff. He does not like the idea of being dependent on oxygen, and his weak condition makes him feel helpless. The physician prescribes bupropion (Wellbutrin SR), 150 mg a day, for depression. Jimmy just wants to go home. He believes that, if he could just get home, all of these problems would resolve. Jimmy is discharged at the end of the week. **[P]**

Episode 12

Jimmy is very happy to be at home in his own bed and with his family. He prefers being cared for by Cecelia and his daughters than by the nurses at the hospital. He is happy to eat the food prepared by his family. He is very discouraged about the oxygen and doesn't want to be dependent. Cecelia places a fan in his room at night to help him rest easier. He goes to outpatient physical and occupational therapy three times a week, and he is slowly regaining his strength. He just can't believe how weak he became while in the hospital. He also goes to the pulmonary rehabilitation clinic this week.

Episode 13

Jimmy continues going to outpatient physical therapy and the pulmonary rehabilitation clinic this week. He hates being attached to the oxygen, but realizes he cannot do without it. Sometimes, he takes it off and sneaks a cigarette, although the idea of smoking turns out to be better than the actual smoking. He begins to lose his desire for cigarettes. **[P]**

Episode 14

No news this week.

Episode 15

Jimmy has completed his rehabilitation and is attempting to get back into his normal daily activities—however, he has had to redefine "normal routine." His energy is gradually improving, but he is unable to do many of his former activities; his son and daughters come by the house every day to help out with whatever needs to be done. Everyone notices his spirits have improved significantly as well—he especially enjoys it when his grandchildren come to the house. Jimmy has finally been able to quit smoking and has vowed to never touch cigarettes again.

Cecelia suggests to Jimmy they go to the Senior Center for bingo, but Jimmy doesn't want to do this because he feels embarrassed about the oxygen. Instead, they decide to spend an evening at their daughter's home.

CECELIA BLEY
Season 1

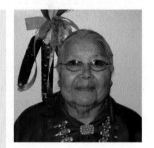

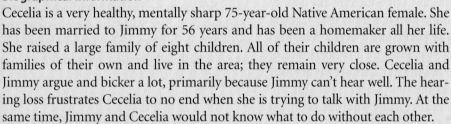

Biographical Information

Cecelia is a very healthy, mentally sharp 75-year-old Native American female. She has been married to Jimmy for 56 years and has been a homemaker all her life. She raised a large family of eight children. All of their children are grown with families of their own and live in the area; they remain very close. Cecelia and Jimmy argue and bicker a lot, primarily because Jimmy can't hear well. The hearing loss frustrates Cecelia to no end when she is trying to talk with Jimmy. At the same time, Jimmy and Cecelia would not know what to do without each other.

Cecelia's only health-related problem is joint pain, which she describes as an annoyance. The joint pain has become increasingly more noticeable over the past few years, but she has never had a medical evaluation for this. She wakes up very stiff and sore in the morning, but usually feels better once the day gets going. Cecelia does most of the general housekeeping, grocery shopping, and cooking. Her primary hobby is making jewelry. She is very skilled at this and, when she was younger, she used to regularly sell her jewelry at shows and to shops specializing in Native American arts. Now that she has gotten older, she only does this on occasion. She gives most of the jewelry she now makes to her daughters to sell for her. Although she likes to spend time in the garden, she limits this activity now because her knees hurt too much. She also enjoys reading and watching television. She is very fond of their two dogs and is an active member of her church.

Episode 1

Cecelia and Jimmy go to the market and then to their daughter's house in the afternoon. While driving in the car, Cecelia has to yell at Jimmy to pull over because he fails to hear an ambulance siren. She often feels frustrated with him because of his lack of concern regarding his hearing.

Episode 2

Cecelia falls in the bathroom after slipping on water from a leaky faucet. She experiences considerable joint pain and hollers out for Jimmy. Because Jimmy is not wearing his hearing aid and is in another room working on the computer, he does not hear her yelling. Cecelia finally gives up yelling for him to help her and gets up slowly herself. She goes into the other room, yells at Jimmy for not helping her, and tells him to fix the leaky faucet. **[P]**

Episode 3
No news this week.

Episode 4
Cecelia's granddaughter asks her to come to her school to talk about her Native American heritage as a presenter during the Cultural Heritage Week at the grade school. Cecelia gives a short presentation to the grade-school children about growing up on a reservation and talks with them about Native American arts and jewelry. Cecelia enjoys having a chance to share her experiences with others.

Episode 5
No news this week.

Episode 6
One of Cecelia and Jimmy's granddaughters has a birthday this week; their entire family will have a party for her at their home over the weekend. Cecelia tells Jimmy about the plans on Wednesday. On Saturday, the family spends the entire day at their home. Jimmy asks Cecelia why he was not told of the party, and Cecelia tells him that he is an old fool for not wearing his hearing aid. Cecelia thoroughly enjoys having her family visit her, but by the time they all go home, her knees and hips are hurting quite a bit—she realizes that she has been up nearly the entire day.

Episode 7
Cecelia goes to a community health fair with her daughter and granddaughter. At the fair, Cecelia has osteoporosis, blood pressure, and glucose screenings, and has her height and weight checked. At one of the stations, Cecelia talks with a nurse about her joint pain. The nurse encourages Cecelia to make an appointment with her health-care provider to have this symptom evaluated and gives her a patient-information flyer on osteoarthritis. After reading the flyer, Cecelia is pretty sure that osteoarthritis is what is causing her pain. Cecelia learns that several over-the-counter medications such as glucosamine, acetaminophen, and ibuprofen are effective for treating arthritic pain. Cecelia's daughter agrees to pick these medications up from the drug store for her to try.

Cecelia also picks up a flyer from a table on smoking cessation. She takes the flyer home and gives it to Jimmy to read. **[P]**

Episode 8
After spending time in her garden this week, Cecelia experiences a great deal of pain in her joints. Her daughter helps her mother by massaging her joints. Cecilia tells her daughter that she is experiencing so much pain that she wants to see a physician to find out if she could benefit from other treatments. Cecelia's daughter calls and makes an appointment for next week.

Episode 9
Cecelia's daughter and Jimmy accompany Cecelia to Dr. Rowe's office, where a history and examination are done. From the history, Dr. Rowe learns that Cecelia's primary symptoms are joint pain and joint swelling. She also learns that Cecelia has had joint pain since her early 40s, but it has become more noticeable and progressively worse in her 60s. Her pain is most severe in the knees and hips—often making walking very painful, especially in the early part of the morning. In the past, Cecelia could get relief by resting, but over the past several years, she has experienced pain with activity and during rest; in fact, she often awakens at night with joint pain. She self-treats with ibuprofen and aspirin. Occasionally, she uses a heating pad over her joints and relates that her daughters help by massaging her joints. After an examination, the physician advises Cecelia to have some lab work and x-rays performed; she is scheduled for these tests in the upcoming week. **[VC]**

Episode 10
Cecelia's son takes her to the outpatient radiology services to have x-rays taken of her knees, hips, and spine; she also goes to the outpatient lab to have blood tests (complete blood count and erythrocyte sedimentation rate) done. Several days later, she returns to Dr. Rowe's office to get her results. She is told that she has joint space narrowing in her joints, a finding that is consistent with osteoarthritis. She is also told that her blood tests were all normal. Dr. Rowe offers Cecelia little more than telling her to do what she has already been doing; basically, she is told to use over-the-counter medications to treat her condition—acetaminophen, ibuprofen, and glucosamine. Additionally, she is advised to increase the period of rest between activities and avoid strenuous movement of her knee and hip joints. Cecelia wonders why she even bothered going to the doctor. **[VC]**

Episode 11
No news this week.

Episode 12
Cecelia has been spending a great deal of time during the past few weeks making jewelry, as she has agreed to go to an art show with her daughter out of town next week.

Fortunately, making jewelry is something she is able to do without causing joint pain. **[P]**

Episode 13

Cecelia shows her jewelry at an arts and crafts fair with her daughter. She enjoys the show and realizes she misses doing this, but also recognizes the amount of work involved in preparing and doing the showing. She has a successful show, but is quite tired from the experience.

Episode 14

No news this week.

Episode 15

Cecelia attends her grandson's music concert at the school. He is thrilled that she and Jimmy come to hear him play. After the concert, Cecelia and Jimmy go to their son's home to visit with family members.

CECELIA BLEY
Season 2

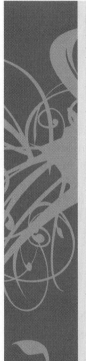

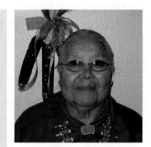

Biographical Information

Cecelia is a very healthy, mentally sharp 75-year-old Native American female. She has been married to Jimmy for 56 years and has been a homemaker all her life. She raised a large family of eight children. All of their children are grown with families of their own and live in the area; they remain very close. Cecelia and Jimmy argue and bicker a lot, primarily because Jimmy can't hear well. The hearing loss frustrates Cecelia to no end when she is trying to talk with Jimmy. At the same time, Jimmy and Cecelia would not know what to do without each other.

Cecelia's only health-related problem is osteoarthritis, which she describes as an annoyance. The joint pain has become increasingly more noticeable over the last few years, and she finally had a formal medical evaluation a few months ago. She was told to treat her condition with acetaminophen, ibuprofen, and glucosamine. Additionally, she was advised to increase the period of rest between activities and avoid strenuous movement to her knee and hip joints.

Cecelia does most of the general housekeeping, grocery shopping, and cooking. Her primary hobby is making jewelry. She is very skilled at this and, when she was younger, she used to regularly sell her jewelry at shows and to shops specializing in Native American arts. Now that she has gotten older, she only does this on occasion. She gives most of the jewelry she now makes to her daughters to sell for her. Although she likes to spend time in the garden, she limits this activity now because her knees hurt too much. She also enjoys reading and watching television. She is very fond of their two dogs and is an active member of her church.

Episode 1

Cecelia and her husband attend a granddaughter's soccer game. It is cold outside, and her arthritis makes walking and moving her hands painful. Jimmy needs to use his inhaler when they return to the car after the game because he is quite short of breath. The cold air bothers both of them. In the car, Cecelia takes an aspirin for her pain.

Episode 2

Cecelia has returned to Dr. Rowe to seek a different treatment, because the arthritis pain is getting worse. Dr. Rowe prescribes Darvocet, 1-2 tablets orally every 4 hours as needed for pain. She is told to be careful and not to take too many, as the medication can be addictive and is constipating. **[VC] [P]**

Episode 3

Cecelia has been worried about what Dr. Rowe said regarding addiction and constipation from Darvocet. She is also very aware of her bowel habits and hates the idea of becoming constipated. For these reasons, she rarely takes the Darvocet, despite the fact that she has been experiencing a great deal of pain and joint stiffness.

Episode 4

No news this week.

Episode 5
Cecelia is frustrated because the dryer is not working properly again and she can't get her laundry dried. Jimmy can fix the dryer, but he does not want to leave the house until the smoky air from the forest fires clears. Cecelia's daughter comes to the house, and they go to a Laundromat together, leaving Jimmy at home. **[P]**

Episode 6
Cecelia cooks a Sunday dinner for her entire family. Her daughters can tell that she is having pain and insist that she sit down while they do the dishes. By the time everyone leaves, Cecelia is very tired and hurting from standing and preparing the meal. She decides to take the Darvocet and risk getting addicted and constipated. **[P]**

Episode 7
Cecelia returns to a follow-up appointment with Dr. Rowe, taking her Darvocet bottle as requested. Dr. Rowe asks Cecelia about her pain and how often she has been taking the pills. Cecelia is reluctant to complain and embarrassed to admit her concerns with constipation and addiction. Dr. Rowe notices how few of the prescribed pills Cecelia has used and begins to inquire further. Cecelia's daughter explains why she has not taken many of the pills. Dr. Rowe counsels Cecelia about appropriate use to minimize her fears about the medicine. **[P]**

Episode 8
No news this week.

Episode 9
Having some of her misunderstandings and fears addressed regarding the pain medication, Cecelia is much more willing to take her pain medicine when she needs it. She has begun to work in her garden more regularly again. Her daughter suggests that they do another art show. Cecelia would like to do it, but the show is out of town, and she is pretty sure Jimmy would rather stay home. **[P]**

Episode 10
Cecelia and Jimmy go to a grandson's soccer game. Cecelia takes some pain medication before she goes, anticipating pain with the walking. She and Jimmy find a comfortable spot from which to watch the game and set up their lawn chairs. She becomes annoyed when some people decide to stand along the sidelines in front of where they are sitting. They pack their stuff up and move to another part of the field. After the game, they go to their son's home for supper.

Episode 11
Cecelia comes down with the flu this week. She is very weak and tired, and has a cough and fever. Cecelia's daughter and granddaughter come to the house to help take care of Cecilia and the household so she can rest. Cecelia's daughters give her plenty of fluids.

Episode 12
No news this week.

Episode 13
Cecelia hears the commotion of a dog and cat fight in the yard and goes outside. She sees that Jimmy is short of breath. She watches him take out some of his nicotine gum and is concerned a short while later when he becomes sweaty and a little pale. She tells Jimmy that the gum is probably not as good for him as he thinks and encourages him to throw it away.

Episode 14
No news this week.

Episode 15
Cecelia, her daughters, and Jimmy go to the Neighborhood Arts and Crafts show. She and her daughters visit each booth and are particularly impressed with the quilts on display. Cecelia has never made a quilt and talks with her daughters about making one. They talk to Pam Allen, the grand prize winner, about quilting designs and the best place in town to shop for quilting supplies. **[P]**

CECELIA BLEY
Season 3

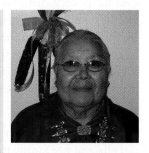

Biographical Information

Cecelia is a very healthy, mentally sharp 76-year-old Native American female. She has been married to Jimmy for 57 years and has been a homemaker all her life. She raised a large family of eight children. All of their children are grown with families of their own and live in the area; they remain very close. Cecelia and Jimmy argue and bicker a lot, primarily because Jimmy can't hear well. The hearing loss frustrates Cecelia to no end when she is trying to talk with Jimmy. At the same time, Jimmy and Cecelia would not know what to do without each other.

Cecelia's only health-related problem is osteoarthritis, which she describes as an annoyance. The joint pain has become increasingly more noticeable over the last few years, and she finally had a formal medical evaluation last year and was told to treat her condition with acetaminophen, ibuprofen, and glucosamine. A few months ago, the pain really interfered with her activities, and she went back to see Dr. Rowe at the Neighborhood Clinic. Her pain medications were adjusted, and Cecelia has had some improvement.

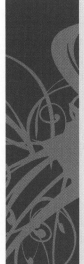

Episode 1
Cecelia's daughter tells her she heard an announcement on the radio about free flu shots offered at the Neighborhood Clinic. She recommends that both of her parents get the vaccine, as they are older and considered to be at high risk for the flu. Cecelia agrees that this is a good idea and plans to go when the shot clinic is offered. Jimmy goes along, but decides not to get the shot.

Episode 2
Cecelia and her daughters spend an afternoon working on their quilts. Cecelia finds the work enjoyable, but it causes her hands to be sore. She takes ibuprofen and feels a bit better.

Jimmy frequently coughs during the night lately, waking Cecelia. She gets annoyed, not only because it wakes her up, but also because Jimmy sleeps right through it. She figures he sleeps through it because he can't hear anything.

Episode 3
No news this week.

Episode 4
Cecelia attends an all-day function at the church, making lunches for the Neighborhood Homeless Shelter. One of the ladies comments to Cecelia that she looks tired. She shares with the ladies that her arthritis has been acting up (which is true). She does not mention that the real reason she is tired is because Jimmy's coughing at night wakes her frequently.

After spending the entire day on her feet, she takes two Darvocet tablets and puts her legs up when she gets home.

Episode 5
Cecelia continues to be kept awake at night with Jimmy's coughing. She knows he is not feeling like himself because of his limited activity. He can hardly do anything without waiting a long time to catch his breath. She has repeatedly tried to get him to see the doctor, but he does not think he is that sick.

Episode 6
Cecelia is glad to see that Jimmy seems to be feeling better. She is very annoyed about the fact that they have no water service. It is a significant disruption to her routine. She hears the National Guard is distributing bottles of water, so Cecelia goes with her daughter and son-in-law to get some water for the house.

Episode 7
This week, Cecelia notices that Jimmy is eating and drinking very little, and he has shortness of breath with limited activity. Cecelia wakes from sleep hearing Jimmy cough and gasping for air; he is very anxious and gets no relief with his inhaler. Jimmy does not argue with her when she tells him they must go see a doctor, but he refuses to go in an ambulance. He insists they go in their car. She calls one of her daughters and her son to help her take Jimmy to the Neighborhood Hospital Emergency Department, where he is treated by Dr. Gordon and later admitted to intensive care. **[P]**

Episode 8
Cecelia is very distressed about Jimmy's condition. She and her family stay at the hospital and visit him whenever they are allowed into the ICU. She tries to get as much information as she can from the doctors and nurses, but everybody is so busy. She has a hard time understanding everything that is happening. **[P]**

Episode 9
Jimmy has taken a turn for the worse. The physicians tell Cecelia and her family that Jimmy's condition is very serious, and they want to know what she might want to do if his heart stops. She has not had this conversation with Jimmy before and is confused about what to do. In her tradition, families don't talk about death. She doesn't want to talk to her children about it either. She is angry that the doctors are discussing the possibility of Jimmy dying; she would rather they attended to him in every way and not speak of such things. She doesn't like having to be asked these questions. She prays often for his healing. Cecelia worries about the care Jimmy is receiving. She has read in the newspaper about the nursing strike and wonders if the nurses caring for Jimmy know what to do. She wonders if the reason he got worse is because of the nursing care. **[P]**

Episode 10
Cecelia continues to remain with Jimmy every day. She is relieved that her prayers have been answered. Although she is glad he has improved enough to be moved to a step-down unit, she is a bit worried that they will not monitor him as closely as they were able to in the ICU. She also does not know if the nurses will care for her husband in the way that they should. She is very tired because of all the time she has spent at the hospital. Cecelia's daughter convinces her to go home and rest for part of the day while she and her husband stay with Jimmy. **[P]**

Episode 11
Cecelia worries about how down Jimmy is; he does not seem to care about getting better. She wishes there was something she could do to lift his spirits. Cecelia meets with the discharge planner to discuss Jimmy's needs once he leaves the hospital.

Cecelia shares her concerns with the staff about Jimmy's mood; she learns the physician has prescribed an antidepressant. Cecelia and her family prepare to bring Jimmy home from the hospital. The medical supply company comes to the home to install grab bars in the showers and deliver home oxygen. Cecelia and her son and daughters are taught how to use the oxygen tanks. Cecelia is thankful for her children, who will help her take care of Jimmy once he comes home. **[VC]**

Episode 12
Cecelia and her family are thankful to have Jimmy home, although caring for him is much more work than they anticipated. Cecelia is glad the physical therapist taught them how to help Jimmy get up and is thankful that the nurses taught them about oxygen therapy and his medications. Cecelia's children are at the house regularly and take Cecelia and Jimmy to all of his outpatient appointments.

Episode 13
Cecelia is encouraged by the progress she sees Jimmy making with rehabilitation. His spirits seem to be better, and he is taking a greater interest in the activities around him. She also notices Jimmy is not smoking much—she knows he tries to "sneak" a cigarette on occasion, but doesn't let on that she knows this.

Episode 14
No news this week.

Episode 15
As Jimmy's condition has improved, Cecelia has been able to get more rest. She finally has a chance to get back to the quilts she and her daughters started months ago, and her daughter has talked about getting enough jewelry made for an upcoming show. With all of the activity, Cecelia has let the garden go these past few months and is not sure she will get back to it this season.

JAMES HOUSEHOLD

JAMES FAMILY STORY OVERVIEW

Character	Season 1	Season 2	Season 3
NORMA JAMES	Mrs. James is a widow who lives alone and is somewhat socially isolated. She has type 2 diabetes, atrial fibrillation, and hypertension. She sees multiple physicians and takes multiple medications. Early in this season she has a diabetic ulcer on her foot. She becomes acquainted with Karen, a nurse at the local Senior Center, and begins to go there regularly.	Mrs. James has a mild stroke during this season. She has initial affective aphasia, problems swallowing, and weakness to the right side of her body. She has a feeding tube and Foley for a short while, and develops a UTI. She experiences depression over her situation. She spends time at the rehabilitation hospital and eventually returns home in the care of her son, Brian.	Mrs. James makes remarkable progress at home in the care of her son, Brian. Eventually she becomes independent enough that Brian is able to return to his home. The ordeal has resulted in the reestablishment of a positive relationship between Mrs. James and her son.

CONCEPTS   *Communication, Coping, Infection, Interpersonal relationships, Intracranial Regulation, Metabolism, Mobility, Mood, Nutrition, Pain, Perfusion, Tissue Integrity, Sensory/Perceptual*

NORMA JAMES
Season 1

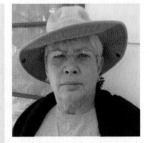

Biographical Information

Norma James is a 65-year-old widow who lives alone. Although she has lived in the Neighborhood for years, she is somewhat socially isolated. She has two adult sons with whom she has limited contact—they live out of the state and rarely call. There are only a few individuals Mrs. James considers friends; she does not particularly like many people and prefers the company of her six cats. She has a long history of type 2 diabetes mellitus and hypertension. In recent years, she was diagnosed with atrial fibrillation. She has multiple physicians and takes multiple medications including:

- Glucotrol, 10 mg twice a day
- captopril, 50 mg twice a day
- digoxin, 125 mcg once a day
- Coumadin, 5 mg once a day

Mrs. James has a known drug allergy to penicillin.

Mrs. James does not work; she has very limited savings and relies on Social Security benefits for income. She smokes about $1/2$ pack of cigarettes per day and has been a smoker since she was in her 20s. She drinks alcohol "a couple times a year—usually a glass of wine at a special dinner." Mrs. James does not drive and relies on her friends, neighbors, or the city bus for transportation. She lives near a grocery store and prides herself on being able to get most things she needs without any assistance. She spends most of her time alone at home and occupies herself by watching television, reading, and doing crossword and jigsaw puzzles.

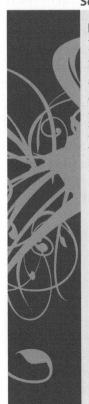

Episode 1

Mrs. James has a sore on her ankle that has been there for the past several weeks. It does not really hurt all that much, but she has been unable to get it to heal. The cashier at the convenience store tells Mrs. James that she should use butter to help heal wounds, because it keeps the wound moist and helps to enhance healing. **[P]**

Episode 2

Mrs. James decided to follow the advice of her friend (the cashier at the convenience store) and has been applying butter to her wound for about one week. The wound does not seem to be getting any better; in fact, it looks a little worse, so Mrs. James stops the butter treatment. She knows she should get an appointment with her primary care provider, but when she calls to make an appointment, she is told that the physician she likes is out of the office on vacation for the next 2 weeks. She has heard about a nurse clinic at the Neighborhood Senior Center not far from her home, but has never been to the center because she does not perceive herself to be old. Mrs. James decides to continue treating the wound herself. **[P]**

Episode 3

Mrs. James' wound continues to look progressively worse; it now has a yellowish drainage, and the skin around the wound has become red. Her foot also now hurts when she walks on it. She goes to the emergency department (ED) early in the morning. After sitting in the waiting room for 4 hours, Mrs. James tells the ED receptionist that she has better things to do than sit in a waiting room all day. She decides to go to the Senior Center just this once to see if the nurse at the clinic will look at her leg.

At the Senior Center Nurse Clinic, Mrs. James meets Karen, a geriatric clinical nurse specialist. Karen takes a short history and checks Mrs. James' vital signs and glucose levels. Mrs. James is unable to recall all of the medications that she takes. After looking at the wound, Karen tells Mrs. James that she must see her physician. Karen makes an appointment for that day and arranges a ride for Mrs. James through the Senior Center. Before leaving, Karen suggests to Mrs. James that she come back to see her next week and bring a list of medications that she takes. Mrs. James also learns from Karen that free lunch is served at the Senior Center.

At her physician's office, Mrs. James is told that her foot is infected and will require antibiotic treatment and dressing changes. The office staff arranges for Mrs. James to have a home health nurse make daily visits for IV antibiotic therapy and dressing changes for 10 days. The nurse and physician both note that her blood pressure and glucose level are somewhat elevated, but they assume the change is related to the infection and pain. **[VC]**

Episode 4

Mrs. James completes her 10-day dose of antibiotic therapy. The wound is no longer painful and is beginning to heal. She has a follow-up visit at her primary care physician's office and is instructed to continue with daily wound care. The office nurse talks with Mrs. James about the need for medication adherence to limit the effects of her diabetes. The nurse asks her if she has any problems with her medications. Mrs. James says she has no problems—she just doesn't always take her medication. **[P]**

Episode 5

No news this week.

Episode 6

Mrs. James decides to go back to the Senior Center Nurse Clinic to see the nurse because she likes Karen and wants to show her that her leg is healing. Karen checks her vitals and glucose level, noting that both are elevated. Karen looks at the leg and can see that the wound is healing. Mrs. James forgets to bring the list of medications she is currently taking, so Karen talks with her about how she obtains her medications and how she keeps them organized. Karen gives Mrs. James a diabetes and foot care brochure and asks her to bring a list of the medications she takes on her next visit. Mrs. James is in a hurry to leave so she can get to the free Senior Center lunch. **[VC]**

Episode 7

Mrs. James was planning to go back to the Senior Center this week to see the nurse, but she didn't like what was on the lunch menu for that day. She is scheduled for another follow-up visit at her physician's office, but elects not to go because it is raining hard on the day of her appointment and she does not want to be out in the weather. **[P]**

Episode 8

No news this week.

Episode 9

Mrs. James is on her way out the door to go to the Senior Center for lunch and to see the nurse when one of her cats gets out. She spends the next hour waiting by the window for the cat to come back. She is worried that the cat will be killed by a car or a dog and is mad that she is going to miss the lunch that day. When the cat comes back to the front door, Mrs. James is relieved and decides she needs to stay home the rest of the day to take care of her cats. **[P]**

Episode 10

Mrs. James finally makes it back to see Karen at the Senior Center Nursing Clinic. Her vital signs are checked (blood pressure, 126/92 mm Hg; blood glucose, 124 mg/dL), and Karen asks Mrs. James about her medication list (which she has not brought along with her). When examining Mrs. James' feet, Karen notices that her shoes are in poor shape; the edges of her shoes have been cut down and covered with cotton balls and tape. The nurse talks to her about the need for shoes that fit and suggests that she check at the Senior Center for help with obtaining properly fitting shoes. Karen also notes that the wound on her leg has almost completely healed.

Mrs. James goes to the Senior Center with the intention of getting lunch, but instead wanders into a leather craft class. She sits down and begins to work with the leather. She listens to some of the other women in the class and is annoyed at all their chatter, especially one lady named Mary Martin. She likes the leather craft activity, but does not like interacting with the women there. **[P]**

Episode 11

Mrs. James gets a notice in the mail from the city, stating that the bushes in her front yard are encroaching on the street and blocking the view. The notice states she has 30 days to cut back the branches or pay the city to remove the brush and potentially face a city fine. This makes Mrs. James very upset, because she knows she can't just go out and cut down bushes at her age. She asks a neighbor to help her cut the bushes back. A few days later she sees a teenager in her yard doing the work, but Mrs. James does not go out to talk to him or thank him. She wonders if he is in a gang and is not sure if he can be trusted. **[P]**

Episode 12

No news this week.

Episode 13

Mrs. James runs out of her Glucotrol, and when she calls the drugstore to get it refilled, she is informed that her prescription has expired. Mrs. James goes to the Senior Center Nursing Clinic the following day to see Karen and explains her situation. Vitals and blood glucose are measured (blood glucose, 192 mg/dL). Karen calls the physician's office and arranges for a small refill to be available to her until she comes in for an appointment. While on the phone with the physician's office, the nurse is able to get a list of Mrs. James' medications and dosages, as well as the names of her cardiologist and gynecologist. Karen also sees that Mrs. James is still wearing the same shoes as the last visit.

Karen also talks with Mrs. James about her prescription drug benefits. Mrs. James indicates she received something in the mail some time ago, but did not understand what it was and threw it away. **[VC]**

Episode 14

No news this week.

Episode 15

Mrs. James has become a regular at the Senior Center on days the nurse is in the clinic. She has come to trust Karen and, in fact, considers her a friend. Over time, she has become more open to discussing personal matters. Mrs. James tells Karen in detail things about her cats and some of her neighbors. When questioned about her sons and whether they are available to help, Mrs. James explains that her sons don't like her very much, but they would help her if she needed them to. She goes on to mention that they are very busy and they know she does not need their help. **[VC]**

NORMA JAMES
Season 2

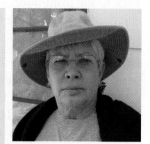

Biographical Information

Norma James is a 65-year-old widow who lives alone. Although she has lived in the Neighborhood for years, she is somewhat socially isolated. She has two adult sons with whom she has limited contact—they live out of the state and rarely call. There are only a few individuals Mrs. James considers friends; she does not particularly like many people and prefers the company of her six cats. She has a long history of type 2 diabetes mellitus and hypertension. In recent years, she was diagnosed with atrial fibrillation. She has multiple physicians and takes multiple medications including:

- Glucotrol, 10 mg twice a day
- captopril, 50 mg twice a day
- digoxin, 125 mcg once a day
- Coumadin, 5 mg once a day

Mrs. James has a known drug allergy to penicillin.

Mrs. James does not work; she has very limited savings and relies on Social Security benefits for income. She smokes about $1/2$ pack of cigarettes per day and has been a smoker since she was in her 20s. She drinks alcohol "a couple times a year—usually a glass of wine at a special dinner." Mrs. James does not drive and relies on her friends, neighbors, or the city bus for transportation. She lives near a grocery store and prides herself on being able to get most things she needs without any assistance. She spends most of her time alone at home and occupies herself by watching television, reading, and doing crossword and jigsaw puzzles.

In recent months, Mrs. James has been going to the Neighborhood Senior Center regularly.

Episode 1

The Senior Center is sponsoring a weekend trip by bus to a nearby national park. Although a fee is required, the cost is minimal. Karen (the nurse at the Senior Center) tells Mrs. James about the trip and suggests that she go on the outing. Mrs. James tells Karen that she has already seen all those parks before, and if she were to go on a bus trip, she would have to listen to all the women chatter. She tells Karen, "It's bad enough to listen to them at lunch. I can't imagine listening to them for days." Mrs. James also reminds Karen that she could never leave her cats alone for that length of time. **[P]**

Episode 2

Mrs. James goes to the drugstore to get her prescriptions refilled. When she gets there, she is told that her co-payment for the prescriptions (Coumadin and digoxin) is $20. This makes Mrs. James very angry. She demands

to know why the co-pay has changed and is told it is due to changes in the insurance plan. Although she has the money, Mrs. James decides not to pick up the prescription. Instead, she goes to the grocery store to buy a new carton of cigarettes and then to the Senior Center for lunch. She dreads it when she walks into the Senior Center and sees Mary Martin, the lady who talks too much. She glares at Mary as she walks past her and sits at a table by herself so she doesn't have to listen to Mary talk. **[P]**

Episode 3

No news this week.

Episode 4

One of Mrs. James' cats dies this week. Mrs. James is so devastated that she does not leave the house for several days. She buries the cat in her backyard near the graves of her other deceased cats. She covers up the area with rocks to prevent a dog from coming along and digging her kitty up. **[P]**

Episode 5
No news this week.

Episode 6
On Tuesday morning, Mrs. James wakes up at about 7 a.m. She does not feel right, but is not sure why. Her right arm feels tingly and somewhat numb. She feeds her cats and decides to go back to bed. At 9 a.m., she wakes up again. When she tries to sit up, her right arm feels very heavy. When she tries to stand up, her right leg also feels heavy, making it difficult to walk; she can't seem to get her leg to support her.

Mrs. James wonders if the diabetes has caused her blood glucose levels to drop. She navigates to the kitchen and checks her glucose, noting it is 137. She decides to eat some breakfast, thinking she will feel better soon. Mrs. James begins to get worried when her symptoms don't subside. At about 10:30 a.m., she calls her neighbor on the phone, explains the situation, and asks her to come over to help her. The neighbor tells Mrs. James to call 9-1-1 for an ambulance and that she will come over as soon as she can. Mrs. James does not want to call 9-1-1 because ambulances charge too much; she decides to wait for her neighbor to take her to the hospital.

The neighbor arrives at Mrs. James' home at about 10:50. By this time, Mrs. James is talking, but not making any sense. The weakness on her right side has become even worse, to the point at which Mrs. James is unable to walk. The neighbor (believing Mrs. James called 9-1-1) is hopeful the ambulance will show up soon. By 11 a.m., the neighbor decides to call 9-1-1 and ask about the ambulance; she learns that a previous call was not made. An ambulance arrives shortly thereafter and takes Mrs. James to Neighborhood Hospital. She arrives in the emergency department about 11:35. She is treated by Dr. Gordon, who determines that she is having a stroke. Mrs. James is admitted to the medical-surgical unit. [MR] [P]

Episode 7
Mrs. James remains at Neighborhood Hospital. She has had a difficult week. Because of swallowing difficulty, a feeding tube was placed, and tube feeding was initiated. She has ongoing issues with nausea and abdominal fullness. Additionally, she has been experiencing diarrhea; she has had two episodes of fecal incontinence because she was unable to get the nursing staff to answer her call light. She is unable to ambulate independently at this time.

Mrs. James also develops an elevated temperature and confusion before anyone notices that the urine in her Foley bag is cloudy. A urinalysis (UA) and culture and sensitivity (C&S) test confirm that she has a urinary tract infection.

She has become very depressed and has taken a very passive role in her care; she wants the nurses to just take care of all of her needs. She continues to experience expressive aphasia and is embarrassed about the way she sounds. Mrs. James' son, Brian, comes to see her at the hospital this week. She barely speaks to him the entire time he is there. He only stays for a few days to take care of a few things at her home. Brian leaves his contact information with the nursing staff in case they need to contact him for anything. Mrs. James feels angry about the entire situation, and she is unhappy with the general inconsistency in the care she has received. One of the nurses she really does not like is Bobby. She does not find him to be nice or caring at all. [P]

Episode 8
This week, Mrs. James is transferred to the Neighborhood Rehabilitation Center. Because of ongoing swallowing difficulties, a percutaneous endoscopic gastrostomy (PEG) tube is inserted for continued tube feedings shortly before she is transferred.

At the rehabilitation center, she works with physical, speech, and occupational therapists. She continues to have little to no motivation for improvement. Mrs. James is pleased when Karen (the nurse from the Senior Center) comes to visit her. She tells Karen what a horrible experience this has been. Karen, who is aware that Mrs. James has been very passive, tells her she needs to work on getting better so she can go home to take care of her cats. If she fails to improve, she might be placed in a nursing home. Mrs. James tells Karen that the cats are probably all dead by now and that there is no point in going home. Karen assures Mrs. James that her son, Brian, placed them in a boarding facility and that they are being well cared for. This information provides a spark in Mrs. James, and she now has a reason to get better; her cats need to be rescued from the inhumane treatment they are probably receiving at the boarding facility. [P]

Episode 9
Mrs. James remains at the Neighborhood Rehabilitation Hospital. She is making excellent progress and has regained much of her mobility. She continues to work with the staff to regain her ability to independently carry out activities of daily living (ADL) skills.

Episode 10
Mrs. James remains at the Neighborhood Rehabilitation Hospital and continues to progress in her mobility, speech, and swallowing.

Episode 11

Arrangements are being made for Mrs. James to be transferred home. Because of her ongoing care needs, her son, Brian, has agreed to spend up to a month with his mother in the role of caregiver while she makes the transition home.

Brian James has returned to The Neighborhood and spends several days making the necessary arrangements for her discharge. Among the arrangements are making home modifications (such as rails and a seat for the shower), obtaining equipment (wheelchair, walker, and grab bars), making appointments for follow-up physician visits and ongoing outpatient physical therapy, and figuring out her medication regimen. Because Mrs. James has prescriptions from several physicians, it takes Brian several days to figure out which are current and which are not. Additionally, Brian finds a box of medications in her home; it seems that Mrs. James has been hording medications for years. Brian throws all the old medications away and buys a pill box to help his mother keep her medications organized. **[P]**

Episode 12

Mrs. James is very glad to come home and thrilled to see her cats. She is so thankful that Brian rescued them. Although she is glad Brian has come to help her, she immediately begins to criticize many of the things he has done. She really did not want those ugly bars placed in the shower—he should have asked her first. She is also angry when she learns that he threw her box of medications away and that he won't buy her cigarettes. At the same time, Mrs. James does not understand why her sons have ignored her for so many years.

Episode 13

No news this week.

Episode 14

Mrs. James' son remains at her home caring for her, taking her to her various appointments and enduring a constant barrage of criticism. He is highly motivated to get his mother back to functional independence so he can go home. **[P]**

Episode 15

No news this week.

NORMA JAMES
Season 3

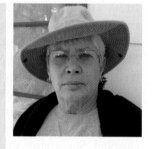

Biographical Information

Norma James is a 66-year-old widow who lives alone. Although she has lived in *The Neighborhood* for years, she is somewhat socially isolated.

Mrs. James has a history of type 2 diabetes, hypertension and atrial fibrillation. She recently experienced a stroke and spent several weeks in acute care and rehabilitation. Her current medications are:

- Glucotrol, 10 mg twice a day
- captopril, 50 mg twice a day
- digoxin, 125 mcg once a day
- Coumadin, 5 mg once a day

Mrs. James has a known drug allergy to penicillin.

Mrs. James is currently recovering from her stroke. Her son, Brian James, has been helping her to regain basic living skills so that she can continue to live in her own home. Before her stroke, Mrs. James smoked 1/2 pack of cigarettes per day. She has not smoked since the stroke—primarily because her son refuses to purchase cigarettes for her.

Up until this recent stroke, Mrs. James' contact with her sons was very limited. There are only a few individuals she considers friends; she does not particularly like many people and prefers the company of her five cats. She does not drive and relies on her friends, neighbors, or the city bus for transportation. She lives near a grocery store and has always been able to get most things done without assistance.

Episode 1

Mrs. James has become accustomed to having her son, Brian, help her with things around the house. He literally takes care of everything for her, and she has come to expect him to do everything for her. Although she is very appreciative of his efforts, Mrs. James has a hard time openly acknowledging this and usually praises him through the eyes of her cats. "You are a very good cat master," she tells him. **[P]**

Episode 2

Mrs. James has finished her outpatient physical therapy. Brian tells his mother that he will be leaving soon, but before he goes, he wants her to prove to him that she is safe living on her own. Brian levels with his mother and tells her that, if she is unable to do so, they might have to consider assisted living options. Mrs. James is furious with this and is determined to show Brian that she is capable of living on her own and that she does not need him. **[VC]**

Episode 3

Mrs. James, accompanied by her son, Brian, walks to the grocery store to do some shopping. It is her first time to the store since her hospitalization. Brian evaluates her ability to get to the store, make purchases, and get home from the store. He is impressed by her determination and stamina, despite changes in mobility. Mrs. James decides not to even try to buy the cigarettes she craves; she figures he will be leaving soon enough. Next, they go to the drugstore to get fresh refills on all of her medications.

At home, Mrs. James makes all three meals for several days in a row, takes care of all the household chores, and is able to get to the toilet, dressed, and bathed without any assistance. She has learned to keep her medications organized and checks her glucose twice a day. During this week, she gives hints to Brian that he could help out, but he just sits and watches her. Mrs. James wonders aloud how she ever raised such a lazy son. **[P]**

Episode 4

Brian heads home this week after the long stay with his mother. Mrs. James is deeply saddened to see him go, but keeps a stiff upper lip when he leaves. She tells him she is tired of having him there and wants the house to herself now; she has many things to do. Brian knows his mother all too well and gives her a hug as he goes out the door. **[P]**

Episode 5

Mrs. James readjusts to her new life. She is able to do most things, but it takes her longer. She finds the house quiet and lonely since Brian has left, although her cats keep her company. Mrs. James has avoided going to the Senior Center because she believes everyone will talk about her. Her son Brian calls her to ask how things are going; she tells Brian she is just fine and doesn't need anything. **[P]**

Episode 6

No news this week.

Episode 7

Mrs. James decides to go see Karen, the nurse at the Senior Center. She is glad no one is with the nurse when she arrives. Karen measures her blood pressure at 120/78 mm Hg and her glucose at 122 g/dL. Mrs. James enjoys visiting with her for 15 minutes before being interrupted by "a stupid old man" who wants to see Karen. Mrs. James wanders out to the main room and finds a group of ladies playing cards. They invite her to join them. Mrs. James tells them she can only stay for a few minutes because she has other things to do, but ends up staying for the entire afternoon. They suggest she join them again the following week. **[P]**

Episode 8

Mrs. James decides not to join the ladies at the Senior Center for cards, but she goes for lunch twice this week. She wonders why she has not heard from Brian lately and decides to call him. They talk for a short while, and Mrs. James tells him about the ladies asking her to join them in card games. Brian encourages her to join them again sometime soon.

Episode 9

No news this week.

Episode 10

Mrs. James sees Karen at the Senior Center again this week. She is annoyed when Karen asks her about her medications and glucose measurements because she just wants to visit. However, because she is self-managing her disease better, Mrs. James is able to recall her medications and her most recent glucose readings. She isn't sure when she should be going back to see her physicians, however. Karen checks her blood pressure and finds it to be 118/82 mm Hg; her glucose is 116 g/dL. **[P]**

Episode 11

Mrs. James sees the card-playing ladies at the Senior Center this week and is again invited to join them. She spends most of the afternoon playing cards and finds that she can beat them easily because they spend all their time talking to one another as opposed to paying attention to the cards in their hands. **[P]**

Episode 12

No news this week.

Episode 13
No news this week.

Episode 14
Mrs. James is invited to spend a week at the home of her son, Brian, and his family. Brian has offered to drive to her home, board her cats in a kennel, and then drive her to his home several hours away. Mrs. James is reluctant to leave

her home and her cats. However, because it has been years since she last visited with her grandchildren, she is anxious to see them. Mrs. James agrees to visit Brian and spends the rest of the week getting ready to go. **[P]**

Episode 15
Mrs. James is out of town visiting her son, Brian, this week.

JOHNSON HOUSEHOLD

JOHNSON FAMILY STORY OVERVIEW

Character	Season 1	Season 2	Season 3
YVONNE JOHNSON	Yvonne is a presumably healthy single mother who experiences unexplained mild to moderate generalized symptoms of joint swelling, pain, and fatigue. Several trips to her family physician do not reveal a cause of the problem. The story describes how these unexplained symptoms begin to affect her personal life.	Yvonne's symptoms continue to progress during this season. She begins to experience problems associated with work, and the symptoms impact her relationship with her son. After researching her symptoms on the Internet, she finally demands to be seen by a specialist, who diagnoses her with a connective tissue disorder.	Yvonne is referred to a nephrologist, who determines that she has renal insufficiency associated with SLE. Yvonne's health continues to decline. She loses her job and struggles to find adequate income and health insurance benefits.
RANDALL JOHNSON	Randall is in good health. His story focuses on typical teen-related behaviors related to school, sports, and his social life. He is frustrated with mother, because he perceives her as being lazy.	Randal remains in good health and is active in school and sports. He hates the fact that his mother is always feeling sick, even though she looks fine. He gets a car during this season and must get a job to pay for car insurance and gas.	Randall remains healthy. The story focuses on typical adolescent behaviors and the impact of his mother's illness on his life.

CONCEPTS   *Elimination, Family Dynamics, Fatigue, Immunity, Interpersonal Relationships, Pain, Role Performance.*

YVONNE JOHNSON
Season 1

Biographical Information

Yvonne Johnson is a 35-year-old African American female. She is a single parent to her 15-year-old son, Randall. Yvonne never married Randall's father and has always resented him because he left her for another woman when Randall was an infant. He lives in a nearby town and sees Randall several times a year. He sends Yvonne child support on a semi-regular basis. Yvonne has had relationships with men off and on, but is not currently involved with anybody at this time.

Yvonne completed a Bachelor's degree in marketing 5 years ago, but has been unable to break into the marketing field locally. Instead, she has been working full time as an Administrative Assistant for a large company. She is really not satisfied in her current job, because she wants to be in the marketing field and, in her opinion, she is underemployed. The positive aspects of her current job are excellent health insurance and other benefits and the close proximity of work to her home. Although other opportunities are potentially available in other cities, she has lived in the Neighborhood most of her life and is not

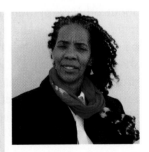

Continued

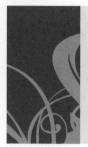

interested in leaving. Her parents and siblings live nearby, and she maintains a close relationship with them.

Over the past 4 years, Yvonne has noticed mild swelling in her hands and feet every morning. The symptoms began subtly not long after graduating from college and getting a job. She has always attributed the symptoms to her sedentary lifestyle and being somewhat overweight. More recently, she has been experiencing pain along with the swelling in her hands and feet.

Episode 1

No news this week.

Episode 2

Yvonne spends Saturday afternoon at her parents' home, helping her mother make centerpieces for an upcoming banquet. She shares with her mother that she has had pain in her hands for the past couple of months that she just can't seem to explain. Her mother tells her there is no reason that a healthy young woman should have pain and swelling in her hands at her age, and that she should see a doctor about it. Yvonne decides her mother is probably right. The only health care provider she has seen in the past 10 years has been a nurse practitioner in a women's health office for her yearly pelvic exams. She makes an appointment with a family practice physician on her medical plan. **[P]**

Episode 3

Yvonne has her appointment with Dr. Rowe, a family practice physician. She shares with Dr. Rowe that she has had pain in her hands for the past several months. When asked about other symptoms, she mentions the swelling in her hands and feet for the past 4 years. Dr. Rowe believes the pain is occupational in nature (typing) and suggests that she take ibuprofen. Dr. Rowe notices that Yvonne's blood pressure is slightly elevated (134/92 mm Hg), but attributes this to her race and diet. She suggests that Yvonne try to lose a little weight and reduce her salt intake. **[VC]**

Episode 4

Yvonne has been exceptionally busy at work and has been frustrated with the lack of administrative support in the office. She feels that there are too many expectations of her and not enough time to complete all of the tasks she is assigned. Yvonne has hinted to her boss that perhaps another person should be hired, but her boss seems to just ignore her. Yvonne attends the parents' night open house at the high school and visits with Randall's teachers. All of the teachers share with her that Randall is progressing well in school.

Episode 5

Yvonne has had another exceptionally busy week at work and frequently feels tired. Her hands continue to hurt, and the swelling in her feet and hands also continues. At work, Yvonne has her annual evaluation. She is told by her boss that she has been doing excellent work, but her boss is not willing to hire another office assistant. Yvonne's boss mentions administrative reorganization changes that are planned for next year and hints that she might be considered for a promotion. She is encouraged by the fact that her job situation has the potential to improve.

Over the weekend, Yvonne has a garage sale at her home, along with her sister and mother. She makes over $400 and is thrilled to get rid of so much stuff. After the garage sale, she feels very tired and elects not to go to her sister's house for dinner. Her sister criticizes her for feeling tired, pointing out that their mother has more energy than she does. **[P]**

Episode 6

No news this week.

Episode 7

Yvonne has been trying to follow Dr. Rowe's advice for the past 3 months. Despite the fact that she has lost about 5 pounds, has avoided salty foods, and has been taking ibuprofen three times a day, she continues to have pain in her hands and swelling in her hands and feet. She also wonders if the symptoms are really associated with her work. She takes Randall for his annual sports physical examination and hopes to talk to Dr. Rowe while there. She learns that Dr. Rowe is out of the office, but is told that she is more than welcome to make an appointment. Yvonne considers this, but does not act on it. **[VC]**

Episode 8

No news this week.

Episode 9

Randall is trying out for the baseball team after school every day this week. Yvonne goes to work early so that she can leave in time to watch the tryouts. After practice, she takes Randall home and makes him dinner. She feels quite tired after a long day of work and all the running around after work. **[P]**

Episode 10
No news this week.

Episode 11
It has now been several months since Yvonne saw Dr. Rowe. She begins to notice that she has stiffness in her hands in the morning, as well as continued hand pain and swelling in her hands and feet. She also does not feel rested when she wakes up and often needs to lie down when she gets home from work. She does not have the same energy on the weekends that she used to have. She continues to be unhappy in her current job and decides the symptoms are related to job dissatisfaction in her current position. She would quit, but thinks she might get the promotion at work if she just sticks it out. **[P]**

Episode 12
On one afternoon this week, Yvonne goes to Randall's baseball game after work. Following the game, she is too tired to cook and stops for a hamburger on the way home. Randall tells her that it is okay with him to eat hamburgers and suggests they do this after every game.

Episode 13
On Saturday, Yvonne watches Randall play in a baseball tournament all day. She wakes up on Sunday absolutely exhausted, and when she looks in the mirror, she notices a splotchy rash across her face. She also experiences increased pain in several of her joints, which really worries her. She decides to rest all day on Sunday (despite protests from her son) and expects to feel good by Monday morning. However, she continues to feel progressively worse. On Monday morning, she calls in sick to work and tries to get an appointment with Dr. Rowe. Dr. Rowe's office is unable to see her until the end of the week. Yvonne is advised to go to the Urgent Care Clinic or the emergency department (ED).

Yvonne's elects to go to the ED. Upon arrival, her blood pressure is 134/92 mm Hg. Yvonne tells the ED physician, Dr. Gordon, about the red rash on her face, her excessive fatigue, and her other symptoms, including swelling and pain in her joints. She mentions that her finger joints and hip joints are hot, and that the swelling in her lower legs has been present for 8 months. Dr. Gordon does not notice a rash on Yvonne's face because of her dark skin pigmentation. Based on her other symptoms, he suggests that Yvonne make an appointment with her primary care physician for a full work-up to rule out a virus or arthritic condition. To keep her comfortable in the meantime, he gives Yvonne a 14-day prescription for prednisone in a decreasing dose. Yvonne gets the prescription filled that day and immediately begins to feel better. **[VC]**

Episode 14
Yvonne finishes the prednisone prescription. She feels great! The swelling and pain are completely gone, and she has more energy than she has had in months. She feels so good that she decides she does not need to make an appointment with Dr. Rowe. **[P]**

Episode 15
No news this week.

YVONNE JOHNSON
Season 2

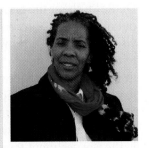

Biographical Information
Yvonne Johnson is a 35-year-old African American female. She is a single parent to her 16-year-old son, Randall. Yvonne never married Randall's father and has always resented him because he left her for another woman when Randall was an infant. He lives in a nearby town and sees Randall several times a year. He sends Yvonne child support on a semi-regular basis. Yvonne has had relationships with men off and on, but is not currently involved with anybody at this time.

Yvonne completed a Bachelor's degree in marketing 5 years ago, but has been unable to break into the marketing field locally. Instead, she has been working full time as an Administrative Assistant for a large company. She is

Continued

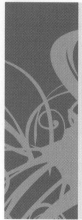

really not satisfied in her current job, But is hopeful for a promotion. The positive aspects of her current job are excellent health insurance and other benefits and the close proximity of work to her home. Although other opportunities are potentially available in other cities, she has lived in the Neighborhood most of her life and is not interested in leaving. Her parents and siblings live nearby, and she maintains a close relationship with them.

Yvonne has seen Dr. Rowe during the past year because of fatigue and pain and swelling in her hands and feet. Most recently, she was seen by a physician at the Emergency Department. He gave her a prescription for prednisone, and this seemed to have cured her. She has felt great ever since. Because she felt so good, she did not keep her appointment with Dr. Rowe, believing that whatever it was that was bothering her has finally been resolved.

Episode 1

Work continues to be frustrating for Yvonne. Reorganization rumors are rampant, and many of her coworkers are concerned about their jobs. Yvonne remains hopeful that the reorganization will result in a promotion for her. For this reason, she has been putting extra effort into her work.

Episode 2

Because Randall went out of town to see his father, Yvonne takes the opportunity to paint his bedroom, a project she has wanted to do for months. **[P]**

Episode 3

Yvonne wakes up one morning this week feeling exhausted. When she gets out of bed and stands up, she experiences intense pain in her hips. Her hands are also red, swollen, and painful. She also notices generalized swelling over her entire body. She realizes the symptoms are back and calls her family practice physician, Dr. Rowe, insisting that she be seen that day. She calls in sick from work.

At Dr. Rowe's office, the medical technician measures Yvonne's blood pressure at 136/94 mm Hg. She tells Dr. Rowe about the current symptoms and how they came out of nowhere. She also tells Dr. Rowe about her previous visit to the ED. Dr. Rowe orders several diagnostic blood tests and sends her to the outpatient lab to have them drawn. She asks Yvonne to return the following day. Yvonne has the blood drawn and spends the rest of the day in bed. She calls work and tells them she might not be in for several days. Although she knows there is nothing she can do about it, she worries about the impact of missing work again.

The following day, Yvonne sees Dr. Rowe again. Dr. Rowe shares with Yvonne that some of her lab results are abnormal. Dr. Rowe tells Yvonne that many people have these abnormal results, and it is probably nothing; however, it could be related to a connective tissue disorder. Dr. Rowe gives Yvonne prescriptions for hydrochlorothiazide, 25 mg to be taken once a day for blood pressure control, and ibuprofen 800 mg to be taken three times a day for joint pain. She tells Yvonne to "watch things" for a while and see what happens. Yvonne wonders just what exactly she is supposed to watch. **[VC]**

Episode 4

Yvonne begins feeling better soon after taking the medications prescribed by Dr. Rowe. She takes the medications as directed, and within a few days, the pain and swelling are completely gone. Because she missed several days of work last week when she was sick, Yvonne works late each day in an attempt to catch up. She begins to worry about the number of sick days she has taken and the impact this may have on her performance evaluations. Yvonne gets up enough energy to drive over to Randall's best friend, Charles', home to take pictures of the boys with their dates before the school dance. **[P]**

Episode 5

No news this week.

Episode 6

Yvonne continues to feel good and is completely pain free. She is able to focus on work and prepares for a major presentation; she is hopeful that her presentation will be noticed by the company managers. One of her coworkers asks her if she plans to be sick again the week she gives her presentation, which makes Yvonne furious. After work, she goes to the high school basketball game to watch Randall play.

Episode 7

Yvonne has a discussion with Randall about getting a car. He wants a car of his own to drive, but she can't afford to buy him a car and pay his car insurance. In addition, Yvonne is not so sure she wants him running all over town anyway. She tells Randall that, if he wants a car, he can buy one for himself. Yvonne knows he won't be able to earn the money anytime soon.

Episode 8

No news this week.

Episode 9

Yvonne has a performance evaluation at work this week. She is told that she is capable of excellent work. The managers point out that every time she misses work, she tends to fall behind, and her coworkers end up having to do extra work to make up for her absence. They tell her she is still being considered for a promotion, but they would like to see these issues addressed. Yvonne tells them she thinks her illness is over, and that the medications she took seemed to have cured whatever was wrong with her. Yvonne decides she should be in each morning a bit early and stay a little later in the evenings to show that she is committed to the job.

On Friday night, Yvonne watches Randall play in a basketball game. After the game, Randall fails to come home by his midnight curfew. Yvonne is angry when he finally comes in at 1:30 a.m. He tells her it isn't his fault, because he doesn't have a car to drive himself home. **[VC]**

Episode 10

Yvonne's best friend calls this week and asks her if she would like to go to the beach with her next week over the 3-day weekend. Yvonne knows Randall is planning to visit his father and agrees to go.

Episode 11

Yvonne and her friend go on a 3-day beach vacation. She has a great time, but feels very tired by the time she gets home on Sunday afternoon. On Monday, she continues to feel tired at work. Initially, she thinks it is a case of "vacationitis," but then she notices the rash across her face again. Over the course of the next 2 days, the fatigue does not resolve, and she begins to experience joint pain and swelling again. Yvonne recognizes these symptoms and also notices that she has been forgetting details and "feeling foggy." She takes the rest of the week off from work to rest, but she does not improve.

Frustrated with the ongoing problems, Yvonne does an Internet search for "fatigue and joint pain" and comes across Web sites that describe rheumatoid-type problems. She enters a rheumatology support bulletin board, posts her symptoms, and asks for advice. Many people respond to her posting, telling her that she should see a rheumatologist. **[P]**

Episode 12

This week, Yvonne continues to feel poorly. She misses 2 days of work, but makes herself go to work the other days. She finds that trying to get to work and keep up with her projects is exhausting. She tries to go to work a little late and to go home early to compensate for the exhaustion, but the schedule is just killing her. Yvonne also overhears some of her coworkers talking about her and her lack of productivity. Because of this, she decides to make an appointment with Dr. Rowe again.

Randall tells Yvonne that he is getting a car from his father. She is angry with Randall's father for not talking with her about it first, but is too tired to get into an argument with anybody. She tells Randall the car insurance is very expensive and that he will have to help pay for it. **[P]**

Episode 13

Yvonne sees Dr. Rowe this week. Dr. Rowe recommends another prescription for steroids and raises the possibility that she is depressed, making the suggestion that antidepressants might be helpful. Yvonne becomes angry and insists there is something more wrong with her than depression. She tells Dr. Rowe what she learned by searching the Internet and reminds her that the symptoms have been coming and going now for quite some time and getting worse. She demands that Dr. Rowe refer her to a rheumatologist, and Dr. Rowe agrees to this. **[P]**

Episode 14

Yvonne has missed several days of work during the past couple of weeks because she is so tired and feels poorly. When she does get to work, she has a hard time getting much done. She is not thrilled that Randall has his own car now and makes it clear he will have to pay for part of the car insurance. She wishes Randall did not have to work on top of all his other activities, but knows she really cannot afford his insurance right now. She is hopeful that, with a promotion at work, her income will improve. **[P]**

Episode 15

It takes several weeks for Yvonne to see the rheumatologist. She has missed work about one-half of that time and is worried about the amount of time she has missed. At the rheumatologist's office, a detailed family history reveals that Yvonne's maternal aunt had rheumatoid arthritis, and her grandmother had hypothyroidism. The rheumatologist repeats many of the same diagnostic tests previously ordered by Dr. Rowe. Yvonne tests positive for anti-DNA antibody, anti-Smith antibody, and antinuclear antibody (ANA). An initial diagnosis of undifferentiated connective tissue disease is made. The rheumatologist tells Yvonne that this is a common initial diagnosis for people who have symptoms of autoimmune illness, and the specific diagnosis will become clear over time although it is likely that she has systemic lupus erythematosus (SLE). Because of the amount of protein in her urine, the rheumatologist also tells Yvonne she probably has renal insufficiency and refers her to a nephrologist. Yvonne is not sure exactly what this means, but knows it has something to do with her kidneys. The rheumatologist gives her a prescription for hydroxychloroquine (Plaquenil), 400 mg two times a day, and ibuprofen, 800 mg three times a day. Yvonne is told to come back and see the rheumatologist again next month. **[P]**

YVONNE JOHNSON
Season 3

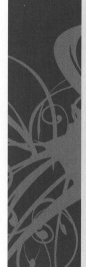

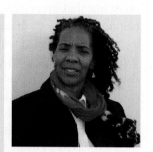

Biographical Information

Yvonne Johnson is a 36-year-old African American female. She is a single parent to her 16-year-old son Randall. She does not date, primarily because Randall has not reacted well to her having relationships with men. Her parents and siblings live nearby, and she maintains a close relationship with them.

Yvonne has recently been diagnosed with an undifferentiated connective tissue disease and has been told it is most likely systemic lupus erythematosus (SLE). The rheumatologist she has been seeing has prescribed a maintenance dose of hydroxychloroquine (Plaquenil), 400 mg once a day, and ibuprofen, 800 mg three times a day. Yvonne is scheduled to see a nephrologist to evaluate her renal function. She is motivated to adhere to her recommended treatment regimen.

Yvonne continues to work as an Administrative Assistant, but has had a difficult time keeping up with the job demands. Because of her illness, she has missed a lot of work. Although she once believed she might get promoted, at this point, she is just concentrating on keeping her job.

Episode 1
No news this week.

Episode 2
Yvonne has an appointment with the nephrologist this week. She is scheduled for outpatient urine and blood tests, and a renal biopsy to rule out lupus nephritis. She has the biopsy at the Neighborhood Outpatient Surgery Center at the end of the week.

Yvonne misses 2 days of work this week to accommodate the appointments. Because she has missed so much work, she is reassigned to another position in the company—a position that is clearly a demotion. She finds many of the individuals who were once friendly and helpful to her now avoid her. Yvonne knows they don't understand how she feels. **[P]**

Episode 3
Yvonne meets with the nephrologist again this week. She is told that the laboratory tests show protein in her urine and an elevated creatinine level. These tests, along with the biopsy results, suggest she has progressive glomerulonephritis and renal insufficiency, and confirm a diagnosis of lupus nephritis. The nephrologist tells Yvonne that she has chronic kidney disease and is at risk for developing end-stage renal disease. To help preserve her renal function, the nephrologist prescribes a steroid burst of prednisone with a tapering dose, cyclophosphamide (Cytoxan), and azathioprine (Imuran). Because her blood pressure is elevated, despite taking hydrochlorothiazide, the physician adds metoprolol to her medication regimen. Yvonne tells the physician that she finds all of this information overwhelming and confusing. She is referred to the Neighborhood Patient Education Center for further patient teaching. **[VC]**

Episode 4
Yvonne leaves work early for an appointment with a nurse educator at the Patient Education Center. At the center, Yvonne learns about her disease process, her medications, diet (low protein, low salt), and self-management strategies

for lupus and renal insufficiency. She finds the session helpful and finally begins to understand the severity of her illness. Yvonne agrees to return for additional sessions with the nurse educator. **[P]**

Episode 5

Yvonne is very concerned when she learns that Randall's best friend, Charles, almost ran over and killed a young boy who was riding his bike. Yvonne reminds Randall that he needs to be careful when driving.

Episode 6

Yvonne finds that the new medications are helping somewhat, but she continues to experience joint pain and fatigue. She has great difficulty keeping up with her household and job responsibilities. Although she continues to go to work, she often feels crummy and misses work frequently. Yvonne has been unable to go to Randall's baseball games because of the need to avoid sun exposure. They have an argument, and she comes to understand that Randall is angry with her for being sick.

Episode 7

Yvonne has a follow-up appointment with the nephrologist. Her urine output has decreased somewhat, and she is feeling puffy. Based on additional tests, she is told that her kidney disease has progressed, as evidenced by a further reduction of her creatinine clearance. Although her BUN and creatinine levels are borderline normal, she is told she is going to need dialysis treatment in the future. The goal at this point is to continue to preserve her kidney function as long as possible. Yvonne is taught how to measure her urine output and instructed to reduce her daily fluid intake to 600 ml plus the measurable urine output from the day before. She is also told to measure her weight daily and report increases in weight over 4 pounds.

Yvonne notices Randall is out every night with his new girlfriend. She worries about the time they are alone and tries to talk with him about being careful with her and avoiding sexual contact, but this results in another argument.

Episode 8

Yvonne is fired from her job this week, with her employer citing poor quality of work as the reason for termination. She is devastated, because she knows she needs the health insurance coverage—not only for herself, but also for Randall. She signs up for COBRA coverage and is shocked at the cost of the monthly premiums. She realizes she will not be able to afford to pay the premium, particularly if she is out of work. She has prepaid her insurance until the end of the next month, so she is hopeful she can find another position before she has to pay for the COBRA coverage. **[P]**

Episode 9

Yvonne spends the entire week looking for work. She feels crummy and is sure this is impacting her presentation to potential employers. She does not want to share with them what is wrong with her, for fear that they will not be interested in hiring her. Yvonne feels fortunate that her mother and siblings are supportive of her situation and have promised to help her in any way. **[P]**

Episode 10

Yvonne is excessively tired this week, to the point at which she is unable to look for a job. She sees her physician and is found to be anemic and hypocalcemic. Her blood pressure remains within normal limits. She is given a subcutaneous injection of Epogen. **[P]**

Episode 11

No news this week.

Episode 12

Yvonne is feeling noticeably more energetic than in weeks past. A follow-up visit with her physician confirms that her RBC, hemoglobin, and hematocrit levels are elevated in response to the Epogen. Yvonne is able to get a temporary position; although there are no benefits, she at least has some income for the time being. She realizes that she will not easily be able to get a permanent job. At the suggestion of a friend, she applies for Social Security disability. She is overwhelmed with the process. **[P]**

Episode 13

Yvonne talks at length with Randall's father about her inability to get full-time employment and her inability to make ends meet. She asks him if he can help her out with additional child support so that she can better provide for Randall. He accuses Yvonne of wanting the money to pay for her medical bills and tells her that if he sends any additional money, it will be sent directly to Randall. He also suggests that Randall live with him to finish out his high school years. **[P]**

Episode 14

Yvonne receives notification that she has been turned down for the Social Security disability, because she has not had documented disability long enough and she is currently employed by the temporary agency. Yvonne can't believe it. She has to work to keep from losing her home, but if she works, she can't get disability. She does not understand how anybody gets disability benefits within such a system.

Episode 15

Yvonne has become excessively fatigued again and short of breath this week. She has experienced a 6-pound weight gain in the past 3 days and notices excessive swelling in her legs. Yvonne makes a call to her nephrologist, fearing the worst. **[P]**

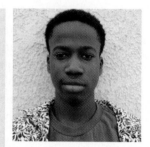

RANDALL JOHNSON
Season 1

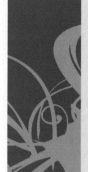

Biographical Information

Randall is a healthy, athletic 15-year-old African-American male. He lives with his mother Yvonne in a small but comfortable home. Randall is very close to his mother, but does not like it when she dates men. His father and stepmother live in a nearby town; although he visits his father several times a year, he does not feel particularly close to him.

Randall is in his first year of high school. He is an excellent student, is very athletic, and has many friends. He plans on playing basketball and baseball for the high school team. He is looking forward to taking driver education and getting his driver's license soon.

Episode 1

No news this week.

Episode 2

Randall spends most of the weekend hanging out with his best friend, Charles. They go to the mall to meet some friends and then to the golf course to hit balls on the driving range. Randall does not know how to play golf, but thinks he might like to learn how to play. **[P]**

Episode 3

Randall spends a 3-day weekend with his father. When he comes home, he tells his mother that it gets boring at his Dad's house because he doesn't have any friends there to hang out with. His father keeps trying to teach him some basics of woodworking in his workshop, but Randall is completely disinterested.

Episode 4

Randall asks his mother to attend the parents' night open house at school this week. He knows she will be pleased with his grades this past quarter because he has worked hard and has made all 'A's and one 'B.' He also is excited for her to meet his favorite teacher, Mrs. Graham. **[P]**

Episode 5

Randall helps his mother, aunt, and grandmother have a garage sale. He does not particularly like doing the work,

but his mother promises to give him $25 for helping. He notices his mother is tired after the garage sale, but figures she is just old and out of shape. **[P]**

Episode 6

No news this week.

Episode 7

Randall sees a nurse practitioner at the Family Practice clinic for a physical examination. He hates having a physical exam, but knows it is required for him to play high school sports. Randall mentions to the nurse that he would prefer it if his mother were not in the room during the exam. The nurse practitioner asks Yvonne if she would mind staying in the waiting room during his examination; Randall is relieved that his mother agrees to this. All of his physical examination findings are within normal limits for his age. **[VC]**

Episode 8

No news this week.

Episode 9

Randall tries out for the baseball team this entire week. At the end of the week, he is thrilled to learn that he has earned a starting position on the Junior Varsity Squad. Randall goes to his friend Charles' house, where they have a celebration cookout for the other kids who made the team. **[P]**

Episode 10

Randall has baseball practice every evening this week to get ready for the season opener. Following practice on three of the evenings, he goes to the gym with his friends to lift weights and does not get home until well after 9 p.m. He then has to start homework. Randall is irritated with his mother when she suggests that he not lift weights in the evening. She obviously does not understand the need for strength building to improve his hitting. **[P]**

Episode 11

Randall's baseball team loses their first game this week. Randall is very disappointed in the loss and feels that, if he played better, his team would have won. **[P]**

Episode 12

Randall has an uneventful week at school. During the weekend he goes to the high school dance with his guy friends. He sees one of the cheerleaders, Kristina Martin, at the dance with Jared Williams (the quarterback of the high school football team). He wishes he could date cheerleader girls like Kristina.

Yvonne allows him to go out, but worries about his safety because his friend just recently obtained his driver's license. Randall thinks his mother is too protective and that he can take care of himself. The boys spend the evening cruising on one of the main streets in the Neighborhood with some of the other local high school kids; he gets home by 11:30 p.m.

Episode 13

Randall plays in a 2-day baseball tournament over the weekend. His mother promises to watch all of the games. After going to all of the Saturday games, she says she is too tired to go to any of the Sunday games. Randall tells her that he really wants her to come and watch and is disappointed when she declines. At one of the games, he hits a home run and is angry that she is not there to see it. **[P]**

Episode 14

No news this week.

Episode 15

Randall and his friends go out for pizza after a baseball game. While out with his friends, Randall learns that Jeremy's (one of the guys at school) parents are out of town, and he is having a party. Randall knows the party would be a lot of fun, but also knows his mother would be incredibly angry if he went. He tells his friends that he has other plans and goes home instead. **[P]**

RANDALL JOHNSON
Season 2

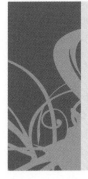

Biographical Information

Randall is a healthy, athletic 16-year-old African-American male. He lives with his mother Yvonne in a small but comfortable home. Randall is very close to his mother, but does not like it when she dates men. His father and stepmother live in a nearby town; although he visits his father several times a year, he does not feel particularly close to him.

Randall is in high school. He is an excellent student, is very athletic, and has many friends. He plays on the high school basketball and baseball teams. He has been taking driver's education and will soon be getting his driver's license.

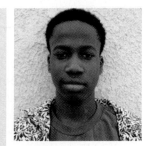

Episode 1

Basketball season started this week. Randall and his friends stay after school each afternoon for practice. He comes home just before dinner and then completes his homework in the evening. **[P]**

Episode 2

Randall spends a 3-day weekend with his father. He tells his father that he can't come to visit again for a while because his basketball games start next week, and he'll be playing basketball every weekend. He suggests to his father that he come to see him play basketball.

Episode 3

One morning this week, Randall is surprised by how ill his mother looks. She tells him she feels pretty bad and is going to stay home from work and see the doctor. She asks him to get a ride to and from school, because she does not want to get out and drive any more than she must—she is feeling a lot of pain. Randall wonders why his mother is sick again. **[P]**

Episode 4

Randall and his best friend Charles go to the school dance with two of the girls from school. The girls spend all afternoon getting ready for the dance. In contrast, Randall and Charles hang out together until about an hour before they are scheduled to pick up the girls. Randall's mother comes by Charles' house to take their pictures. Randall is glad she is feeling better.

Episode 5

No news this week.

Episode 6

Randall gets his driver's license this week. He tells his mother he wants a car. Yvonne tells him they will have to talk about it, but in the meantime, he can borrow her car once in a while. Yvonne watches him play basketball over the weekend. **[P]**

Episode 7

Randall continues to bug his Mom about getting a car. He thinks he should be able to have one; most of his friends have been given a car by their parents. Yvonne tells Randall she can't afford to buy him a car or pay for the car insurance; if he wants a car, he'll have to get a job and buy one. Randall knows it will be near to impossible to save enough money to buy a car any time soon. **[VC]**

Episode 8

No news this week.

Episode 9

Because his mother worked late on Friday evening, Randall needs to catch a ride to his basketball game with Charles. After the game, he hangs out with his friends and does not come home until after 1:30 a.m. Yvonne is furious with him for coming home so late. Randall tells her he had no choice because he was with Charles, and Charles was driving. He tells his mother that, if he had his own car, he could come home on time.

Episode 10

Randall's basketball season has come to an end. They lost a game in the state basketball tournament in the opening round. He is disappointed that they didn't win, but does not dwell on it. He begins to think about try-outs for the track and field team. **[P]**

Episode 11

Randall spends a 3-day weekend with his father. He complains to his father about not having a car to drive. His father tells him that he will buy a car for him, and Randall can pay him back during the summer. Randall thinks this is awesome.

Episode 12

Randall notices his mother is feeling bad again; she spends a lot of time just lying around on the couch. Sometimes, she doesn't even make dinner, instead asking him to make himself a frozen pizza. He tells his mother that he is going to get a car soon from his father, and she tells him he is going to have to help pay for the car insurance. Randall tells his mother he is going to be on the track and field team, but will get a part-time job. **[VC]**

Episode 13

Randall gets a part-time job at a fast-food restaurant. His manager promises to be flexible with his work schedule to accommodate his track and field season. Randall is very pleased with the arrangement.

Episode 14

Randall's father comes through with a car for him. It is a late-model sedan, but he is thrilled to have it. He meets with the insurance agent and is surprised at the cost of car insurance, but decides it's worth it to be able to have his own car. He figures out how many shifts a week he needs to work to pay for his portion of the insurance. **[P]**

Episode 15

Randall is adapting to his new schedule of school, track team practice, homework, and working a few hours several evenings a week. He quickly finds that working at a fast-food restaurant is not a great job, but he's happy to make the money. He is aware that his mother has been going to the doctor a lot, but does not ask her much about it.

RANDALL JOHNSON
Season 3

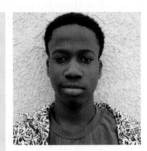

Biographical Information

Randall is a healthy, athletic 16-year-old African-American male. He lives with his mother Yvonne in a small but comfortable home. Randall is very close to his mother, but does not like it when she dates men. His father and stepmother live in a nearby town; although he visits his father several times a year, he does not feel particularly close to him.

Randall is a high school student and keeps a very busy schedule. He is an excellent student, plays on several high school sports teams, and most recently has started a part-time job at a fast-food restaurant to pay for a car and auto insurance. He has very little free time. He knows his mother has been sick, but has not talked with her very much about it.

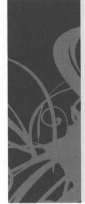

Episode 1

No news this week.

Episode 2

Tryouts for the baseball team are taking place this week. Randall literally goes from school to practice to work and does not get home until after 10:30 p.m. four nights this week. Although his mother tells him he can't maintain that schedule or his grades will suffer, Randall is confident he can keep up with everything. He wonders about the number of days his mother misses at work.

Episode 3

Yvonne tells Randall that the doctor finally knows what is wrong with her, and she is going to have to take many medications and change her diet. Randall does not quite understand what is wrong with her, but he is aware she is always tired and looks swollen at times. He hopes the medications will make her better. **[P]**

Episode 4

Randall makes the varsity baseball team this year and is thrilled. He shows his mother his schedule and tells her he hopes she can make it to his games this year. Randall's grades in school are beginning to be affected by his busy schedule—he does not share with his mother that he has a 'C' in three of his classes, fearing that she will make him quit work. He is not willing to quit working, because having his own car to drive is more important to him than making 'A's in school. This week, Randall goes to the formal high school dance with Natalie, a girl he has had a crush on for several months. They have a great time, and she agrees to be his girlfriend.

Episode 5

Randall's best friend Charles was speeding in his car when he accidentally hit a kid riding a bike. Charles is freaked out by the incident and calls Randall. Randall talks to Charles and goes with him to the police department for questioning. Randall feels badly for Charles when his parents arrive. They are angry with him for wrecking the car, being careless, and almost killing a little boy. Randall thinks it is pretty pointless to yell at Charles about what happened—he already feels badly enough. **[P]**

Episode 6

Randall is angry with his mother and argues with her when she tells him she is going to miss another baseball game. He tells her that all she ever does is lie around, and he wishes she would quit being sick all the time.

Randall and Charles make a visit to Neighborhood Hospital to visit Marcus Allen, the boy Charles injured with his car. Charles tells the boy how sorry he is for what happened. The boy's Mom is very rude at first, but eventually she warms up to them. **[VC]**

Episode 7

Randall spends most of his spare time with his new girlfriend Natalie. During the evenings that he is not working, Randall is at her house. His mother verbalizes concern about the time they spend together. Randall becomes angry with his mother and perceives that she does not want him to do anything but come home and watch her lying around on the couch.

Episode 8

Randall finds his mother crying in the living room after coming home from a baseball game. She tells him she has been fired from her job because of her illness and is not sure what they are going to do. She tells Randall that they may have some tough times ahead. Randall does not think it's fair that they fired his Mom just because she is sick. At the same time, he feels angry with her for letting it happen. **[P]**

Episode 9

Randall's grandmother unexpectedly picks him up from school after baseball practice and tells him he is having dinner with her. He initially protests, telling his grandmother he has plans with Natalie, but his grandmother tells him to get on his cell phone and let Natalie know his plans have changed for the evening.

Randall's grandmother outlines what is going on with his mother in a way that he better understands. She points out to him that he is being very unfair in his assessment of his mother, who is doing the best she can. Randall's grandmother tells him to let her know if there is something he needs, and she will help him get it. She also suggests he talk to his father and let him know what's going on—maybe he can help out somewhat. Randall feels badly about some of the things he said to his mother in the previous weeks, but still does not comprehend the seriousness of his mother's illness.

Episode 10

Randall helps his mother around the house this week. She is very appreciative of his efforts. He asks Natalie to come to his house on the evenings he is not at work. Randall retrieves his report card out of the mailbox, because he doesn't want his mother to see it. He knows it will just make her upset, and he does not want her to worry about him anymore. He figures that, as long as he is passing, what she doesn't know won't hurt her. **[P]**

Episode 11

No news this week.

Episode 12

No news this week.

Episode 13

Randall's father suggests that he come to live with him, since his mother is having such a tough time. Randall tells his mother and his father that there is no way he is going to move. He is not interested in changing schools, leaving his girlfriend, or leaving his mother. He tells his Dad that he is paying for all of his car insurance at this point, and it might take longer to pay him back for the car than they had originally agreed. **[P]**

Episode 14

No news this week.

Episode 15

Baseball season has come to an end. Yvonne did not see Randall play a single game, but at this point, he is accepting of this. He worries about his mother and elects to not go out for the track and field team so that can help her more around the house and pick up additional shifts at work. He hopes to work enough hours to help his mother through the rough times that lie ahead.

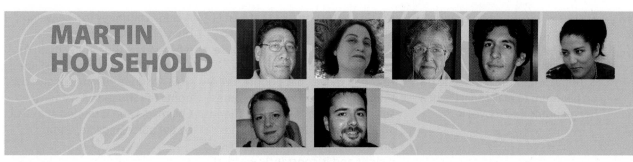

MARTIN HOUSEHOLD

MARTIN FAMILY STORY OVERVIEW

Character	Season 1	Season 2	Season 3
GILBERT MARTIN	Gil is a healthy adult male with chronic back pain and hyperlipidemia. He tries to watch his diet and is compliant with medications. Gil is a very hard worker and wants to take care of everyone. He allows his mother to move into home after his father's death, which creates tension in the household and with his wife.	Gil has ongoing issues with chronic back pain. He allows his son, Mark, and grandson, Tyler, to move in (without consulting with Helen), until Mark can catch up on his bills. He does this not only for Mark, but also for the sake of his grandson. Gil is devastated when Anthony experiences psychotic episodes.	Gil continues to have ongoing issues with chronic back pain. The family home becomes chaotic with so many people in the home, Mark's devastating injury, and Anthony's mental illness.
HELEN MARTIN	Helen is Gil's wife. She is unhappy when Mary comes to live with them, finding her presence to be disruptive to the family. Helen is obese and has had cholelithiasis; she attempts to manage her condition through diet and weight loss.	In addition to the mounting chaos in her home, Helen has acute cholecystitis and eventually has a laparoscopic cholecystectomy. She has a great deal of post-op nausea. Helen is angry with Gil for allowing Mark and Tyler to move into the home. She is also very distraught about Anthony and his mental illness.	With Mark's injury, Anthony's mental illness, and her mother-in-law living in the home, Helen has anxiety attacks and is diagnosed with an anxiety disorder. She becomes further distraught when Tracie decides to move out of the house.
MARY MARTIN	After being recently widowed, Mary moves in with Gil's family. She is a "busybody," and moving into the household disrupts the family. Mary is in good health, although she has cataracts and glaucoma, and is found to have osteoporosis.	Mary is very critical of Helen when Anthony has mental health problems, however, she is very supportive of Anthony. She continues to have problems with her vision.	Mary finally decides to have cataract surgery. Following surgery, she starts driving again. She attempts to help Anthony and takes care of Mark after his accident.
ANTHONY MARTIN	Anthony is Helen and Gil's son. He is in his final year of high school, is a loner, and does not participate in many activities. He begins to display some odd behavior during this season, but it goes unnoticed by his parents.	Anthony moves out of house and into college housing. He has a psychotic episode requiring hospitalization and is diagnosed with schizophrenia. He tries to go back to school, but has a second episode and drops out of school. He moves back home.	Anthony is in outpatient treatment, but is not compliant with his medications. He has a suicide attempt, another hospitalization, and more outpatient treatment. Eventually he leaves home after constant fighting with his parents and becomes homeless.

KRISTINA MARTIN

Kristina is Gil and Helen's daughter. She is a typical high school sophomore who is on the cheerleading squad and considered popular She is furious when she is asked to give up her room to make space when her grandmother moves in.

Kristina hates the fact that her older stepbrother and nephew Tyler have moved into the house and hates it even more when Anthony moves back home. Everything in Kristina's world becomes so crazy. She goes out with friends and stays out late at night. She goes to parties. She begins to lose weight and is constantly worried about being fat. She also becomes sexually active with Jared.

Kristina continues to lose weight, but Helen and Gil are so overwhelmed by the family situation that they don't notice. Tracie notices Kristina's weight loss and confronts the situation. Kristina gets Chlamydia and is treated at a clinic by the nurse midwife, Carol.

TRACIE AMES

Tracie is Helen's daughter from a previous marriage. She attends a local college and lives at home to save money. She does not appreciate Mary moving into the home and frequently feels angry at her because of the way Mary treats her mother.

Tracie is disgusted with her stepbrother Mark, but she adores his son Tyler and spends a great deal of time with him. Tracie is very concerned for her brother Anthony, but does not understand why he just doesn't take his medications.

Because of all the household chaos, Tracie moves in with her boyfriend. She takes Tyler with her because of Mark's situation. Her move makes Helen very sad.

MARK MARTIN

Does not live here yet

Mark is Gil's son from a previous marriage. He is a single parent to Tyler, his 2-year-old son, and experiences significant financial problems. Mark and Tyler move into Gil and Helen's home when Anthony goes to college. Mark spends most of his free time partying; he does not take much responsibility for Tyler.

Mark is involved in a motor vehicle crash after drinking and driving and suffers a spinal cord injury. He is treated at the acute care hospital and spends time at a rehab hospital before being discharged into the care of his parents. Complications experienced include a sacral decubitus ulcer, autonomic dysreflexia, and depression.

TYLER MARTIN

Does not live here yet

Tyler is Mark's 2-year-old son. Tyler and Mark move into Gil and Helen's home. Tyler is healthy, but has severe dental caries. The story revolves around getting Tyler appropriate referral and treatment and getting him up to date with immunizations. Tyler enjoys spending time with Tracie.

Tyler has an allergic reaction after eating peanuts, which requires a trip to the ED. He is too young to understand the severe injuries his father has suffered, but is not too young to realize that his father is not around. He is especially close to Tracie and goes to live with her when she moves out of the house.

CONCEPTS   *Altered Thought Process, Anxiety, Coping, Elimination, Family Dynamics, Immunity, Infection, Inflammation, Interpersonal Relationships, Interpersonal Violence, Metabolism, Mobility, Mood and Affect, Nausea, Nutrition, Pain, Role Performance, Self Image, Sensory/Perceptual, Sexuality, Sleep, Stress, Tissue Integrity*

GILBERT MARTIN
Season 1

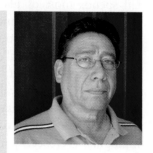

Biographical Information

Gilbert Martin is a 52-year-old Hispanic male who is married to Helen. They have been married for 18 years. Gil has a son (Mark) from a previous marriage, a stepdaughter Tracie (whom he has raised since she was 3), and two teenage children with Helen (Anthony and Kristina). He considers his marriage excellent, although he knows Helen does not get along with well with his mother and oldest son, Mark. Because Gil's father recently passed away, he spends a lot of time helping his mother manage her home.

Gil works as a local delivery truck driver for a construction company. His job includes assisting with the loading and unloading of materials off the truck. He has been in this position for over 20 years. Although he finds the pay to be competitive and has health insurance, he gets no paid vacation.

Gil considers himself to be in good health, with one exception—he has chronic back pain, which frequently makes him miserable. He usually manages the pain with over-the-counter analgesics, but he has a prescription for oxycodone with acetaminophen (Percocet), which he takes when the pain becomes severe; however, he is unable to take the Percocet on days he works. Gil also has a medical diagnosis of hyperlipidemia, for which he takes atorvastatin (Lipitor) 20 mg/day. He sees his physician once a year for cholesterol, triglycerides, and liver function tests. Gil has also been encouraged to eat a low-fat diet.

Episode 1

Gil spends the entire weekend at his mother's home, helping her pay bills and performing other various chores. She has been a widow for 6 months and does not seem to be managing her situation very well. She tells Gil that she is just too old to do these things alone and wishes his father were still alive to take care of her. Gil feels sorry for his mother and knows she must be very lonely.

Episode 2

While at his mother's house this week, Gil suggests to his mother (Mary) that maybe she should consider living with them. Mary immediately jumps at the opportunity to do so and tells Gil that is exactly what she would like to do. Gil made the comment as a suggestion to think about and did not expect his mother to react the way she did.

When he gets home, Gil tells Helen that his mother wants to move in and that they should make room for her. He is disappointed in her reaction, but attributes her behavior to not feeling well and going "through the change." Gil makes arrangements for his mother to move in during the upcoming weeks and plans to help her sell her home. [VC]

Episode 3

Gil tells Kristina and Tracie that they'll need to share a bedroom to make space for their grandmother. Gil spends several days helping his mother move. Mary moves to their home and brings with her more possessions than there is room in the house. He fills the garage with her boxes. Helen comments to Gil that there is now no room to park the cars. Gil experiences back pain for several days.

Episode 4

No news this week.

Episode 5

Gil is happy to see his mother involved with cooking meals. He knows this makes her happy, and he wants her to feel welcome in their home. He also has always loved his mother's cooking and is happy to see some of his favorite dishes (even though he knows the meals are not optimal, considering his hyperlipidemia). When Helen complains to him about his mother sabotaging her diet, he suggests that she eat low-fat foods for breakfast and lunch, and limit what she eats at dinner.

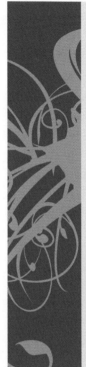

Episode 6

Gil spends most of his evenings at his mother's home doing home repairs and getting it ready for sale. On Thursday evening, he strains his back while moving furniture. He is in a great deal of pain and considers going to the emergency department, but decides not to, because he knows he will have to wait for hours to be seen. Instead, he takes a sick day on Friday and spends the next 3 days lying down, using a heating pad, taking oxycodone with acetaminophen (Percocet) pain medication, and drinking a lot of beer to treat his back strain. He is aware that Helen gets frustrated with his ongoing back pain, especially this time, because it was caused by him taking care of his mother. By Monday morning, he is able to go back to work, but he is still uncomfortable. **[P]**

Episode 7

Gil is still suffering from back pain this week. Each day he goes to work and then comes home, takes pain medication, lies on the couch to watch TV, and drinks a few beers. Gil's mother Mary tells him she wants to get a bone scan. He makes an appointment for her to see Dr. Rowe, the family physician. **[P]**

Episode 8

Kristina tells Gil that Grandma is willing to let her use her car, but only if it is OK with him. He confirms this with Mary and decides it wouldn't hurt to let Kristina drive that car—it would also get her to stop bugging him about getting her a car. Helen is angry with Gil over this decision. Gil recognizes she has been moody and again believes this is all related to her menopause. **[P]**

Episode 9

Gil spends the evening lying down on the couch watching TV with a heating pad applied to his back. He is angry with Anthony when he returns home from college night without Kristina, and tells him that, no matter what, he must look out for his sister.

Episode 10

No news this week.

Episode 11

Gil finally has his mother's house ready to put up for sale. He is hopeful that she will be able to get a good price for the home so she will have her own spending money.

Episode 12

Gil and Helen ground Kristina for staying out past curfew after the high school dance. Gil backs Helen on this decision, but wonders if Helen is being too tough on their daughter and blowing it all out of proportion.

Episode 13

Gil strains his back at work again this week while unloading his trailer. Because he is in severe pain, he goes to the emergency department, gets a narcotic pain injection and a prescription for a smooth muscle relaxant, and is told to follow up with his primary care provider. He has to take several days off from work and is relieved that it is classified as a workmen's compensation injury, so that he gets paid despite being off from work.

Episode 14

No news this week.

Episode 15

Gil manages to get Mary's house sold. He had hoped she would receive a nice sum of money to use for personal expenses, but as it turns out, he is barely able to sell it for enough to pay off the mortgage and real estate broker fees.

GILBERT MARTIN
Season 2

Biographical Information

Gilbert Martin is a 53-year-old Hispanic male who is married to Helen. They have been married for 18 years. Gil has a son (Mark) from a previous marriage, a stepdaughter Tracie (whom he has raised since she was 3), and two teenage children with Helen (Anthony and Kristina). He considers his marriage excellent, although he knows Helen does not get along with well with his mother and oldest son, Mark. Because Gil's father recently passed away, he spends a lot of time helping his mother manage her home.

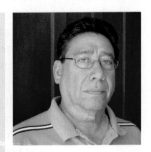

Continued

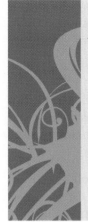

Gil works as a local delivery truck driver for a construction company. His job includes assisting with the loading and unloading of materials off the truck. He has been in this position for over 20 years. Although he finds the pay to be competitive and has health insurance, he gets no paid vacation.

Gil considers himself to be in good health, with one exception—he has chronic back pain, which frequently makes him miserable. He usually manages the pain with over-the-counter analgesics, but he has a prescription for oxycodone with acetaminophen (Percocet), which he takes when the pain becomes severe; however, he is unable to take the Percocet on days he works. Gil also has a medical diagnosis of hyperlipidemia, for which he takes atorvastatin (Lipitor) 20 mg/day. He sees his physician once a year for cholesterol, triglycerides, and liver function tests. Gil has also been encouraged to eat a low-fat diet.

Episode 1

Gil's oldest son Mark (from a previous marriage) has fallen on hard times. He has been attempting to raise his 2-year-old son (Tyler) alone and has been experiencing significant financial difficulty. Gil wants to help his son and grandson out. Because Anthony has moved out of the house to go to school, Gil suggests that Mark and Tyler move in with them, temporarily allowing Mark to catch up on some of his bills. Gil cannot understand why Helen is so angry about this. **[VC]**

Episode 2

Gil is sympathetic to Helen's abdominal pain. He can tell she is very uncomfortable and encourages her to go see the doctor about it. He overhears his mother telling Helen about Goldenseal and recalls that his mother had her gallbladder removed when she was about 40.

Gil talks with Kristina about his concerns regarding her dates with Jared. He understands that she really likes him, but is concerned about the obvious differences between high school and college-aged students. Gil tells Kristina that, if she is going to see Jared, he wants her word that she will not go into his dormitory room. Kristina assures her father that she won't do anything like that.

Episode 3

Gil truly loves children and finds it enjoyable having a young child in his house again. While playing with Tyler, Gil takes the opportunity to look at Tyler's teeth (based on Mary's concerns); he, too, notices that Tyler's teeth appear to be in bad shape. When he mentions this to his son, he learns that Mark is aware of the problem, but does not have the money to take him to a dentist.

Gil hurts his back while doing some work around the house and ends up lying on the couch for the next couple of days taking pain pills and nursing a bottle of scotch. **[P]**

Episode 4

Gil goes to the hospital to be with Helen for her surgery. He is amazed that they took her gallbladder out, and all she has to show for it is four Band-Aids on her abdomen. He feels sorry for her, as she keeps getting sick all evening, and he feels helpless for not being able to do anything for her. Kristina, Mark, Mary, and Tracie all come to the hospital that evening to visit.

Episode 5

No news this week.

Episode 6

Gil receives a phone call from a woman named Louise, who introduces herself as a psychiatric clinical nurse specialist. She informs Gil that Anthony was admitted to the hospital the day before, following an acute psychotic episode. Gil demands to know why he wasn't called earlier and asks multiple questions about his son's state of mind. Louise suggests they make a visit to the hospital so they can meet in person and see Anthony.

When Gil and Helen arrive at the hospital, both are anxious and afraid of what they might find. They learn that Anthony has been admitted to a locked acute care unit. Louise takes them into Anthony's room, where they find him hiding under the covers.

Gil and Helen talk with Louise for a time before participating in a team meeting. During the meeting, Gil asks what has happened to Anthony. The psychiatrist tells Gil and Helen that they are still gathering information, but it appears that Anthony had some type of psychotic break. Gil does not fully understand what "psychotic break" means, and the psychiatrist explains that Anthony had a break with reality. Helen and Gil find the meeting very emotionally difficult. Gil goes home and shares a 12-pack of beer with his son, Mark.

Episode 7

Gil is very glad Anthony is coming back home. He is sure that the stress of going away to college contributed to his breakdown and is confident that, if he lives at home in comfortable and familiar surroundings, the problem will go away. Gil talks to Mark and explains that it is very important for Anthony to feel comfortable at home. He asks Mark if he can let Anthony have his room back and is relieved that Mark agrees to do this.

Episode 8

Helen tells Gil that Mark is not living up to his parental responsibilities with Tyler. She points out that he works, stays out late, sleeps in during the morning, and lets everybody else take care of Tyler. Gil admits that Mark is out a lot, but also reminds Helen that helping him take care of Tyler is what families do. He agrees to talk with Mark about being more responsible, but also perceives that his wife is overly anxious and stressed out because of Anthony.

Episode 9

Gil hurts his back again this week while moving boxes in the garage. He is unable to complete the task and asks Mark to finish the project. Mark willingly does so, and Gil considers the fact that having Mark around the house is actually helpful.

Episode 10

Gil is aware that his wife is increasingly anxious. She tosses and turns in bed at night, keeping him awake. She has a hard time getting things done around the house. Gil suggests to Helen that she go see a physician to help her feel less anxious and settle down.

Gil is very concerned when Anthony decides to return to school. He tries to discourage Anthony from doing this, but it is clear to him that Anthony already has his mind made up.

Episode 11

Gil sees Anthony this week and is relieved that his son seems to be doing fine. He begins to think that he was wrong for discouraging him to return to school.

Episode 12

Mark tells Gil that his truck is finally paid off and he has caught up on all his credit card debts. He asks Gil if he can stay a bit longer to save for a down payment on a house. Gil is proud of Mark's progress and does not consider his request to be unreasonable. He wishes his wife could see the progress Mark has made, as opposed to always being critical of him.

Episode 13

Gil gets another disturbing call from the hospital. Anthony has been arrested for indecent exposure and attempted assault on a police officer, and has been admitted to a hospital inpatient psychiatric hospital again. Gil and Helen go to see their son and are confused about what might have happened. **[P]**

Episode 14

Gil welcomes Anthony home and encourages him to do everything he is asked to do in the therapy sessions. He assures Anthony that he has the support of his family, but that he also needs to take measures to take care of himself.

Episode 15

Gil is notified by the insurance company that Anthony has almost maxed out his coverage for psychiatric services. Gil is glad that Anthony has nearly completed his intensive outpatient program.

GILBERT MARTIN
Season 3

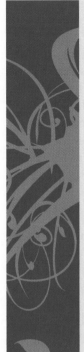

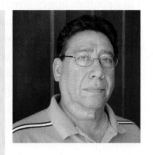

Biographical Information

Gilbert Martin is a 53-year-old Hispanic male who is married to Helen. They have been married for 19 years. Gil has a full house. His mother Mary, oldest son Mark, grandson Tyler, stepdaughter Tracie, and two children with Helen (Anthony and Kristina) are all currently living in his home. Mark and Tyler will be moving soon into their own home. He is primarily concerned about his son, Anthony, who has been recently diagnosed with schizophrenia, and is attempting to help him adjust to living with this illness.

Gil works as a local delivery truck driver for a construction company. His job includes assisting with the loading and unloading of materials off the truck. He has been in this position for over 20 years. Although he finds the pay to be competitive and has health insurance, he gets no paid vacation.

Gil considers himself to be in good health, with one exception—he has chronic back pain, which frequently makes him miserable. He usually manages the pain with over-the-counter analgesics, but he has a prescription for oxycodone with acetaminophen (Percocet), which he takes when the pain becomes severe; however, he is unable to take the Percocet on days he works. Gil also has a medical diagnosis of hyperlipidemia, for which he takes atorvastatin (Lipitor) 20 mg/day. He sees his physician once a year for cholesterol, triglycerides, and liver function tests. Gil has also been encouraged to eat a low-fat diet.

Episode 1

Gil and Helen have been very attentive to Anthony; they want to support him as much as possible. Gil is happy to see him working and making such good progress.

Episode 2

No news this week.

Episode 3

Gil takes his mother to the outpatient surgery center for the first of two cataract surgeries. He is glad that everything goes smoothly and hopes his mother's vision improves.

Gil is happy to see Mark and Shelly looking for a home to buy. He likes Shelly and thinks she is good for Mark. In his mind, she has helped him settle down and will be a good mother for Tyler. Not only will he be glad to see Mark regain his independence, but he is also looking forward to having fewer people in the house.

Episode 4

Gil is devastated when he gets a phone call from the hospital, informing him that Mark has been involved in a serious car accident. He goes to the hospital immediately. When he arrives at the hospital, he is told by the emergency department charge nurse that Mark is in serious condition. Gil asks to see him but his request is denied. The charge nurse tells Gill that Mark is in the trauma room and he would just be in the way. He is told to take a seat in the waiting room.

Hours later, Gil is further devastated when he learns that Mark has a spinal cord injury and is paralyzed from the waist down. He is so distraught that, after meeting with the physicians, he goes home and gets drunk. Helen is angry with him for drinking, because this is what caused Mark to be in the condition that he is in. **[P]**

Episode 5

Gil takes a week off from work to be with Mark. He attempts to be supportive, but is aware of the difficulties that lie ahead for his son. Gil is not surprised by Mark's anger in response to fully understanding his injuries. Gil prides himself on being able to help his family members in times of need, but realizes that, in this particular case, he is completely helpless.

Episode 6

Gil continues to visit his son at the rehabilitation hospital. He can see that Mark is depressed; he knows that Shelly is no longer in his life and that Mark is having difficulty finding anything to look forward to.

Episode 7

Gil becomes angry when Anthony tells him that he wants to stop taking his medications. Gil cannot understand why in the world Anthony would even consider such a thing, especially in light of what happened the last time he stopped taking his medications. Perhaps it is because of the stress associated with Mark's injuries, but Gil tells Anthony that the family is supportive of him—but only if he agrees to treatment. If Anthony does not undergo treatment, he is just going to have to find someplace else to live.

A couple hours later, Gil has to break Anthony's door down, because it's locked and Anthony does not respond to his mother. Gil sees that his son has taken an overdose of medication and calls for an ambulance. Helen becomes upset, pale, and sweaty. She tells Gil that she has chest pain, and her neck feels like it is swelling shut. Gil really has his hands full and doesn't know if he should attend to Helen or Anthony. Gil feels terrible and blames himself for Anthony's suicide attempt and Helen's near heart attack.

Episode 8

No news this week.

Episode 9

Gil is glad Anthony is out of the hospital and wants to ensure his success with outpatient therapy. He tells Anthony that he is sorry for making him upset and just wants him to be better. Gil notices that, although Anthony talks with him, there is little emotion in his voice. He feels so sad about the conditions of both of his sons. He buries his feelings and tries to just focus on work.

Episode 10

Gil takes several days off from work at the end of the week to make the necessary arrangements for Mark's discharge home. He obtains a specialty bed and makes phone calls to arrange for a home health nurse to help with Mark's wound care. After Mark comes home, Gil hurts his back while trying to move him into bed. He must elicit Anthony's help to get him moved. Gil spends the next several days trying to rest his back before going back to work.

This week, Tracie decides to move out of the house. Gil knows this makes Helen very upset. Although he hates to see her go, he recognizes that the household has been in total chaos and understands her decision to leave.

Episode 11

Gil overhears Anthony yelling at his mother about taking his medications. He finds Helen in tears. Gil and Anthony have another confrontation about Anthony's lack of compliance with his medications. Gil tells Anthony that he just doesn't have any additional energy to deal with him, and if he doesn't want help, he is out of the house—he just can't take anymore! Anthony gathers a few things and storms out of the house. Gil asks him where he will be, but Anthony does not answer. Gil notices that Anthony left his medications in the bathroom.

Episode 12

Gil learns that Anthony has been staying with a friend from high school. He attempts to call to find out how he is doing, but cannot reach him. Gil worries about both of his sons and his wife, and wishes he could make everything okay again. He does not know how to express what he is feeling—he feels the need to be "man of the house" and not show his emotions. Gil is glad that Kristina and Tracie have not had any problems.

Episode 13

No news this week.

Episode 14

Gil thinks about Anthony and Mark constantly. He is glad to see Tracie step up to take care of Tyler and makes a point to spend time with Tyler each day. It is important to him to have a close relationship with his grandson, and he appreciates Tracie's efforts to bring him over each day.

Gil also notices that Kristina has not been running around with her friends as much and is glad that she is home more. He is particularly glad that she has not been going out with Jared. [P]

Episode 15

Gil learns that Anthony is staying in one of the homeless shelters in the downtown area. He is devastated to know that one of his children is on the streets, but doesn't know what else to do. He knows he cannot bring him back into the house at this time, but worries constantly about him.

HELEN MARTIN
Season 1

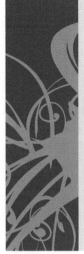

Biographical Information
Helen Martin is a 48-year-old White female who is married to Gil. They have been married for 18 years. Helen has a daughter (Tracie) from a previous marriage, and she has two teenage children with Gil (Anthony and Kristina). She has been relatively happy in this marriage; her primary frustration with Gil is that he always wants to take care of everybody and has a hard time saying no. She thinks he is almost generous to a fault. Helen has never gotten along well with Gil's adult son, Mark, or Gil's mother Mary. She also frequently feels frustrated with Gil, because he always is complaining of back pain.

Helen works as a teller at a bank. Although she finds her job monotonous, she appreciates the steady income. Helen is overweight and has tried to lose weight most of her adult life. She frequently diets and, in fact, has lost a great deal of weight in the past, but just can't seem to keep it off. She blames menopause for her most recent weight gain.

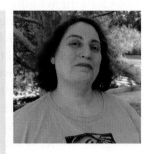

Episode 1
Helen experiences indigestion following a few meals this week. She takes an antacid, believing the problem is just heartburn. She also experiences hot flashes. **[P]**

Episode 2
Gil tells Helen that his mother wants to move in and that they should make room for her. Helen is furious with this decision for several reasons: Gil did not first consult with her, they don't have room for her, they cannot afford another person in the house, and Helen has never gotten along well with her mother-in-law.

Helen continues to have indigestion following meals; it does not occur following all meals, just sometimes. The discomfort is usually located in the upper right side of her abdomen, and sometimes it is quite painful. The pain can last for up to a couple of hours and then subsides. Occasionally, she feels nauseous as well. To top it off, Helen experiences several episodes of hot flashes. **[VC]**

Episode 3
Helen's two daughters are angry and fighting because they have to share a bedroom to accommodate their grandmother. Helen thinks this is very unfair to both the girls.

Helen continues to experience pain and indigestion after meals; in fact, the weeks have become more frequent. She decides to make an appointment to see her physician about the symptoms.

Episode 4
Helen has not slept well this week. She has a hard time falling asleep, because she worries about everything—the kids, money, problems at work, and recent problems on the national level affecting the country. Often times, she gets up and paces about the house, trying to turn her mind off. About the time she falls asleep, she is woken up by Mary watching TV in the den during the middle of the night. She asks Mary to keep the volume down so that the family is not disturbed. She also awakens at times because of hot flashes.

Helen sees her family physician, Dr. Rowe, this week for indigestion. Based on Helen's symptoms, Dr. Rowe suspects that Helen has cholelithiasis and orders an ultrasound scan of the abdomen. The ultrasound confirms the presence of gallstones. The physician tells Helen that she has two options: (1) conservative therapy that would involve dietary modification (a low-fat diet and a reduced-calorie diet to promote weight loss); or (2) surgery to remove her gallbladder. Helen decides to try dietary modification. The Dr. Rowe refers her to the Neighborhood Patient Education Center for further information. She is encouraged to use over-the-counter analgesics for pain.

Episode 5
Helen goes to the Patient Education Center and receives dietary counseling from a nurse educator. She is taught about low-fat food options and is given sample menus and cooking techniques to minimize fat. Helen is very

motivated to go on this diet to avoid the pain, and she looks forward to losing some weight.

Helen agrees to Mary's request to prepare dinner three times a week. Helen shares with Mary what she learned at the Patient Education Center, with an expectation that the meals would be prepared based on this dietary plan. She becomes angry when she finds that Mary essentially ignores her requests and is frustrated because the rest of the family members comment on how good dinner is when Grandma cooks. She believes that Mary is intentionally is sabotaging her dietary efforts. **[P]**

Episode 6
Helen comes home one day after work this week and is unable to find anything because Mary has rearranged the entire kitchen. Helen feels angry and invaded. Mary defends her actions by claiming that Helen's kitchen was very disorganized and that she is just trying to help the entire family.

Episode 7
Helen becomes frustrated when she finds that Mary continues to rearrange things in the house and clean things that were already clean. Helen also notices that Mary is often unaware that the dishes she washes and puts away are still dirty, so Helen ends up rewashing dishes.

She has given up fighting with Mary over the dinner menu and decided to take Gil's advice and limit fat intake at other meals, eating only small portions when Mary cooks. **[P]**

Episode 8
Helen is angry when she learns that Mary and Gil have given Kristina permission to use the car. She does not feel it is appropriate for Mary and Gil to make such decisions without her input. But, at this point, if she were to put a stop to it, she would end up looking like the "bad guy." Helen is so frustrated with this that she eats a large, fatty meal and ends up having 2 hours of indigestion, pain, and nausea as a result. She also has trouble sleeping that night. She blames Gil and Mary for the pain and loss of sleep.

Episode 9
Helen panics when Anthony fails to bring Kristina home after a school function. She tries to call Kristina's cell phone, but it is turned off. She becomes frantic and is sure somebody has abducted Kristina. Helen gets in the car and drives to the school to see if she can find her. On the way to school, she becomes increasingly anxious and begins to experience shortness of breath and tightness in her chest and throat. The closer she gets to the school, the worse the symptoms become. Helen's symptoms reach the point at which her heart is pounding in her chest and she feels like she is suffocating; she then breaks out in a cold sweat. Helen pulls over to the side of the road and begins to cry. She tells herself to calm down and that everything surely will be all right. After a few minutes, Helen composes herself and continues driving to the school. When she gets to the school, she finds the college fair is over and nearly everybody has left. By the time she gets back home, Kristina is at home watching TV. Helen screams at her and wants to know where she was and why she didn't answer her phone. She tells Kristina that she almost had a heart attack and that her gallbladder acted up because of this situation. **[VC]**

Episode 10
No news this week.

Episode 11
No news this week.

Episode 12
Helen is worried about Kristina when she fails to come home by 1 a.m. following a school dance. She attempts to call Kristina's cell phone, but it is turned off. She paces the house and alternately worries that Kristina has been in a wreck or that she is up to no good with her date. She feels a subtle tightness in her chest and slight shortness of breath, which she attributes to her gallbladder problems. When Kristina comes home, Helen grounds her for staying out one hour past her curfew. Helen feels frustrated because Tracie and Anthony never behaved in this way. **[P]**

Episode 13
No news this week.

Episode 14
No news this week.

Episode 15
Helen begins to experience indigestion and pain again. She knows that she has not stuck with her low-fat diet very well. She is hopeful that the symptoms will subside with better eating habits. **[P]**

HELEN MARTIN
Season 2

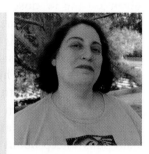

Biographical Information

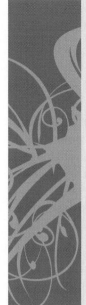

Helen Martin is a 48-year-old White female who is married to Gil. They have been married for 18 years. Helen has a daughter (Tracie) from a previous marriage, and she has two teenage children with Gil (Anthony and Kristina). She has been relatively happy in this marriage; her primary frustration with Gil is that he always wants to take care of everybody and has a hard time saying no. She thinks he is almost generous to a fault. Helen has never gotten along well with Gil's adult son, Mark, or Gil's mother Mary. She also frequently feels frustrated with Gil, because he always is complaining of back pain. Helen has had recent stress in her marriage because Gil's mother Mary is now living with them. Helen's son, Anthony, has recently left home to attend college nearby.

Helen has been experiencing ongoing abdominal pain due to gallstones. She has been trying to manage the problem through dietary modification, but this effort has not been successful. Helen is overweight and has tried to lose weight most of her adult life. She frequently diets and, in fact, has lost a great deal of weight in the past, but just can't seem to keep it off. She blames menopause for her most recent weight gain.

Episode 1

Helen is furious with Gil for suggesting that Mark and Tyler move into their home. Helen and Mark have never gotten along very well, so she is very resentful that Gil gave Mark permission to live with them. Helen thinks that Mark is a loser because he cannot seem to keep a job, and the party scene is more important to him than looking for work or raising Tyler. She believes Mark should have to figure out a solution to his own problems. Helen is also angry with Kristina for staying out late again. Helen grounds her, but recognizes that this punishment has not been terribly effective with her in the past.

Episode 2

Helen has an abrupt episode of intense abdominal pain and vomiting. She becomes sweaty and feels that her heart is racing. At first, she thinks she is having a heart attack, but then she concludes the pain is probably being caused by her gallbladder. The pain lasts about an hour and then subsides. She has given up hope that conservative treatment will resolve anything. She has an appointment with Dr. Rowe the following day, who refers her to a surgeon. After meeting with the surgeon, Helen decides to go ahead with surgery to remove her gallbladder. She is scheduled to have the surgery in a couple of weeks. Helen talks with Anthony this week. He tells her that he elected not to go to the football game. Helen wishes her son would interact more at school. She frequently feels anxious about his well-being. **[P]**

Episode 3

No news this week.

Episode 4

Helen is anxious all week, worrying about her surgery—almost to the point of not being able to do basic tasks around the house. She goes to the hospital 2 days before the surgery for preoperative testing and blood work. On the day of surgery, she arrives at the hospital about 6 a.m. She is in the surgical suite by 10 a.m. and has a laparoscopic cholecystectomy performed. The surgery goes smoothly, with no complications.

When Helen begins to wake up in the post-anesthesia care unit, she experiences a great deal of pain and nausea. She is given morphine and ondansetron to treat her symptoms. She is transferred to the surgical unit when she is mostly awake, and her vital signs are stable. She has no bleeding at the surgical site, her respiratory rate is 18, and her oxygen saturation is 97%.

Helen continues to have problems with pain and nausea throughout the afternoon and evening, and has several episodes of emesis. On the surgical unit, she is given a 4-mg IV dose of ondansetron, which seems to do little for the nausea. She is also given 4 mg of morphine, which effectively eases her pain. She is unable to eat her dinner and has several more episodes of emesis during the evening. The pain and nausea make Helen increasingly anxious, to the point at which she is tearful. Helen is then given a 25-mg dose of promethazine, which helps her to relax and relives her nausea. She finally falls asleep about 3 a.m. The next morning, despite the fact that she has slept only a few hours, Helen feels much better. The nausea is gone, she has minimal pain, and she is able to eat. Her IV is discontinued, and she is discharged by mid-afternoon the day following her surgery. **[P]**

Episode 5

Helen takes this week off from work to recover from her surgery. She spends a great deal of time with Tyler and actually finds the time quite enjoyable, although she would never admit this to anyone. She frequently feels anxious while at home about what might be going on at work. She does not leave her home often during her week off. **[P]**

Episode 6

Gil informs Helen that Anthony has been admitted to the psychiatric unit at the hospital. Helen becomes very anxious and does not know what to think. She feels her heart racing and starts to cry. A while later, after having a chance to settle down, Helen goes with Gil to see Anthony. Upon arriving at the unit, Helen and Gil go into Anthony's room and find him hiding under the bed sheets. Helen approaches the bed and calls his name softly. Anthony peeks his head out from underneath the sheets and starts to cry uncontrollably. Helen cries also. Gil attempts to console Helen, but she continues to cry.

Louise, the clinical nurse specialist, asks Gil and Helen to accompany her to the day room. Helen wonders what she might have done to cause Anthony to act in this way. Louise obtains a family history from Helen and Gil; during this interview, it is revealed that Helen's maternal aunt spent many years at a psychiatric facility. She reports that her aunt was a bit "weird," but couldn't give further details.

Helen and Gil later participate in a family meeting involving Louise, the psychiatrist, and Anthony. Both Helen and Gil find the meeting very difficult emotionally.

Episode 7

Helen is glad that Anthony has moved back home. At the same time, she hates the commotion it has caused. Mark and Tyler are now sleeping in the family room, and the house feels very crowded and chaotic.

Episode 8

Helen is quite aware of Mark's late-night partying and talks with Gil about this. Although she does not come out and say it, she resents having to take care of Tyler. She is not interested in raising another child. She points out to Gil that the rest of the family (including herself) should not be responsible for taking care of Tyler just because Mark wants to party all the time. These recent changes in her household and going through menopause have placed quite a strain on Helen's marriage with Gil. These stressors make Helen feel anxious.

Episode 9

Helen continues to feel anxious about many things, including Anthony, Kristina, Mark, and Gil. Her symptoms have gotten so bad that just leaving the house makes her feel anxious; for this reason she feels demoralized. Helen asks Tracie to accompany her to the grocery store.

Episode 10

Helen's anxiety escalates when Anthony returns to school. She is sure he is in for further problems and is tearful when he goes, despite her objections. Helen feels paralyzed at times with her anxiety. She is unable to work two days this week. Helen is glad Mark has taken Tyler to get his teeth checked.

Episode 11

No news this week.

Episode 12

Helen notices Kristina has been looking thin and asks her about her weight. Kristina tells her Mom she lost a few pounds, but it really has been no big deal and denies that there are any problems. Helen fails to notice that Kristina's grade report came in the mail. **[P]**

Episode 13

Helen is devastated when she learns that Anthony has been readmitted to the hospital. She is angry with him when she learns that he quit taking his medications. She feels her heart is racing, and it is very hard for her to settle down. Gil again suggests she go see a doctor. Helen is worried that she might have a heart problem and avoids making the appointment out of fear of having an anxiety attack at the physician's office.

Episode 14

Helen is relieved when Anthony is discharged from the hospital and comes back home. She is determined to help him keep up with all of his medications. She worries that he will have another "episode." She tells Gil that Mark needs to move out and get his own place. Gil tells Helen that Mark is planning to move soon.

Episode 15

Helen's anxiety has reached the point at which she only goes out to go to work. She does not like going out because she is fearful of having an anxiety attack in public. She asks Tracie to go with her nearly everywhere she goes. Tracie tells her mother she needs to get checked out by a doctor. **[P]**

HELEN MARTIN
Season 3

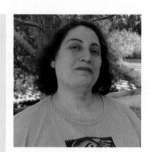

Biographical Information

Helen Martin is a 49-year-old White female who is married to Gil. They have been married for 19 years. Helen has a daughter (Tracie) from a previous marriage, and she has two teenage children with Gil (Anthony and Kristina). Up until lately, she has been relatively happy in this marriage; however she has been feeling frustrated with Gil because he allowed his mother Mary and then his adult son, Mark, and Mark's son Tyler to move into their home. Helen has never gotten along well with Mark or Mary, so these changes have been difficult.

Recently, Helen had a cholecystectomy for treatment of gallbladder disease. More recently, she has been frequently experiencing anxiety. Much of the anxiety has been due to her concern for Anthony and issues with her daughter Kristina. She has not formally seen a physician for the condition, although several of her family members have suggested she do so. Helen works as a teller at a bank. Although she finds her job monotonous, she appreciates the steady income and benefits, including family health insurance.

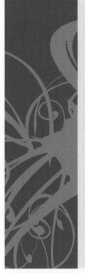

Episode 1

Helen is very attentive to Anthony. She pays close attention to his mood and affect to be sure not to miss something. She makes sure he takes his medications every day and helps him to get to work on time. She is glad he has a job to go to every day and is hopeful that he is on the road to recovery.

Episode 2

Helen is glad to hear that Mark and Shelly are planning to buy a house. Mark has been living with them too long already, and she can't wait to see him leave.

Episode 3

No news this week.

Episode 4

Helen is upset when she learns of Mark's accident. She is angry with him for driving his truck drunk and shocked to learn his injuries have left him paralyzed. She wonders how he will ever be able to care for himself and how he will be able to raise Tyler. Helen is furious when Gil comes home from the hospital after seeing Mark and gets drunk. **[P]**

Episode 5

Helen and Gil spend a great deal of time at the hospital with Mark this week. Helen is worried about the long-term consequences of Mark's injuries. Although they have never been close, and despite the fact that he brought this on himself, Helen feels very badly for Mark. She wonders what lies ahead for not only his life, but Tyler's life as well, which causes her to worry almost constantly.

Episode 6

No news this week.

Episode 7

Helen is upset with Gil for yelling at Anthony. She hears him slam his door and decides it is best to leave him alone for a while. After a couple of hours, Helen gently knocks on the door. Anthony does not respond, and she attempts to enter his room, but he has locked the door. She knocks louder, and he still does not answer. Gil finally forces the door open, and Helen sees Anthony lying on the floor, stuporous and incoherent. She sees a large (500-count), empty bottle of Tylenol in the trash can. They call 9-1-1.

Finding Anthony on the floor causes Helen to have a severe anxiety attack. She begins to experience severe chest pain. When the paramedics arrive, they tell her she needs to be seen in the emergency department (ED) as well. In the ED, Helen reports nausea, chest pain, shortness of breath, neck tightness, diaphoresis, and palpitations. She has a cardiac work-up, which is negative. She sees a cardiologist in the ED, who orders Holter monitoring for one week to rule out a dysrhythmia. Helen is also given a prescription for 0.5 mg of lorazepam (Ativan) to take when she has anxiety. **[P]**

Episode 8

Helen sees the cardiologist this week, who determines she has no evidence of cardiac disease. After taking a thorough history and learning about the recent events within Helen's family, the cardiologist refers her to a psychiatrist about a possible anxiety disorder. Helen is told she cannot get in to see the psychiatrist for 3 months, so instead agrees to make an appointment with a psychiatric clinical nurse specialist (CNS). Helen has been taking the Ativan and finds it helps her to feel better.

Episode 9

Helen sees the psychiatric CNS this week. Helen tells the nurse that the Ativan definitely helps, but she also feels like she is "on a seesaw"—up and down, feeling good, feeling anxious, then needing more medications. The nurse takes a thorough history and orders a fasting glucose and lipids. **[P]**

Episode 10

Mark is discharged from the rehabilitation hospital this week. It has been quite an ordeal getting ready for him to come home. Helen is glad to have the Ativan to keep her anxiety under control. She feels very down about the fact that she is now responsible for caring for a depressed paraplegic man and his son. The one positive thing, however, is that her mother-in-law Mary has made it clear that she is going to help take care of Mark. For the first time since she has moved into their home, Helen is glad to have Mary's help.

Things get worse for Helen when Tracie announces that she has decided to move out of the house. Helen is so upset by this that she cries uncontrollably for hours. She feels overwhelmed and as though her life is spinning out of control. Tracie is the one solid person that Helen knows she can count on. Helen sees the clinical nurse specialist again this week. She is started on a prescription of Zoloft 50 mg daily and buspirone 20 mg daily. **[P]**

Episode 11

Helen feels stressed from attempting to help care for Mark and is getting into regular arguments with Anthony about taking his medications. She does not know how much more she can take of all this. She is devastated when Anthony has an argument with Gil and storms out of the house.

The clinical nurse specialist has increased Helen's Zoloft dose to 100 mg once a day. Helen is feeling better on the medications and is less anxious. The CNS recommends personal and family counseling. Helen would love to go, but just does not think there is any way she can afford the time or the cost. **[VC]**

Episode 12

Helen worries all week about Anthony and keeps hoping he will come back home. Helen's friend, Martha, calls to tell her that Anthony is living with her son's friend, Jason. Helen gets Jason's phone number and tries to call, but is not able to reach Anthony. Helen also misses having Tracie and Tyler at the house. She wishes Tracie and Anthony would both come home. **[P]**

Episode 13

Helen is pleased to see Tracie bring Tyler over to visit Mark every day. She can see how happy Tyler is with her and how good Tracie looks. Helen realizes it is probably good for Tracie and Tyler to be out of the house, despite how much she misses them.

Episode 14

Mark makes his first unassisted transfer from the bed to a wheelchair this week. Helen is glad to have something positive to think about. She wishes she knew how Anthony was doing.

Episode 15

Helen is devastated to learn that her son, Anthony, is living in a homeless shelter. She pleads with Gil to go get him and bring him home, but Gil tells Helen that they cannot have that disruption in their home. Helen blames Gil for driving Anthony away.

MARY MARTIN
Season 1

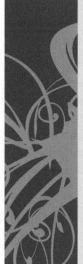

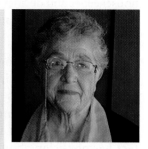

Biographical Information

Mary Martin is a 75-year-old female who was recently widowed. She and her husband were married for 52 years when he died from cancer 6 months ago. She has a limited income, because her husband's pension terminated when he died. She receives $752 each month in Social Security benefits. Mary has not adjusted well to being alone. Her son, Gil, visits her frequently and helps her manage her home.

Mary does not see particularly well. Otherwise, she is in excellent health; the only health-related problems she is aware of are cataracts and glaucoma, for which she sees an ophthalmologist on a regular basis. The only prescription drug that she uses is latanoprost ophthalmic solution (Xalatan) to manage her glaucoma (her dose is 1 drop in each eye once a day), and her only complaint about the eye drops is the cost. Although she has a car and driver's license, she does not drive very often due to problems with night vision. She prefers to get friends and family members to take her where she needs to go.

Episode 1

Mary is happy that Gil spent most of his time with her this past weekend. Not only does she enjoy his company, but she appreciates the fact that he takes care of things for her. Although it has been 6 months since her husband died, she has not become comfortable living alone. She tells Gil that she wishes his father were still alive to take care of her. To pass the time and combat loneliness, she spends a great deal of time at the Neighborhood Senior Center.

Episode 2

Mary bakes cookies for Gil this week and then calls him to invite him over for a treat. She wishes he would spend more time with her because she feels so lonely. While Gil is visiting, she tells him that she has such a hard time managing her home. Gil tells her that perhaps she should think about staying with them for a while. This is exactly what Mary has been hoping for, and she immediately agrees that moving in with his family would be the best thing to do. Although she is not fond of Gil's wife Helen, she loves her son and her grandchildren and knows she will be much happier living with them. She quickly begins making plans to move.

Episode 3

Mary moves into Gil and Helen's home this week. She is unaware of the disruption that her moving in has created within the household. She has many possessions she wants to bring with her to Gil's home, but space is somewhat limited. Several boxes of her possessions are placed in the garage, with the understanding that she will go through the boxes and determine what she wants to keep and what she wants to give away. Mary agrees to let Gil clean up her home in order to list it for sale.

Episode 4

Mary is still in the process of fitting into the family. She has the house to herself during the daytime and feels a bit out of place, at times even wishing to be back in her home. At night she has trouble sleeping and frequently goes out to the den to watch television during the middle of the night.

Episode 5

Mary loves to cook and is actually very good at it. Mary tells Helen that she will make dinner for the family 3 nights a week. Helen agrees to this and asks Mary to try to keep dinners low in fat because she is trying to stay on a diet. Mary decides that Gil probably does not get enough to eat, and she knows what his favorite foods are. Mary liked Gil's first wife much better and is not too concerned about cooking foods consistent with Helen's request—she is much more interested in preparing dinners that her son likes. She is very pleased that all of the family members (except Helen) comment on how good her dinners are. Mary also spends time this week at the Senior Center with her friends and goes out to get her hair and nails done.

Episode 6

This week Mary decides the kitchen cabinets need to be cleaned and reorganized; she proceeds to rearrange the entire kitchen to suit her needs. Mary thinks Helen is a lazy housekeeper and decides it is a good thing she is living with them to help them out and take care of her son Gil. **[P]**

Episode 7

Mary goes to the community health fair with her friend. While at the fair, she has a bone density screening performed and is told that she possibly has low bone density—a finding commonly associated with osteoporosis. The health fair nurse suggests that she contact her physician about getting a full bone scan so her condition can be evaluated further. When Gil comes home from work that evening, she tells him she needs to have a bone test done and would like him to arrange this for her. **[P]**

Episode 8

Mary hears the argument between Kristina and her parents about the car. When Kristina asks Mary if she may drive her car, Mary decides it would be fine—but only if she promises to take care of the car and only if her father approves it.

Mary goes to the Senior Center twice this week for lunch and to play cards with her friends. She tells her friends that she must take care of her son because her daughter-in-law is lazy and does not cook properly. During lunch she notices her friend Beatrice eating two pieces of cake. Mary reminds Beatrice that she should not eat this way.

At the end of the week, Mary sees Dr. Rowe and tells her about the health fair. She asks Dr. Rowe about getting a bone test. **[VC]**

Episode 9

Mary has an appointment for the bone scan this week; following her scan, she asks Gil to take her to the beauty salon to have her hair and nails done. Later in the week, she observes Helen cleaning the house and determines that it is not being done correctly. She often follows behind Helen and repeats the cleaning so that the house is cleaned properly. **[P]**

Episode 10

In a follow-up visit with Dr. Rowe, Mary is told that her bone scan shows evidence of decreased bone mineral density that is consistent with osteoporosis. She is told to increase her activity for weight-bearing exercise, increase her calcium intake to 1,500 mg per day, and take vitamin D supplements. She is also given a prescription for alendronate (Fosamax). Dr. Rowe also tells Mary that new research points to a link between osteoporosis and celiac disease, and suggests that she be screened. Mary agrees to the screening, and serologic autoantibody testing is performed.

Mary also goes to the Neighborhood Senior Center this week and attends a leather craft class. During the class, she tells all the ladies about the medical tests, her new medication for osteoporosis, her new exercise regimen, and all the events happening at her home. **[VC]**

Episode 11

Mary receives a phone call from the physician's office, informing her that her blood tests were negative for the presence of celiac disease. Mary does not really understand what celiac disease is, but is relieved to know that she doesn't have another condition to worry about. She walks around the block early every morning this week for weight-bearing exercise. **[P]**

Episode 12

No news this week.

Episode 13

Mary continues her walking routine. She also gets involved in some of the exercise classes offered at the Neighborhood Senior Center. **[P]**

Episode 14

Mary has an appointment with her ophthalmologist this week, who notes that her cataracts continue to worsen and recommends she consider surgery. Mary does not admit the fact that she is afraid to have surgery on her eyes. She tells the doctor she might have the surgery at some point, but is too busy to do it right now. The physician gives Mary a new prescription for her eyeglasses, which will help her vision at least for a little while. Mary is told to increase the amount of light and use reading glasses or a magnifying glass for reading.

The physician also notes that Mary's intraocular pressure has increased since her last visit. She is asked how often she uses the latanoprost (Xalatan) eye drops. Mary admits to the ophthalmologist that she only uses the drops on Mondays, Wednesdays, Fridays, and Sundays, as opposed to every day. Mary explains that she does this because the drops are expensive and this regimen makes the drops last longer. The office nurse assists Mary with finding a prescription assistance program to help defer the cost of the eye drops. **[P]**

Episode 15

Mary is angry that somebody hit her car in the school parking lot while Kristina was driving. She tells Kristina she understands that the accident was not her fault, but she needs to take good care of the car. Mary is disappointed, but not really surprised, to learn that she only is getting $12,500 from the sale of her house.

MARY MARTIN
Season 2

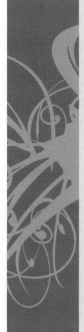

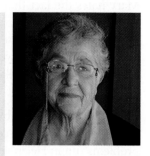

Biographical Information

Mary Martin is Gil Martin's 75-year-old mother. About one year ago, Mary's husband of 52 years died from cancer. Because she was feeling so lonely Mary jumped at the opportunity when Gil suggested that she move in with his family. It is Mary's perception that Gil and his family need her because she can cook and clean for them. She has never felt that Gil's wife Helen was a good housekeeper. Mary has a limited income because her husband's pension terminated when he died. She receives $752 each month in Social Security benefits.

Mary does not see particularly well. Otherwise, she is in excellent health; the only health-related problems she is aware of are osteoporosis, cataracts, and glaucoma, for which she sees an ophthalmologist on a regular basis. The only prescription drugs and over-the-counter supplements that she uses include alendronate sodium (Fosamax), calcium, and latanoprost ophthalmic solution (Xalatan) to manage her glaucoma (her dose is 1 drop in each eye once a day). Her only complaint about the eye drops is the cost. Although she has a car and driver's license, she does not drive very often due to problems with vision. She prefers to get friends and family members to take where places she needs to go.

Episode 1

Mary is thrilled at the news that her oldest (and favorite) grandchild is moving in with them. She has always been fond of Mark and is glad he is finally getting a chance to live with his father. She tells Helen that Gil has done the right thing by letting Mark and Tyler live with them. She tells Kristina that she should be happy to share a room with her sister; when she was growing up, she tells Kristina, she had to share a room with four of her sisters. Mary offers to babysit her great-grandchild, Tyler, whenever Mark needs her to. **[P]**

Episode 2

Mary notices that Tyler has no toys or books. She asks Kristina to drive her to her hair appointment and then to the discount store, where she buys Tyler toys, puzzles, and books.

Mary spends time with her friends at the Neighborhood Senior Center, telling them in detail all about her granddaughter Kristina dating a college boy, about the fact that Mark and Tyler have recently moved in with them, and how her daughter-in-law is so intolerant of other people's misfortunes. As she talks, she notices a small, white-haired woman walk by and scowl at her. She asks the ladies at the table who the woman is; although a few ladies say they have seen the woman before, nobody knows her name.

When Helen has her gallbladder attack this week, Mary tells her that she should just take Goldenseal (*Hydrastis canadensis*) instead of having surgery. Mary swears this is the way her gallbladder problems were cured when she was 44 years old. **[P]**

Episode 3

Mary overhears Tracie commenting to Tyler about the condition of his teeth. With her bad eyesight, Mary really never noticed the condition of his teeth before. Later in the day, she is shocked at how bad they are—or at least what she can see. She mentions it to Mark and can tell by his response that he is unaware of the problem. Mary tells her son Gil that somebody needs to talk with Mark about Tyler's teeth. **[VC]**

Episode 4

Mary takes over most of the household duties when Helen goes to the hospital for her surgery. She enjoys being in charge and making dinner for everyone. Mary has another visit with the ophthalmologist this week. She tells her doctor that her vision is foggy and that it has become hard to see clearly, even with the eye glasses. The physician indicates that a stronger prescription of eye glasses will help for now, but that she really needs to consider having the cataract surgery. **[P]**

Episode 5

Mary hates the fact that Helen is home all this week and feels irritated when she complains about her pain. Mary prefers to have the house mostly to herself during the daytime when Helen is at work. Mary listens to the local news and wonders if they will ever get the forest fire put out. **[P]**

Episode 6

Mary is very saddened by the problems Anthony has been experiencing. When it comes to light that mental health problems run in Helen's side of the family, Mary is quick to point out that it is obvious where Anthony's problems have come from. She gets a friend to pick her up to join the ladies at the Neighborhood Senior Center. Mary embellishes all the things happening in her household this week. **[P]**

Episode 7

Mary is somewhat annoyed initially when Anthony moves back home because Mark and Tyler have "taken over" the family room; this interferes with Mary's late-night TV watching. In the mornings, she encourages Mark to sleep in. She gladly takes care of Tyler because it makes her feel useful.

Mary talks Tracie into driving her to get her hair and nails done. On the way home, she asks Tracie to stop at the mall. At the mall, she buys Tracie some badly needed new shoes in appreciation for her time.

Episode 8

Mary overhears Helen sharing her concerns with Gil about Mark's late-night schedule. Mary tells Gil that he should not give Mark too hard of a time for being out late; she points out to him that she likes taking care of Tyler, and it all seems to work out just fine. Mary tries to talk with Anthony, but can tell he is just not interested. She bakes him his favorite cookies to try to cheer him up. **[P]**

Episode 9

No news this week.

Episode 10

Mary is hopeful that Anthony's return to school is successful. She believes he has had such a hard time in life because of Helen and believes that being away from her is what he really needs. Mary spends time at the Neighborhood Senior Center playing cards, although it is getting more and more difficult for her do to so because of her vision. **[P]**

Episode 11

No news this week.

Episode 12

Mary decides that her eyesight has gotten bad enough that she should go back and see the ophthalmologist. She asks Tracie to help make an appointment for her because she has trouble seeing. She makes an appointment, but cannot be seen for a couple of weeks.

Episode 13

Mary feels so sorry for Anthony and feels badly for her son Gil. She wishes that Anthony did not inherit the mental problems from his mother and wishes something could be done about it. Mary talks with Kristina about Anthony and tries to point out that he cannot help what is happening to him.

While playing cards at the Neighborhood Senior Center this week, Mary tells all of her friends about Anthony. She denies that he has mental health problems and does not believe he needs the prescribed medications. She tells the ladies, "If he is crazy, it must be Helen's fault, because we don't have those kinds of problems on our side of the family." **[P]**

Episode 14

Mary makes an effort to help Anthony. She wants everything to be okay for him. She tells Anthony over and over again that everything will work out and that he needs to let his father help him. Mary does not feel a bit guilty about the fact that she has a bedroom to herself, while Mark and Tyler have to sleep in the family room; instead, she finds the arrangement annoying because it interferes with her late-night television viewing.

Episode 15

Mary is very supportive of Anthony; she just thinks he is who he is. It is obvious to her that those people at the university don't understand him and are just mean. In her mind, Anthony would never hurt anyone.

Mary has an appointment with the ophthalmologist. He confirms that her vision has indeed become worse and tells her she really needs to have the cataract surgery. Mary has been very resistant to this, but is now realizing that her loss of vision is impacting her quality of life. She talks with the doctor about the fear she has about having eye surgery. The physician points out that, without the surgery, she will lose her sight—essentially, she has nothing to lose and everything to gain. Mary tells the physician she will consider it.

Later in the week, Mary is at the Neighborhood Senior Center and tells her friends about possibly having cataract surgery. Three of the ladies tell her that they have had it done, and it really is no big deal. Mary tells them that she heard people can go blind from the surgery and is scared to do it. They suggest she talk to Karen Williams, the nurse in the clinic at the Senior Center. Mary talks with Karen about having surgery. Karen assures her it is a very common procedure, and it could potentially improve the quality of her life by improving her vision. **[VC] [P]**

MARY MARTIN
Season 3

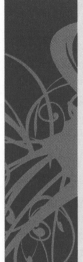

Biographical Information

Mary Martin is Gil Martin's 76-year-old mother. About 18 months ago, Mary's husband of 52 years died from cancer. Mary has been living with Gil and his family for about one year now. It is Mary's perception that Gil and his family need her because she can cook and clean for them. She has never felt that Gil's wife Helen was a good housekeeper. Mary has a limited income because her husband's pension terminated when he died. She receives $752 each month in Social Security benefits.

Mary does not see particularly well. Otherwise, she is in excellent health; the only health-related problems she is aware of are osteoporosis, cataracts, and glaucoma, for which she sees an ophthalmologist on a regular basis. The only prescription drugs and over-the-counter supplements that she uses include alendronate sodium (Fosamax), calcium, and latanoprost ophthalmic solution (Xalatan) to manage her glaucoma (her dose is 1 drop in each eye once a day). Her only complaint about the eye drops is the cost. Mary's vision has been getting increasingly poor; for this reason she has been contemplating having cataract surgery.

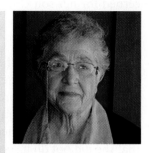

Episode 1

Mary hears Tyler crying and investigates the problem. Even with her poor eyesight, she can see that the child is covered in hives and his lips are swollen. She asks Mark about this, and he tells her he did not notice it. Mary tells Mark to take Tyler to a doctor immediately.

Mary returns to the ophthalmologist this week and tells him she has decided to go ahead with the surgery. The ophthalmologist tells Mary that they will do surgery on one eye first and then wait 4 to 6 weeks before performing surgery on the other eye.

Episode 2

No news this week.

Episode 3

This week, Mary has her first cataract surgery. The day before surgery, she asks Kristina to take her to the church so she can pray to the Virgin Mary for her health. She also sees Father John and asks him for a blessing.

Gil takes Mary to the Neighborhood Outpatient Surgery Center for the cataract surgery on her right eye. She is instructed to put ketorolac tromethamine ophthalmic solution (0.4%) and gatifloxacin ophthalmic solution (0.3%) in her eyes 4 times a day for 2 days following the procedure. She stays awake during the procedure; anesthetic eye drops were used, so she did not feel anything at all. After the surgery, she is sent home with a bandage and eye shield over her eye. She is told to wear it until she returns to the office in the morning for a postoperative check. Mary does not experience any pain or problems that afternoon or evening.

The following morning, she is examined by the ophthalmologist, who tells her that everything looks great. Mary is amazed at how bright and brilliant colors are; she notices immediately that the "foggy" sensation is gone. Mary is instructed to use the eye drops that were given to her preoperatively, along with prednisolone acetate (1.0%) eye drops 4 times a day for a week; the following week, she is told to use the ketorolac and prednisolone eye drops twice a day for another week. **[P]**

Episode 4

Mary is devastated about Mark's accident. She cannot believe Mark will never walk again. She refuses to believe that Mark was responsible and is sure somebody else must have caused the accident and left the scene. On the other hand, Mary tells Gil that the people who had the party should be sued for getting Mark drunk.

Episode 5

Mary goes with Gil and Helen every day to see Mark at the hospital. She takes prayer cards and brings him a statue of the Virgin Mary to help him heal. She prays the Rosary for him with the hopes of a full recovery. She asks Father John to include Mark in his prayer intentions at Sunday mass. **[P]**

Episode 6

No news this week.

Episode 7

Mary is very upset about Anthony's suicide attempt. She worries about Anthony and wishes there was something she could do for him. She blames Helen for upsetting him to the point of wanting to kill himself. She is very concerned for her son Gil, considering the toll all this stress must be having on him.

Episode 8

Gil takes Mary in for her second cataract surgery—this one on the left eye. She experiences the same exact course of events as with the previous surgery and has no problems with her postoperative recovery. Mary is so pleased with the outcome of her surgery that her only regret is that she did not do it sooner. **[P]**

Episode 9

Because Mary feels her vision is greatly improved, she decides to start driving again. She tells Kristina that she wants to have her car back. Kristina does not think this is fair and tells Mary that she needs the car for school and cheerleading. Mary is also somewhat angry to see that Kristina has not done a good job caring for the car. It is full of trash, and there are many stains on the seats and carpet. **[P]**

Mary learns that one of the church parishioners, Pamela Allen, died this week. She signs up to take food to the family. She bakes a chicken casserole and takes it to the Allen's home. She talks briefly with Clifford Allen. The conversation with Clifford causes Mary to reflect on her husband's death from cancer. Mary feels very sad for the rest of the week.

Episode 10

When Mark is discharged home, Mary decides to make him her new project. She wants to take care of him and is willing to do whatever it takes to help him recover. She tells Mark she will make him whatever he wants to eat, recognizing that he has been eating poorly since the accident. It makes Mary very sad to see Mark in the condition that he is in. She cannot bear the thought of her precious grandson confined to a bed and wheelchair.

Mary watches with great interest when the home health nurse comes to see Mark. She asks the nurse many questions so that she can take good care of him. Being Mark's primary caregiver makes Mary feel very useful, but the amount of care he requires is somewhat overwhelming.

Episode 11

In addition to having great concern for Mark, Mary is deeply concerned about Anthony. She does not directly criticize her son Gil, but she blames Helen for driving Anthony away and out of the house. She believes that he would be okay if everybody could just be more patient with him.

Episode 12

No news this week.

Episode 13

Every day, Mary talks to Mark about the people at church who are praying for him, and explains that the Virgin Mary and Jesus are there to help him get better. She does everything she can think of to get him to eat and is disappointed when he doesn't. She has been meticulous about taking care of his wounds and is pleased at the progress that she can see.

Episode 14

Mary is delighted when Mark transfers himself out of bed and into a wheelchair without assistance for the first time. She recognizes this as a major milestone and is hopeful it will encourage him enough to become more independent.

Episode 15

Mary makes a point of driving by the parks and through the downtown areas every day this week hoping to see Anthony. She knows he is out on the street somewhere and wants to find him so she can bring him home. Mary is embarrassed by the fact that her grandson is homeless and does not mention it to her friends at the Neighborhood Senior Center. It is, in her opinion, completely unacceptable for one of her family members to be homeless. **[P]**

ANTHONY MARTIN
Season 1

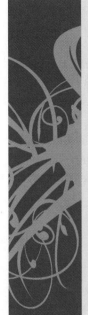

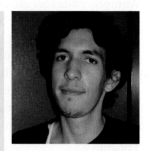

Biographical Information

Anthony is the 17-year-old son of Helen and Gil Martin. He lives with his parents and two siblings, Tracie and Kristina. He gets along with his family, but still feels somewhat isolated. His parents are not aware that he feels this way and perceive him to be a quiet, serious child. He tends not to interact with family members very much and prefers to isolate himself in his bedroom.

Anthony is in his senior year of high school. Although he is an excellent student (has a 3.9 GPA), he does not participate in any school-related activities, with the exception of science fairs, and has only a few friends. He rarely socializes, because he is more comfortable being alone. Many of the kids at the high school consider him to be weird, but he is never teased or bullied—for the most part, he just blends in with the other kids. His typical routine involves going to school, coming home, and then working part-time; three nights a week, Anthony bags groceries at the local grocery store. He gets along well with his coworkers; in fact, the cashiers (who tend to be middle-aged women) like it when he works, because they perceive him to be very polite.

Anthony is in excellent health and, with the exception of dental exams, has not needed health-related care since entering high school.

Episode 1
Anthony is somewhat annoyed with his sister, Kristina, because she was named captain of the cheerleading squad this week and has been talking about it nonstop. He doesn't understand how she can't see that cheerleading is a trivial and worthless activity. When Kristina asks Anthony if he would like to see some of her cheers, he tells her, "When I get bored enough, I'll let you know." He wonders why she wants to talk to him about cheerleading. **[P]**

Episode 2
No news this week.

Episode 3
There is a lot of commotion at the house this week— Anthony's grandmother has moved in, and the girls are fighting because they now have to share a bedroom to make room for their grandmother. Anthony is relieved that he won't have to share his space. He hears his mother yelling at his father about the situation. Anthony likes his grandmother and does not think her moving in is that big of a deal.

Episode 4
Anthony's bedroom is adjacent to the den. In the middle of the night, he wakes up to the sound of the television coming through his heating vent. He goes into the den and finds his grandmother watching a movie. Mary tells him that she has had trouble sleeping at night ever since his grandfather died. Anthony wonders why his grandmother sits in the room next to his during the middle of the night.

Episode 5
Anthony likes his grandmother's dinners—the food is quite good, although he wonders if she does something to his food. He does not understand why his mother has to argue so much with his grandmother. Although he finds his job boring, he is relieved to go to work so he doesn't have to listen to the arguing. On the nights that he is home, he mostly stays in his room and listens to classical music. **[P]**

Episode 6
No news this week.

Episode 7
Anthony starts exploring college opportunities. Because of the limited financial help his parents can offer, he knows he will need to get an academic scholarship or settle for attending the local college, which he would like to avoid. His mother has verbalized that she thinks he should stay at home and go to the local college like Tracie. Anthony submits applications to several colleges and scholarship programs. He knows he wants to get a degree in mathematics, but is not yet sure exactly what he wants to do.

Episode 8

Anthony enters an exhibit in the school science fair, hoping to win one of the top three exhibit awards and the opportunity to show in the state science fair. If he were to place at the state science fair, he would win an academic scholarship to one of the large universities in the state. He does not tell his parents about the science fair, because he would rather go alone. He is disappointed that he does not win one of the three best entries.

Episode 9

Anthony attends a college fair night at the high school. His sister, Kristina, wants to go along with him. He is mostly annoyed with this, but agrees to take her. Anthony visits most of the booths and picks up a few more applications. He does not see Kristina at all after they get there. When he is ready to go, he looks for her everywhere. After searching for 30 minutes, he just goes home. When he gets home at 9 p.m., Helen and Gil are angry with him for not bringing Kristina home.

Anthony goes to his room, angry that his parents blamed him for Kristina's actions. After Kristina comes home, Mary tells Anthony not to worry about it. She points out that his mother got hysterical over nothing. Anthony is indifferent to his grandmother's attempts to make him feel better. **[VC]**

Episode 10

No news this week.

Episode 11

Anthony receives acceptance letters to several colleges. Although he has been offered scholarships from the large university in the state, he knows they will not total enough for him to be able to attend. A small college about 45 minutes away from home has offered him a scholarship that would not only pay for his tuition and books, but would also pay for him to live on campus. As much as he wants to go to the big university, he decides this is his best option and commits to the small college.

Episode 12

A girl at school asks Anthony to the formal school dance. Anthony is not interested in girls and does not want to go to a high school dance. He tells the girl he has other plans and cannot go. **[P]**

Episode 13

No news this week.

Episode 14

Anthony takes his grandmother to the eye doctor this week so that his parents don't have to take off from work. While waiting for her, he reads a magazine article about the damaging effects of sun to the skin. Anthony begins to think about radiation from space and becomes very concerned. He does not share his concerns with anyone, but when he gets home, he places foil over the windows in his bedroom to block radiation from entering. **[P]**

Episode 15

No news this week.

ANTHONY MARTIN
Season 2

Biographical Information

Anthony is the 18-year-old son of Helen and Gil Martin. He recently graduated from high school and was accepted into a college nearby with an academic scholarship that pays for his tuition and dormitory. He just moved into the dormitory and has a roommate named Jeff. He gets along fine with Jeff, although they are really not friends. Anthony is taking a full, typical freshman curriculum and hopes to earn a degree in mathematics. Because he tends to be a loner, he does not feel particularly close to many individuals; he prefers not to interact much with the college kids.

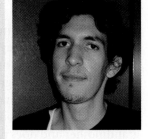

Episode 1

Anthony has recently moved from his home into the college dormitory. On Saturday, there is a large party on campus that is sponsored by the student life center and dormitory. His new roommate Jeff and several other guys invite Anthony to join them, but he declines, explaining that he has homework to do. Anthony leaves the dormitory and goes to the library so that nobody will bother him.

Episode 2

The biggest football game of the year is held at the college this week. Recognizing that he is not socializing much, Anthony's roommate Jeff suggests that he go to the game with the guys. Anthony tells Jeff that he doesn't like large crowds and prefers to stay at the dormitory. That afternoon, Anthony has the dormitory practically to himself. He likes the fact that it is quiet, but wonders what those people who are still in the building are doing.

Episode 3

No news this week.

Episode 4

Many of the students in Anthony's political science class have decided that Anthony is "peaced out." Several times he has verbalized his opinions about government conspiracy theories involving mind control, radiation poisoning, and aliens that listen in on conversations on earth. He also has begun to dress in mismatched or poorly kept clothes. Anthony also suspects that his roommate Jeff has been spying on him. In addition, he wonders if his parents have implanted a radio transmitter in his head and are reading his thoughts. **[VC]**

Episode 5

Anthony tells Jeff that he has been receiving secret messages from the television, newspaper, and radio about a government conspiracy occurring on campus. Jeff thinks his roommate is "wacko" and puts in a request for a change in roommates; however, he is told that the earliest such a request could be honored would be at the semester break. **[P]**

Episode 6

Anthony's roommate Jeff comes home from classes and finds Anthony hiding under a table. Jeff attempts to coax him out from under the table, but Anthony refuses to come out. Anthony talks in gibberish (using neologisms) and accuses Jeff of plotting to get him expelled from college. Jeff sees that Anthony has a knife, so he immediately leaves the room and summons the residence hall director, who promptly calls the campus police.

Anthony refuses to come out from under the table when the campus police arrive; he becomes agitated and shouts at them. He accuses them of reading his mind and plotting his death. The police observe that he is tightly holding a knife and that his jaw muscles are tightening. Police call for backup and do a "take down." Anthony is combative the entire time—flailing and kicking. He is placed in handcuffs and transported by police to the Neighborhood Hospital emergency department, where he is evaluated, sedated, and then admitted to the inpatient psychiatric unit with an initial diagnosis of acute psychosis. Anthony spends the rest of the week on the inpatient unit.

The following day, Louise, a clinical nurse specialist, obtains Anthony's permission to call his parents and speak to them about his condition. Louise informs Anthony that morning that his parents will be in to see him later. Anthony does not react at all to this news.

When his parents arrive to see him, Anthony is hiding under the sheets in his bed because he is afraid. He begins to cry when he sees his mother. Later in the morning, Anthony participates in a meeting involving Louise, Dr. Jacobe, a psychiatrist, and his parents. During the meeting, Anthony becomes very agitated, gets up, and leaves the room. **[VC]**

Episode 7

Anthony stays at the inpatient psychiatric unit for 5 days. He is started on olanzapine 5 mg once a day; by discharge, his dose is increased to 10 mg per day. He participates in patient education sessions for his medication and attends group psychotherapy. He is discharged home with an outpatient psychiatric appointment the following day. The insurance company authorizes Anthony to participate in intensive outpatient treatment.

Episode 8

Anthony continues to live at home and completes his outpatient therapy sessions. The sessions are effective, as evidenced by his increased attention to hygiene, ability to carry on conversations, reduced agitation, and lack of hallucinations. He is expected to follow up with Dr. Jacobe, the psychiatrist, on a monthly basis. He continues to take the olanzapine and is now up to a dose of 15 mg daily. Anthony is anxious to return to school, but is strongly advised to take a semester break before going back to school. He is somewhat overwhelmed by the constant commotion at home and spends most of his time in his room.

Episode 9

No news this week.

Episode 10

Despite the fact that he has missed nearly a month of school, Anthony wants to return to college. He speaks to an academic counselor, who informs him that the date to withdraw from classes has passed, but in some cases they can approve an administrative withdrawal. She encourages him to talk with his instructors. She also tells him that in some cases they can do an administrative withdraw. Anthony informs his parents that he is going to go back to school; he is confident that he can catch up and is sure his instructors will work with him. Gil, Helen, and Mary all attempt to dissuade him, as does the psychiatrist. Against everyone's advice, Anthony goes back to school.

Episode 11
Anthony does not like the way the medication makes him feel and decides to take a lower dose than was prescribed. Without telling anyone, Anthony cuts back on the amount of medication he is taking. **[P]**

Episode 12
This week, voices from the television begin to tell Anthony that medications are poisonous. Anthony stops taking his medication. **[P]**

Episode 13
While walking to a late morning class, two girls spot Anthony lying naked in the grass near the center of the main campus. They are frightened by this and call the campus police. When the campus police confront Anthony, he accuses them of trying to kill him, and he becomes combative. A large crowd gathers to watch the naked student battling with the officers. The police transport Anthony to the emergency department. Anthony is delusional and accuses the nurses of inserting electrodes into his head. He is restrained, placed in seclusion, and

sedated. He eventually calms down to the point at which he is compliant. Anthony is admitted to the inpatient psychiatric facility.

Later the same day, Anthony refuses to take the medication given to him by a nurse because he thinks it is poisonous. He is argumentative at first, but quickly becomes combative and hits the nurse in the head with his fist. Security is called to assist and, against his wishes, Anthony is restrained, sedated with haloperidol (Haldol) and lorazepam (Ativan), and placed in seclusion. Eventually, he calms down and is released from the restraints. However, even after calming down, he continues to refuse medications. It becomes necessary for Dr. Jacobe, the psychiatrist, to file for the appointment of a conservator to make decisions on Anthony's behalf regarding medications. **[P]**

Episode 14
Anthony spends most of the week in the inpatient psychiatric unit. He is started back on olanzapine 10 mg PO and gradually makes progress. He is discharged home with a referral for 10 days of intensive outpatient therapy.

Episode 15
Anthony continues to go to his daily intensive outpatient therapy sessions with Dr. Jacobe. He makes a great deal of progress. He is notified by the university that he has failed all of his classes and decides he will never try to go back. **[P]**

ANTHONY MARTIN
Season 3

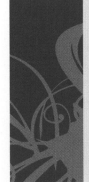

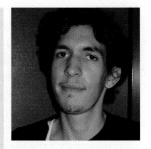

Biographical Information

Anthony is the 18-year-old son of Helen and Gil Martin. He had been enrolled at the local college, but had psychotic episodes and subsequently was diagnosed with schizophrenia. He was hospitalized and then completed intensive outpatient treatment. Currently, Anthony is taking olanzapine 10 mg PO to treat his condition and sees a psychiatrist once a week.

Because of his mental health disorder, Anthony fell behind and failed all of his classes. He has made a decision not to return to college. He has moved back home and now lives with his parents and three siblings (Mark, Tracie, and Kristina), his nephew, Tyler, and his grandmother, Mary.

Episode 1
Anthony returns to his previous job as a courtesy clerk (bagger) at the local grocery store—the same store where Gary Allen works. Although he interacts very little with his coworkers and customers, Anthony is able

to comply with the job description. Anthony's boss would like to see him be more cheerful and friendly toward the customers, but he is aware of Anthony's condition and has been told that a change in demeanor may come with time. **[P]**

Episode 2
No news this week.

Episode 3
Helen makes certain that Anthony takes his medication every day. Despite being on the medication, he becomes suspicious that his supervisor and Gary Allen are talking about him. He reports his suspicions to Dr. Jacobe during an outpatient visit. Dr. Jacobe compliments Anthony for admitting to this symptom and suggests that it may be necessary to change his medication. **[P]**

Episode 4
Anthony is aware that Mark was involved in an accident, but doesn't think about it too much. He spends time in his room wondering if Gary Allen is nearby spying on him.

Despite all of the commotion in the house, Helen makes sure that Anthony gets to his weekly appointment with Dr. Jacobe. He tells Dr. Jacobe that he knows Gary Allen is spying on him and reporting his activities to the boss. Dr. Jacobe changes Anthony's medication to quetiapine (Seroquel). Helen is instructed to give Anthony 25 mg twice a day the first day; 50 mg 3 times a day over the next 3 days, and then 100 mg 3 times a day thereafter. **[VC]**

Episode 5
This week, Dr. Jacobe asks Anthony about his symptoms. Anthony admits that he no longer believes his coworkers are talking about him, but he reports feeling very tired and sedated. The psychiatrist assures him that over time these symptoms will subside. **[P]**

Episode 6
Anthony continues to feel sedated. He is no longer hallucinating, but doesn't like the way the medication makes him feel. **[P]**

Episode 7
Anthony tells his father about the way the medication makes him feel and that he doesn't like taking it. Gil becomes uncharacteristically angry with Anthony and tells him that he *will* take his medications; if he doesn't, he will need to move out of the house. Anthony becomes very upset, runs to his room, and slams the door. He decides it's time to just end it all. He picks up a large bottle of Tylenol and takes all of the pills remaining in it, as well as all of his prescription medication. Later, his mother finds him on the floor in a stupor. An ambulance is called, and Anthony is taken to the emergency department and admitted to the ICU for treatment of a drug overdose. **[VC]**

Episode 8
Anthony returns to inpatient psychiatric treatment and remains in the hospital for 1 week. He has insurance coverage for inpatient treatment, but no longer qualifies for outpatient treatment on his insurance plan. The social worker tries to find an outpatient program for Anthony and helps him apply for Medicaid. Anthony remains in the hospital for 8 days. Now his diagnosis is major depression with psychotic features. He is placed on citalopram (Celexa) 20 mg daily. His antipsychotic medication is changed to risperidone (Risperdal) 1 mg twice a day. The Risperdal is very expensive.

Episode 9
Anthony is discharged home this week and referred to the County Department of Mental Health for follow-up. He can't afford the intensive outpatient treatment anymore, so he is assigned to the mental health clinic and receives an appointment for the following week. During the week, Helen helps Anthony take his medication. He remains calm. **[P]**

Episode 10
Helen and Gil take Anthony to his first appointment at the mental health clinic this week. Anthony agrees to take his medication consistently from now on.

Episode 11
Anthony begins to argue with his mother when she confronts him about not taking his medication. Helen expresses intense frustration and is highly anxious about this. Gil is well aware of the effect this is having on Helen and suggests to Anthony that he move out of the house. Anthony becomes upset, gets up, and storms out of the house. He goes to a friend's apartment and asks if he can stay there for a while. His friend agrees to let him stay there, but has no idea about the problems Anthony has been having. Anthony stops taking his medication.

Episode 12
Anthony is still staying at his friend's house. He has not been going to work, and has not been taking his medication. Not wanting to talk to his parents, he does not return any of their calls.

Episode 13
Anthony begins to exhibit bizarre behavior again. His friend wonders what is going on with him and wonders why he never leaves the apartment.

Episode 14
No news this week.

Episode 15
Anthony has a major argument with his friend, who tells him to move out. Having nowhere to go, Anthony sleeps in a local park. He is still not taking any medication and is now out on the street. **[P]**

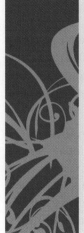

KRISTINA MARTIN
Season 1

Biographical Information

Kristina is the 16-year-old daughter of Helen and Gil Martin. She lives with her parents and two siblings, Tracie and Anthony. She gets along with her siblings, but considers her sister Tracie to be way too serious and her brother Anthony to be a bit strange. Kristina is a fairly typical sophomore who attends the local high school. She is on the junior varsity cheerleading squad at school and has a very busy schedule. Although she has always been close to her family, she feels closest to her circle of friends at school; she is considered popular among the kids at school. Kristina is an average student who usually puts friends and school activities well ahead of school-related work. She has recently completed her driver education class and has a provisional driver's license. She is in excellent health and has not needed health-related care outside of annual physicals to participate on the cheerleading squad.

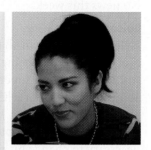

Episode 1

Kristina is named captain of the cheerleading squad this week. She is thrilled, because she knows that as captain she will automatically make the varsity squad next year. She and her friends on the squad spend time after school making posters for pep rally week.

Episode 2

No news this week.

Episode 3

Kristina is furious when she is told to give up her bedroom to make space for her grandmother. She does not think it is fair and asks why her grandmother can't just sleep on the pull-out bed in the den. Kristina moves all of her things into Tracie's room and finds there is not enough space for her stuff. She removes everything on half of the bedroom walls and hangs up her posters instead. She and Tracie have a fight about what should be hung up in the room. **[P]**

Episode 4

No news this week.

Episode 5

Kristina has started taking driver education classes. She is very excited about getting her license so she can drive herself to school and all of her other activities. She asks her parents about getting a car for her and is told she will have to earn the money to buy a car; until then, she will be allowed to borrow one of the family cars when they are not in use. She is not sure how she will ever earn enough money for a car, because she is too busy with cheerleading and other school activities. **[P]**

Episode 6

Kristina tells her mother that she is going to her friend Roslyn's house for a sleep-over with the cheerleading squad. The girls go to the mall and hang out until closing time, and then hang out at the pizza place near the high school until closing time. Then they hang out in the parking lot, talking to some of the guys from high school until 2 a.m., when they are told to go home by the police. Kristina has a blast and thinks it's dumb that cops had to run them off. After all, they weren't doing anything wrong.

Episode 7

No news this week.

Episode 8

Kristina completes her driver education classes. She has a fight with her parents, because she wants to start driving herself to school so she doesn't have to get rides for cheerleading and other activities. In her opinion, she should be given a car to drive. Helen tells her that she has to earn money for her own car—just like Tracie and Anthony have done.

Kristina asks her grandmother if she can use her car, since she does not drive it very much anyway. Her grandmother agrees to this, if it is okay with her father. Gil decides it would be okay and gives her his permission—as long as she takes good care of the car. **[VC]**

Episode 9

Kristina goes with Anthony to the high school career night and college fair. She goes with the intention of meeting up with her friends and hanging out with them. They decide the college fair is boring and leave the school to go to a fast-food restaurant. When Kristina returns to the school, she realizes Anthony has already left, and she has to get a ride home with her friends. She does not get home until 10 p.m. and is surprised to learn that her mother has become so frantic. She tells her friend on the phone later that night, "My mother needs to take a chill pill."

Episode 10
No news this week.

Episode 11
Kristina is asked to the school dance by Jared Williams, a senior and the quarterback of the football team. Kristina knows this is probably going to be the most important night of her life, and she needs to look fabulous. Both her mother and grandmother give her money to go shopping. She spends hours at the mall this week with her friends looking for the perfect dress. Kristina finds a beautiful, low-cut, strapless dress similar to one she saw in a celebrity magazine. She buys the dress a bit small and vows to diet so that she can fit into it. **[P]**

Episode 12
Kristina has practically starved herself during the past couple of weeks so she can fit into the dress she bought for the high school dance. She spends all afternoon getting ready with her girlfriends; they do each other's hair, make-up, and nails. She is happy that she is able to fit into the dress, and her friends keep remarking on how skinny and beautiful she looks. Kristina has a curfew of 1 a.m., but doesn't come home until after 2 a.m. She is grounded for the following week; specifically, she is told not to go anywhere except school and home for 1 week, and she is not allowed to drive. Despite being grounded and not driving for a week, Kristina decides it was well worth it. **[P]**

Episode 13
Kristina takes a pair of Tracie's earrings from her dresser because she thinks they will look good with her outfit. She doesn't bother to ask Tracie, because she figures Tracie will just say no. Kristina predicted correctly that Tracie would be angry with her. She tells Tracie that she is just selfish for not sharing.

Episode 14
No news this week.

Episode 15
This week at school, Kristina runs into another car in the parking lot. Although she does not damage the other car, Kristina ends up with a dent in her grandmother's car. She tells her parents she is not sure what happened to the car, but somebody must have hit it in the parking lot. **[P]**

KRISTINA MARTIN
Season 2

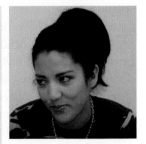

Biographical Information
Kristina is the 16-year-old daughter of Helen and Gil Martin. She lives with her parents, grandmother, sister Tracie, step-brother Mark, and his son Tyler. Her brother, Anthony, recently moved out of the house to attend college. She gets along with her siblings, but considers her sister Tracie to be way too serious and her brother Anthony to be a bit strange. Kristina is a fairly typical sophomore who attends the local high school. She is on the junior varsity cheerleading squad at school and has a very busy schedule. Although she has always been close to her family, she feels closest to her circle of friends at school; she is considered popular among the kids at school. Kristina is an average student who usually puts friends and school activities well ahead of school-related work. She has recently completed her driver education class and has a provisional driver's license. She is in excellent health and has not needed health-related care outside of annual physicals to participate on the cheerleading squad.

Episode 1

Kristina was looking forward to moving into Anthony's room when he moved to college. She becomes angry when she learns that Mark and Tyler are moving into the room instead. Kristina has always gotten along with Mark, although he has never lived with them before. Kristina mainly wishes she could have her own room again.

Kristina gets a call from Jared Williams (the guy she went to the school dance with several months ago), inviting her to go with him to an on-campus party at the college. Jared recently graduated from high school and is now playing on the football team at the local college. In fact, he lives in the same dormitory as Kristina's brother, Anthony. Kristina is excited about going on a date with Jared and hanging out with college kids. She ends up getting drunk that evening. Jared takes her back to his dormitory room and has unprotected sex with her before dropping her off at her home at 2 a.m. Kristina is grounded for one week for being out past her 12:30 a.m. curfew.

Episode 2

Kristina's parents are not happy that she is seeing Jared, suggesting that she date the guys at high school instead. Since she has had sex with Jared, there is no way she is going to stop seeing him now—besides, she likes the idea of going out with an older guy, because it makes her feel older.

Mary asks Kristina to take her to the store to buy toys for Tyler. On the way over to the store, she talks to Kristina about the need to be careful when dating college-aged boys. Kristina thinks her parents and grandmother are just old-fashioned.

Episode 3

Kristina has not been doing well in school lately, because she has been busy socializing instead. She receives a letter from the academic advising office informing her she is close to being placed on probation and will not be allowed to be on the cheerleading squad if her grades don't improve. Kristina is disappointed that Jared does not call her to hang out with him after the college football game this week. She ends up spending time hanging out with her friends instead.

Episode 4

Kristina spends two evenings this week alone with Jared in his dormitory room. She is glad she has not seen her brother, because she doesn't want him to tell her parents that she is on campus with Jared and alone in his dorm room. She brags to her friends that she and Jared are an

item. One of Kristina's friends tells her that Jared is also going out with some girls at the college. Kristina dismisses this, believing that her friend is just jealous that she is dating an older guy. She decides to lose 5 pounds, because she thinks her butt looks big in the mirror.

Kristina is relieved that her mother's surgery went well. She goes to the hospital with Tracie, Mark, Helen, and her Dad the evening following her mother's surgery. She watches her mother get sick and thinks it is gross. She hopes to never have surgery.

Episode 5

No news this week.

Episode 6

Kristina is aware that her brother is in a psychiatric hospital and recognizes how upset her mother and father are over the situation. Kristina doesn't really understand very much about Anthony's problems, but is concerned for him. She does not tell any of her friends about Anthony, because she finds the whole thing embarrassing. Kristina has lost the 5 pounds she set out to lose and is very happy with the way she looks. She likes the compliments from the girls at school about how skinny she is. **[P]**

Episode 7

Kristina finds her home increasingly chaotic with Anthony moving back home and Mark and Tyler living in the family room. She continues to see Jared and has been hitting the college party scene frequently. Her parents are so distracted with Anthony that they don't pay attention to the fact that she is with Jared as often as she is. She has had sex with Jared on several occasions now and is worried about getting pregnant. She asked Jared about using condoms, but he told her he doesn't like the way they feel. Kristina goes to the Neighborhood Community Health Department to get birth control information after learning from her friends that she can get birth control pills there. Carol Ramsey, the nurse at the clinic, talks with her about protecting herself from sexually transmitted infections and pregnancy. Kristina is really only interested in getting birth control pills. **[P]**

Episode 8

Kristina is taking birth control pills, but has heard from her friends that birth control pills cause weight gain. She is worried about getting fat while taking them, so she decides she needs to lose more weight to prevent that from happening.

Episode 9

Jared does not call at all this week and doesn't answer his cell phone or respond to her text messages. She drops by to see him, but he is not in his dorm room. She wonders what the deal is, but turns her attention to her cheerleading and high school friends.

Episode 10
No news this week.

Episode 11
Kristina is glad that Anthony has gone back to school, because Mark and Tyler have moved back into his bedroom. She has not heard from Jared for a while and has been asked out by Ray, one of the guys on the basketball team at the high school. Ray wants to get Kristina drunk, because he has heard she "puts out." They go to a party, and Kristina gets drunk and has unprotected sex with Ray.

Episode 12
Several of the kids at school talk about Kristina after Ray tells many of the guys about the party. Kristina is angry about the rumors and decides that, if she weren't so fat, people wouldn't talk about her. She vows to lose another 5 pounds.

Episode 13
Kristina is embarrassed by the fact that her brother was seen running around naked at the college and got arrested. The kids at the high school hear about the incident and are talking about it. Kristina feels angry with her brother for ruining her reputation. She gets a call from Jared, who tells her that everybody at the dorm thinks Anthony is "peaced out." She is thrilled when he asks her to come by and see him.

Episode 14
Kristina feels sorry for Anthony when he comes back home. She is amazed at how different he looks compared with last year, when he was in high school. Kristina also feels sorry for her mother; she can see that her Mom is constantly nervous and upset. Kristina hates not having any control over all the craziness in her home and wishes there was something she could do to make it stop.

Episode 15
No news this week.

KRISTINA MARTIN
Season 3

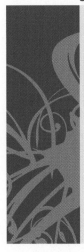

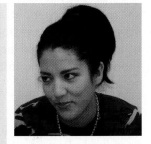

Biographical Information
Kristina is the 17-year-old daughter of Helen and Gil Martin. She lives with her parents and grandmother, her three siblings, Tracie, Anthony, and Mark, and her nephew Tyler. She gets along with her siblings, but she considers her sister Tracie way too serious and is embarrassed by her brother Anthony for being crazy. Kristina is a fairly typical sophomore who attends the local high school. She is on the junior varsity cheerleading squad at school and has a very busy schedule. Although she has always been close to her family, she feels closest to her circle of friends at school; she is considered popular among the kids at school. Kristina is an average student who usually puts friends and school activities well ahead of school-related work. Kristina has recently become sexually active. She is in excellent health and has not had health-related care outside of annual physicals to participate on the cheerleading squad.

Episode 1
Kristina sees Jared every couple of weeks; she would like to see him more, but he tells her he is pretty busy. She has decided that she is definitely going to move into a dorm when she goes to college, because it is so cool.

Episode 2
No news this week.

Episode 3
Kristina has managed to get her grades back up enough so that she is no longer at risk for probation from cheerleading.

She is glad about this because, in her mind, cheerleading is the most important thing she does. **[P]**

Episode 4
Kristina is freaked out when she learns about Mark's accident. She is so worried for him. She goes with her parents and grandmother to see him at the hospital every day.

Episode 5
Kristina sees Jared this week. He tells her that he got Chlamydia from her and that she needs to be tested.

Kristina has heard of it, but is not too sure she knows what it is. She goes back to the community health department and tests positive. She learns from Carol Ramsey, the nurse midwife, that Chlamydia is a sexually transmitted infection. She is given azithromycin (Zithromax) and told to abstain from sex for one week. The nurse talks with Kristina about safe sex practices and encourages her to inform all of her sex partners. Kristina asks the nurse if this means that Jared has been cheating on her. **[VC]**

Episode 6

Kristina finds out that Jared has been dating three other girls at the college. She is devastated to learn this and figures that this is how she got infected with Chlamydia. She is angry and breaks up with him, but feels torn. In some ways, she does not want to see him anymore, but at the same time, she wants to be his girlfriend. She is embarrassed to talk to anybody about what has happened and is afraid her parents will find out.

Episode 7

Kristina is feeling very stressed out about what is happening with her family. When Anthony tries to kill himself, she can't understand it, and she doesn't know how to respond. In many ways, she feels almost invisible. She loses more weight to make herself feel attractive. In the past 6 months, Kristina has lost 20 pounds. She is 5'2" and now weighs 90 pounds.

Episode 8

In Kristina's opinion, her entire world is terrible. Her boyfriend cheats on her and gave her Chlamydia, her mother suffers from anxiety, one brother is paralyzed, and her other brother is crazy. Kristina has become exceedingly thin, to the point at which her friends constantly talk to her about her weight. Her parents have not commented on her weight, and she wonders if they even notice. When her sister Tracie asks her how she is doing and what is wrong, the tears flow, and Kristina shares with her all that is troubling her. She takes comfort in her older sister's concerns and is relieved to have somebody to talk with. Although Tracie encourages her to talk with their mother about these issues, Kristina

elects not to do so, because she perceives that her mother is nearly at a breaking point. She does not want to talk with her father, because she does not want to disappoint him. **[VC]**

Episode 9

No news this week.

Episode 10

Mark comes home from the hospital this week. Kristina no longer looks at his presence in her home as an inconvenience; rather, she is happy to have him there. She helps her mother and grandmother take care of him. Kristina is sad to see Tracie leave this week to move in with John. The pleasure of having a bedroom to herself is minimized by the loss she feels. Kristina makes an effort to put a little weight back on.

Episode 11

Anthony leaves the house after a fight with her parents. Kristina is upset and calls Tracie to tell her what happened. Tracie invites Kristina to spend the night at her apartment with John and Tyler; Kristina chooses to do this over going out with her friends. Tracie comments to Kristina that she is looking better. **[P]**

Episode 12

No news this week.

Episode 13

Jared sends Kristina a text message, asking her to come see him and telling her that he wants to get back together with her. When Kristina reads the message, she calls her sister Tracie and asks her what to do. **[P]**

Episode 14

No news this week.

Episode 15

The kids at school are talking about Anthony. Kristina is angry with many of them, including some of her "friends" on the cheerleading squad. Having them ask her questions about what has happened to him makes her feel embarrassed, and she doesn't really want to talk about it. For the first time in her entire life, she finds herself wishing she weren't the center of attention among her peers.

TRACIE AMES
Season 1

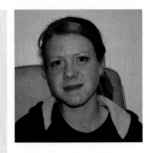

Biographical Information

Tracie Ames is a 20-year-old college student. She is Helen's Martin's daughter and Gil's stepdaughter. Tracie was 3 years old when her mother married Gil, so he essentially has raised her as his own daughter. Although Tracie has had a very positive ongoing relationship with her biological father Rick, she has always lived with her mother and is very close to Helen.

Tracie attends the local college and is working on a degree in English. She hopes to be either a high school or college English teacher when she completes her degree, with a long-range goal of being a writer. She is a very serious young woman and very goal driven; she has been on the Dean's list every semester since beginning school. Tracie has earned scholarships, which help her with tuition, and she lives at home to save money. She would love to live on campus or in an apartment, but to do so would require that she get a full-time job, and she is concerned that this would affect her success in school. Tracie has a part-time student employment position as a writer/editor. She has been in a monogamous relationship with her boyfriend John for one year. He attends the same college and lives in an apartment near campus.

Tracie is in excellent health; she has no medical conditions requiring ongoing care. She watches her weight, exercises regularly, and does not smoke or use illicit drugs or alcohol. She goes for annual examinations each year; the only prescription medication she takes is an oral contraceptive. She does not use any over-the-counter medications on a regular basis.

Episode 1

Tracie attends a political rally on the college campus with her boyfriend John. She has never aligned herself specifically with one political party, but is fascinated with the process and the behavior of individuals at such rallies. Specifically, she thinks many of the individuals are foolish in their behavior and recognizes the many double standards that are presented.

Episode 2

No news this week.

Episode 3

Tracie learns that her grandmother is moving into their home. To make room for her, she is told she will need to share her bedroom with Kristina. Tracie feels it was unfair for Gil to do this without asking her mother, and she is not happy with the situation. However, she recognizes that her grandmother may need some assistance.

Tracie comes home from class and finds that everything she hung up on two walls of her bedroom has been removed by Kristina and replaced with posters of rock groups and celebrities. To make matters worse, Kristina has placed her possessions all over the room and is burning incense. Tracie suggests to Kristina that they need to talk about what it means to share a room; Kristina tells Tracie she is always trying to boss her around.

Episode 4

No news this week.

Episode 5

Tracie is trying to study for a test that will be given the following morning. Her sister is playing rock music in the bedroom and talking on the phone with friends, so she moves to the den. She then hears her mother arguing with her grandmother Mary about the way dinner was prepared. She later hears her mother arguing with Gil about Mary intentionally ignoring her diet. All of the commotion is distracting, so Tracie goes to John's apartment to study for the evening. **[P]**

Episode 6

Tracie continues to be annoyed with her sister Kristina. She finds her to be very immature and self-centered; she seems to think the world revolves around her cheerleading, friends, and driving. She is not sure if Kristina is getting worse, or if these behaviors are just more noticeable now that they are sharing a bedroom. Tracie finds it is very difficult to study and do her part-time editing job at home, so she spends an increasing amount of her time at John's apartment. Mary tells Tracie she should spend more time at home. Helen agrees, but won't say so, as she does not want to support Mary. Tracie has dinner with her father Rick, and tells him about all of the changes that have been occurring at her home. Rick suggests she move out, but does not offer to help her financially with alternative living arrangements.

Episode 7
No news this week.

Episode 8
Tracie overhears her parents arguing about Kristina driving Mary's car and is angry with Gil for allowing her sister to do so. She does not think it's fair and knows that Kristina will not take good care of the car. She also is beginning to see that Mary is manipulative. Tracie does not appreciate the things Mary says and the way she treats her mother. **[P]**

Episode 9
Tracie spends the better part of the week on campus with John working on a school project. She is glad to be out of the house and not listening to the arguments. **[P]**

Episode 10
Tracie and John go out of town with her father Rick for a long weekend at the beach. She has only been to the ocean a few times in her life and is thrilled to go.

Episode 11
No news this week.

Episode 12
Tracie and her mother spend an afternoon together shopping and having lunch. It has been a long time since the two of them shared some time like this. Tracie tells her Mom she misses spending time like that with her. Tracie learns from her mother that she is going through menopause and that she has not been feeling herself.

Episode 13
Tracie sees Kristina wearing her earrings and asks her where she got them. Kristina tells Tracie that she borrowed them and forgot to ask—but didn't think Tracie would mind. Tracie tells Kristina she is not to touch any of her stuff; and Kristina tells Tracie that she is selfish for not sharing. **[P]**

Episode 14
No news this week.

Episode 15
No news this week.

TRACIE AMES
Season 2

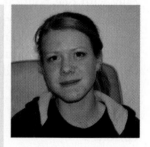

Biographical Information

Tracie Ames is a 20-year-old college student. She is Helen's Martin's daughter and Gil's stepdaughter. Tracie was 3 years old when her mother married Gil, so he essentially has raised her as his own daughter. Although Tracie has had a very positive ongoing relationship with her biological father Rick, she has always lived with her mother and is very close to Helen.

Tracie attends the local college and is working on a degree in English. She would love to live on campus or in an apartment to get out of her very crowded house, but to do so would require that she get a full-time job, and she is concerned that this would affect her success in school. Tracie has a part-time student employment position as a writer/editor. She has been in a monogamous relationship with her boyfriend John for 18 months. He attends the same college and lives in an apartment near campus.

Tracie is in excellent health; she has no medical conditions requiring ongoing care. She watches her weight, exercises regularly, and does not smoke or use illicit drugs or alcohol. She goes for annual examinations each year; the only prescription medication she takes is an oral contraceptive. She does not use any over-the-counter medications on a regular basis.

Episode 1

Gil's 27-year-old son Mark moves into the house with his 2-year-old son Tyler. Tracie is not sure that she agrees with Gil for letting Mark move in with them, but she also recognizes that he has fallen on some tough times. Mainly, she feels sorry for Tyler and is glad that the family might be able to make a difference in her nephew's life.

Episode 2

Tyler quickly becomes attached to Tracie, and she does not mind one bit. She is glad to see him take an interest in books and puzzles, and is happy to read to him in the evenings. **[P]**

Episode 3

Tracie continues going to school in the daytime and spends time with Tyler in the evening. She notices that Tyler's teeth look bad and wonders why Mark hasn't done anything about them. **[P]**

Episode 4

Tracie is glad her mother's surgery went well. She is hopeful that her mother's ongoing abdominal pains will be a thing of the past.

Episode 5

No news this week.

Episode 6

Anthony is hospitalized this week because of his strange behavior, and Tracie is very concerned about him. She is also very concerned about her mother. She recognizes that her mother has been increasingly anxious about everything happening in the family, but this situation with Anthony has been especially difficult for her.

Episode 7

Tracie wonders just how much more chaotic her family could possibly get. With Anthony back home, as well as her grandmother, Mark, and Tyler, the house is quite full. She finds herself spending an increasing amount of time with her boyfriend John. **[P]**

Episode 8

Tracie sees a notice in the paper about a dental screening. She mentions this to Mark and is not surprised when Mark doesn't seem to think taking Tyler to the screening is a priority. Tracie gets Mark's permission to take Tyler herself.

At the screening, Tracie is told that Tyler has "bad teeth" and must be seen by a dentist. Tracie explains that her brother cannot afford a dentist. She is given a referral to the community health services and is told that dental care is offered there on a sliding-scale payment plan.

When asked, Tracie explained that Tyler was given a bottle at night and a sippy cup during the day. Tracie is told that these habits are a huge contributing factor to his poor dental condition and that the family needs to put water in the bottle at night.

Episode 9

Tracie talks with her other family members about the need to stop giving Tyler milk or juice in his bottle at night. They make attempts to do this, but give in when he screams.

Episode 10

Tracie is glad that Mark takes Tyler to the dentist. She suspects Tyler might need to have teeth pulled and can't bear the thought that he might blame her. She is anxious when he comes home and can tell he has been through an ordeal.

Tracie is glad that Anthony made it back to school. She is hopeful that he can put the bad experience behind him and succeed. She is concerned about her mother's obvious problems coping with the situation and wishes she could relax a bit.

Episode 11

Tracie knows Kristina has been out late and has been drinking, because she can smell it on her breath when she comes in at night. She talks to Kristina and suggests she "cool it"; Kristina tells Tracie to mind her own business. **[VC]**

Episode 12

Tracie learns that Mark is going to stay a little longer at the house to save up for his own home. She is almost relieved that he is not yet moving, because Tracie loves Tyler and hates the thought of him moving away from her.

Episode 13

Anthony is readmitted to the hospital this week, because he stopped taking his medication, and his delusions returned. Tracie feels badly for Anthony, but also angry with him for not taking his medication. She does not understand why he would just quit taking it; this relapse is obviously his fault. She is very concerned about her mother's reaction.

Episode 14

Tracie is glad to see her brother back at home, but feels the commotion of the household is back up a notch. No wonder her mother is so anxious! Tracie tells Kristina that she looks like she is losing weight. Kristina denies the weight loss and tells Tracie she is obviously just jealous. **[VC]**

Episode 15

No news this week.

TRACIE AMES
Season 3

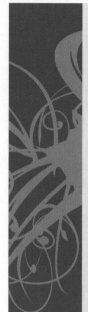

Biographical Information

Tracie Ames is a 21-year-old college student. She is Helen's Martin's daughter and Gil's stepdaughter. Tracie was 3 years old when her mother married Gil, so he essentially has raised her as his own daughter. Although Tracie has had a very positive ongoing relationship with her biological father Rick, she has always lived with her mother and is very close to Helen.

Tracie attends the local college and is working on a degree in English. She would love to live on campus or in an apartment to get out of her very crowded and chaotic house, but to do so would require that she get a full-time job, and she is concerned that this would affect her success in school; she is also concerned how her mother would react. Tracie has been in a monogamous relationship with her boyfriend John for two years. He attends the same college and lives in an apartment near campus.

Tracie is in excellent health; she has no medical conditions requiring ongoing care. She watches her weight, exercises regularly, and does not smoke or use illicit drugs or alcohol. She goes for annual examinations each year; the only prescription medication she takes is an oral contraceptive. She does not use any over-the-counter medications on a regular basis.

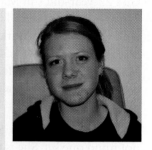

Episode 1

No news this week.

Episode 2

Tracie and John discuss living together. She has decided this is perhaps her best option, but has been reluctant to do so because of her attachment to Tyler. Tracie tells her mother that she is thinking of moving in with John, because the house is so crowded. Helen tells Tracie that Mark is planning to buy a house with his girlfriend Shelly, so there will be more room in the house again soon. Tracie senses that her mother does not want her to move. **[P]**

Episode 3

Tracie is excited for Mark and Shelly to buy a house together, but she is not excited for Tyler to go with them, because she is sure that Shelly does not love Tyler the way she does. Tracie wonders if Mark would agree to let Tyler live with them.

Episode 4

Tracie is in disbelief when she learns that Mark had a serious automobile accident and has permanent injuries. She is further devastated over the impact it has on the entire family. She wonders just how much more chaos her family can possibly take. Tracie and Mary team up to keep the house organized and functional, while Helen and Gil try to manage the problems with Anthony and Mark.

Episode 5

No news this week.

Episode 6

Tracie takes Tyler to see Mark at the rehabilitation hospital. Mark begins to cry when he sees Tyler and tells Tracie that he is depending on her, since there is no way he can ever be a good Dad for his son. Tracie cries along with him and vows to make sure Tyler is always cared for.

Episode 7

Anthony attempts to commit suicide this week. Tracie is very worried about her mother and Gil. She finds them blaming themselves and each other.

Episode 8

It is obvious to Tracie that her younger sister Kristina has been losing weight. She can also tell when Kristina comes in late at night smelling of alcohol that she has been partying. It is also obvious to her that Helen and Gil seem to only be going through the motions, as they deal with so many issues within the family. Although they have never been particularly close, Tracie talks to Kristina about her concerns, not from the perspective of a bossy older sister, but rather out of concern for her health and well-being. To Tracie's surprise, Kristina opens up and shares with her all the problems she has been experiencing, including being sexually active with Jared and getting Chlamydia.

Tracie listens to her sister as she cries about all that has been troubling her. Tracie encourages Kristina to talk with their mother and to stop losing weight.

Tracie talks with her boyfriend John about living together and wants to know if he would agree to letting Tyler live with them as well. Tracie is very happy that John agrees to the idea; in fact, John says he looks forward to spending time with them. **[P]**

Episode 9

Tracie visits Mark at the rehabilitation hospital this week. She shares with Mark her interest in moving out of the house and in with John, and requests his permission to take Tyler with her, promising to bring him over to the house regularly to visit. Mark tearfully agrees to this. He also tells Tracie that Tyler is due for more shots at the community health clinic. Tracie agrees to take him for his shots.

Kristina continues to confide in Tracie and share with her the things that are bothering her. Tracie is happy to finally feel close to her sister, who has always been very self-centered. She realizes that she has the potential to have a positive influence on Kristina and hopes that moving out of the house will not be a deterrent to this. **[P]**

Episode 10

Tracie tells her mother and Gil that she and Tyler are moving to John's house to provide more room for Mark when he comes back home. She is not surprised by her Mom's protests, but did not expect Helen to break down and cry. Gil tells Tracie she should do what she thinks is best; as long as Mark agreed to Tyler living with her, he would support her decision. Tracie feels sorry for her mother, but at the same time recognizes the need to get herself and Tyler away from the constant chaos. **[P]**

Episode 11

Tracie gets a call from Kristina and learns that Anthony has had another fight with Gil and her mother, and he has left the house. She knows her mother is devastated, and Tracie feels a bit guilty about leaving when she did. At the same time, she is enjoying her time with John and thinks that Tyler is adjusting well to his new living arrangement. Tracie invites Kristina to spend the night if she wants to get away from the house.

Episode 12

No news this week.

Episode 13

Tracie takes Tyler to see his father every evening. She can see how depressed Mark is and feels badly for him. She is glad Mark is so positive about Tyler living with her, because she knows deep down that it's the best thing for him.

Episode 14

No news this week.

Episode 15

Tracie finds that going to school, taking care of Tyler, and working is becoming very taxing. Living in an apartment is more expensive than what she imagined. She is glad she is able to rely on her sister Kristina and John to help her with Tyler. She goes to the financial aid and scholarship office at the college to see about possible financial assistance to help her get through this time.

MARK MARTIN
Season 2

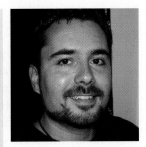

Biographical Information

Mark Martin is Gil's 27-year-old son. Mark is a single parent to his 2-year-old son Tyler. Mark has held a variety of odd jobs while attempting to support himself and Tyler, but has fallen deeply into debt. He has reached the credit limit on all of his credit cards and is struggling to make his car payment, apartment rent, and child care payments. At Gil's suggestion, Mark has moved into his father's house temporarily until he gets caught up on bills. Currently, Mark is working as a security officer for a private security company; he hopes to start taking classes at the local college and work toward a degree, but is not sure what he wants to do with his life. Mark gets along very well with Gil, Anthony, and Kristina, but has never felt close to Helen or Tracie. His father married Helen when he was 10 years old and, even at that time, Mark could tell Helen resented him. Although Mark always lived with his mother, he spent a lot of time with his father's family.

Episode 1

Mark and Tyler settle into Gil and Helen's home. Mark realizes that the house is pretty full and promises Helen he will only stay as long as he has to. He apologizes to Kristina for ruining her plans to move into Anthony's room and thanks her for being so flexible. During the evening, Mark goes to work and leaves Tyler at the house, assuming that nobody will mind taking care of him. He appreciates the fact that his grandmother is also willing to help, but is not sure she can see well enough to care for Tyler adequately.

Episode 2

Mark makes a change to the evening shift so that he can take care of Tyler during the daytime, and his family members can take care of him in the evening while he works. Mark quickly realizes that, between the savings in rent and child care, he can pay off most of his bills within 6 months. This motivates Mark to get along with his family members as well as he can.

Episode 3

Mary mentions to Mark that Tyler's teeth seem to be in bad shape. Mark does not pay much attention to his grandmother; he knows she can't see very well and that she has a tendency to meddle in other people's business. He tells Mary that he already knows about the teeth and it's under control. In truth, Mark has never paid any attention to Tyler's teeth. When Gil asks Mark about Tyler's teeth, Mark tells his Dad that he is aware of the problem, but has been short on cash and not able to afford to take him to the dentist. He also tells Gil that he is not too worried about it, because they are just his baby teeth and they'll fall out eventually anyway.

Episode 4

No news this week.

Episode 5

Mark finds that working the evening shift is great. He can work and then go out and party with friends after work. He often does not come home until 2 or 3 a.m. In the mornings, he gets up to take care of Tyler, but ends up taking a nap most mornings or early afternoons while other family members watch him.

Episode 6

Mark feels badly for his stepbrother, Anthony. He always considered him to be weird, but was really surprised that he flipped out and was admitted to a psychiatric hospital. Mark meets a woman this week at work and parties with her each evening after they get off work. **[P]**

Episode 7

When Mark is told by Gil that Anthony is moving back home, Mark gladly moves out of Anthony's room and takes over the family room. Mark finds that he likes this better anyway, because the family room has more space for him and Tyler. Mark has been partying so much this week that he has stopped getting up in the mornings to care for Tyler. He is perfectly happy to sleep until noon nearly every day, knowing that his grandmother is caring for Tyler.

Episode 8

Tracie tells Mark about a free dental screening and suggests that he take Tyler to it. Mark tells her he has plans with his girlfriend on that day, but gives her permission to take him. Later that day, Tracie tells Mark that Tyler's teeth are in bad shape and he needs to have dental care immediately. Tracie has already made the appointment for Tyler and tells Mark he needs to take him to the appointment. Mark agrees to take care of it.

Gil talks to Mark about coming in so late each night and not taking more responsibility for Tyler. Mark comes home immediately after work for a couple of nights, but is back to his party scene with his girlfriend each night shortly thereafter. On some nights, he spends most of the night with his new girlfriend Shelly, comes in about 6 a.m., and then crashes on the couch in the family room.

Episode 9

No news this week.

Episode 10

Mark is glad to move back into Anthony's bedroom this week. Although he liked the extra room he had in the family room, he hated not having any privacy. Tracie reminds Mark to take Tyler to the community health center for the dental clinic. Mark is not thrilled about taking Tyler because of the cost, but is relieved when he learns the clinic provides services on a sliding-scale payment plan and is willing to help him out with the costs. While taking a history, the nurse asks Mark about Tyler's immunizations. Mark knows he has had "some," but can't remember which ones, and he does not have Tyler's shot records. The staff at the clinic stress to Mark the importance of having his child immunized. Mark is also told by the staff to replace the juice with water in Tyler's sippy cup.

Episode 11

Mark continues to party and spend time with his girlfriend Shelly most nights after work. He knows that between his grandmother, Helen, and Tracie, Tyler is well cared for.

Episode 12

Mark gets his truck paid off this week and has finally been able to pay off most of his credit card debts. He tells his Dad that he would like to stay a little longer to save for a down payment on a house. He is feeling good about getting himself out of debt and celebrates by taking his girlfriend Shelly away on a weekend vacation out of town. **[P]**

Episode 13

Mark and his girlfriend Shelly take Tyler to the park. He is disappointed that Tyler does not want anything to do with his girlfriend. He knows Tyler loves Tracie, but he wants him to love Shelly, too. **[P]**

Episode 14

Mark and Tyler have to move back into the family room when Anthony gets discharged from the hospital. Mark is hopeful that he and Tyler can move out soon. He is thinking about asking Shelly to marry him.

Mark takes Tyler back to the dental clinic for more dental work. The nurses at the clinic also give Tyler immunizations and ask Mark to bring Tyler back in 2 months.

Episode 15

No news this week.

MARK MARTIN
Season 3

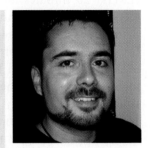

Biographical Information

Mark Martin is Gil's 27-year-old son. Mark is a single parent to his 2 1/2 year-old son Tyler. Mark has been living with Gil and Helen for the past several months because he had fallen deeply into debt and needed help caring for his son. Mark has been steadily working the evening shift as a security officer for a security company. He has recently been able to pay off his truck and credit cards and is currently saving for a down payment on a house. He has a girlfriend, Shelly, whom he hopes to marry in the near future. Mark talks about taking classes at the local college and working toward a degree, but he is not sure what kind of a career he wants to pursue. Mark gets along very well with Gil, Anthony, and Kristina, but has never felt close to Helen or Tracie. His father married Helen when he was 10 years old and, even at that time, Mark could tell Helen resented him. Although Mark always lived with his mother, he spent a lot of time with his father's family. Mark is healthy, although he is a smoker and consumes alcohol on a regular basis. Mark parties after work and does not come home until the early morning hours on a regular basis.

Episode 1

Early in the week, Mark is at home watching a movie. Tyler keeps interrupting him, so Mark gives him some shelled peanuts to eat to keep him quiet. A few minutes later, Tyler is crying; because Mark is busy watching a movie, he fails to notice the hives on his son. Mary points out the problem to Mark and suggests he take Tyler to the hospital.

Mark looks into some of the classes at the local college and is not sure how he can fit in taking classes, taking care of Tyler, and working. He feels a little discouraged and wonders how he can possibly advance out of his security officer job. At the same time, Mark enjoys the guys that he works with. He parties with them three times this week. **[P]**

Episode 2

Mark thinks he has saved up enough money for a down payment on a house. He talks with a real estate agent, Rachel Reyes, who agrees to help him find a small home he can afford. Mark takes Tyler back to the community health clinic for another set of immunizations. He is told to return in 2 months.

Episode 3

Mark and Shelly go out to look at several homes this week with Rachel Reyes, the realtor. Mark and Shelly see several homes they like, but Mark is just unsure about being able to make the house payments. Mark and Shelly have decided to get married at the end of next year, but plan on living together once he has a house to move into.

Episode 4

Mark and several friends from work go to a party 20 miles north of town in the afternoon. He stays there all afternoon and into the evening, and continues to party into the early morning hours. Mark is pretty drunk when he leaves the party at 3:15 a.m. On the way home, while driving on a rural road, Mark crosses the center line in his truck, sees an oncoming car, swerves to avoid the vehicle, and rolls his truck 4 times. Mark is not wearing his seatbelt and is ejected. The driver of the oncoming car sees the accident and calls 9-1-1 for help.

It takes the volunteer emergency medical technicians (EMTs) 20 minutes after the accident to arrive at the scene. Mark is highly intoxicated, but awake. His arms are flailing, and he can answer questions. He is strapped to a backboard and transported to the emergency department (ED) at Neighborhood Hospital, where it is a very busy night. The EMTs tell the ED nurse that Mark is in stable condition.

The ED nurse completes an assessment and realizes quickly that Mark does not have movement or sensation in his lower extremities. She immediately informs Dr. Gordon of the situation and asks him to examine Mark immediately. After an extensive work-up and evaluation, Dr. Gordon diagnoses Mark with a spinal cord injury. A neurosurgeon is called to consult on his case. Because of staff shortages on the neurological unit, Mark stays in the ED on a backboard with spinal precautions for over 8 hours. A nurse is finally able to admit him to the neurological unit. Upon admission to the unit, a large red area is noted on his sacrum.

Mark is told he has fractured vertebrae in his back, and that he severed his spinal cord. He will need to have surgery once the swelling goes down to stabilize the bones in his back. When Mark asks if he will regain feeling and movement in his legs, he is told that, no, the injury will leave him with paraplegia. [P]

Episode 5

Mark is devastated as the reality of his injuries sinks in. He is very angry. Shelly spends a great deal of time at the hospital, and he wonders why she even bothers. He knows they will never buy the house they had dreamed about, and it is unlikely she will want to marry him now. He is scheduled for surgery this week to stabilize the spinal fracture. The skin over the reddened sacral area remains intact. Several people come by to see Mark, but he is not interested in visiting with anybody. [P]

Episode 6

This week, Mark is transferred to a rehabilitation hospital. The day he arrives, the nurse notices a discolored area over his sacrum. By the following day, the discolored area has opened up, revealing a large decubitus ulcer. A large amount of purulent drainage comes from it, and a wound care specialist is called in to consult. The nurses also recognized that Mark is very depressed and unmotivated. He lacks interest in turning or doing any of the rehabilitation exercises. Following a psychiatric consultation and evaluation, Mark is started on bupropion (Welbutrin) for depression. [P]

Episode 7

Mark remains at the rehabilitation hospital. Shelly no longer spends very much time with him. When asked about it, she tells Mark that she has to get on with her life and cannot spend all her time looking at him sitting in a chair. Mark becomes angry with her and tells her to never come back. He is still depressed. [P]

Episode 8

Mark is very depressed. He is not motivated to do anything and frequently has angry outbursts with the nursing staff. When they attempt to point out the benefits of exercise and therapy, he comments that there is no point to doing it. He says his life is essentially over. Occasionally, friends come by to visit, but when they do, Mark does little to interact. [P]

Episode 9

Mark is still at the rehabilitation hospital and is still not engaged in his care. On one afternoon, there is a delay in performing his catheterization. While checking on Mark, the nurse notes that Mark is flushed and has tachycardia. His blood pressure starts to rise. The nurse recognizes the signs of autonomic dysreflexia and knows this is a potential emergency. An in-and-out catheterization is immediately performed on Mark—850 mL of urine is returned with the catheterization. [P]

Episode 10

Mark is discharged from the rehabilitation hospital to Gil and Helen's home. He is to continue outpatient rehabilitation for the next several weeks. Gil and Helen have had to make many modifications to their home to accommodate him. Mark's grandmother Mary lets him know that she is going to take care of him and get him well. Mark appreciates her interest in him, but recognizes she obviously does not understand how he is feeling; she is more interested in seeing him get well than he is.

Episode 11

Mark can hear his father and Helen arguing with Anthony about not wanting to take his medication. Mark feels very angry with Anthony and wishes he would just shut up and take the damn medication. The home care nurse comes to see Mark three times this week for wound care. She reminds Mark about the need to change positions, turn, and eat. Mark has had a poor appetite, partly because he hates having to be dependent for toileting. He hopes to be able to get out of bed and to a real bathroom soon. He continues to work on transfers with a physical therapist in the outpatient rehabilitation clinic. **[P]**

Episode 12

No news this week.

Episode 13

Mark is happy to see his son Tyler nearly every evening. He can see that Tyler is well cared for and that he loves Tracie. He finds himself wishing he could have been a better parent to Tyler and that he could do many things over again. If only he had a second chance.

Episode 14

Mark's decubitus ulcer is nearly healed. This week, he is finally able to transfer himself from the bed to a wheelchair without assistance. He is elated and begins to take an interest in building his upper body muscle strength to facilitate transfers. He can see his grandmother and parents want to help, but finally is beginning to acknowledge that he needs to make more of an effort himself.

Episode 15

Mark hears that his brother is sleeping in the park. He feels angry with his brother for wasting his life. If only he could trade places with him.

TYLER MARTIN
Season 2

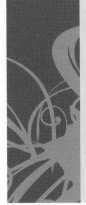

Biographical Information

Tyler Martin is Mark's 2-year-old son and Gil's grandson. Tyler has really only known his father, because his mother began abusing drugs shortly after he was born, and he has not seen her since he was 6 months old. Tyler has been going to various babysitters since he was 1 month old. He and his father have recently moved to his grandparents' home. Tyler loves living there because of all the attention he gets. He also no longer has to go to day care.

Tyler has generally been in good health, although Mark has not consistently taken him for routine infant/child care. He is of normal weight and has a generally good appetite. Tyler still loves his bottle, and each night he is given a bottle of milk or juice to help him go to sleep.

Episode 1

Mark gives Tyler a sippy cup of juice and puts him in front of the TV. Tracie sits down next to Tyler on the couch; Tyler crawls into her lap and falls asleep.

Episode 2

Tyler is enthralled with the toys and books that his great-grandmother has bought him. He immediately sits down on the floor to play with the blocks, with a sippy cup of juice within an arm's reach of him. In the evenings, Tyler sees Tracie studying at the table. He runs to his room to get his new books and holds them up to her to read. **[P]**

Episode 3

Tyler has quickly become very comfortable at Gil and Helen's home. During the daytime, he spends time with his Daddy. In the evenings, he loves the attention from Gil, Helen, Mary, and especially Tracie. He sits in Tracie's lap at every opportunity. Tracie tells Tyler that his teeth look bad and asks him if his Daddy has ever taken him to a dentist. Tyler does not know what any of this means.

Episode 4

No news this week.

Episode 5

During the daytime, while Tracie is at school, Tyler follows his grandmother around almost constantly. She is not usually at home during the day, and he is happy to spend time with her. Tyler likes the fact that Helen plays with him.

Episode 6

No news this week.

Episode 7

Tyler and his Daddy move their stuff into the family room. They sleep on a pull-out bed instead of a regular bed. Tyler sometimes wakes up at night. His Daddy is not at home, but he sees his great-grandmother watching TV. She refills his bottle and tells him to go back to sleep.

Episode 8

Tyler goes to the dental screening clinic with Tracie. At the clinic, a man looks at his teeth and says that they are in bad shape. Tyler wonders how his teeth have been "bad." He is given a toy and a toothbrush, and the assistant shows Tracie how to brush Tyler's teeth.

Episode 9

Tyler is frustrated when Tracie takes his sippy cup full of juice away and gives him water instead. He screams at night for his bottle and does not stop crying until somebody gives him a bottle with juice or milk.

Episode 10

Tyler has a follow-up dental appointment at the community health center. A history is taken, and his height and weight are measured and plotted for 27 months. His length is 91 cm (60th percentile) and weight is 13.2 kg (55th percentile), which are plotted on a growth chart. The dentist finds that two of Tyler's teeth are rotted at the gum line and that he has cavities in five teeth. The two rotted teeth are extracted, which is a frightening experience for Tyler. When they get home, he immediately runs to Tracie to hold him. **[P]**

Episode 11

Tyler hates the fact that his sippy cup has water in it. He screams at the top of his lungs and throws the sippy cup across the room. Mary gets him some juice and puts it in the cup to keep him from crying. **[P]**

Episode 12

No news this week.

Episode 13

Tyler goes to the park with his Daddy. He wants Tracie to go to the park, too, but she is not at home. He does not want the lady with his Daddy to hold him. When she tries to hold him, he cries and kicks his feet until she puts him down.

Episode 14

Tyler has another terrifying experience at the dentist, because he receives very painful shots and has five teeth filled. Because his immunization status is unknown, he is given HBV, DTaP, Hib, IPV, and PCV immunizations during this visit.

Episode 15

No news this week.

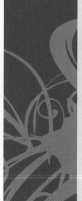

TYLER MARTIN
Season 3

Biographical Information

Tyler Martin is Mark's 2 1/2-year-old son and Gil's grandson. Tyler has really only known his father, because his mother began abusing drugs shortly after he was born, and he has not seen her since he was 6 months old. Tyler and his father have been living at his grandparents' home for the past several months. Tyler loves living there because of all the attention he gets, and he has not had to go to day care. Tyler has become attached to his aunt, Tracie, as a mother figure. He prefers Tracie to all other family members.

Tyler has generally been in good health, although he had bottle mouth (multiple dental caries and rotting teeth), which required extraction of some of his teeth and fillings in others. Tyler also has been behind on his immunizations, and his father has been taking him to the community health center to get caught up on these.

Episode 1

Tyler is bored and wants his Daddy to play with him. Instead, Mark gives Tyler a handful of shelled peanuts to eat. Shortly after eating the peanuts, Tyler begins to cry. His mouth feels funny, and he is itchy all over the place. He runs back to his father crying, but Mark fails to look at him and just tells him to be quiet. After his great-grandmother discovers the problem, Mark takes Tyler to the Neighborhood Hospital emergency department, where he is seen and treated by Dr. Gordon for an allergic reaction. **[P]**

Episode 2

No news this week.

Episode 3

Tyler goes with his father and Shelly to look at homes. Tyler is disinterested in this activity and gets very cranky when he is taken in and out of his car seat at each house. He wants to be home. Mark and Shelly get frustrated with Tyler. **[P]**

Episode 4

Tyler is unable to understand the severity of his father's injuries. He is told by Tracie that his Daddy is sick and at the hospital. Tracie elects not to try to take Tyler to see his Dad until he is in a little less critical state.

Episode 5

No news this week.

Episode 6

Tyler is happy to see his daddy, but does not understand why he is in the hospital and why Tracie and Daddy are so sad. Tyler sits on top of his Dad on the bed and plays with a puzzle; he also shows his Dad the book that Mary bought for him.

Episode 7

No news this week.

Episode 8

No news this week.

Episode 9

Tracie takes Tyler back to the community health clinic for his second round of HBV, DTaP, Hib, IPV, and PCV immunizations. His height and weight are plotted on a growth chart at 33 months. His length is 95 cm (60th percentile) and weight is 14.4 kg (60th percentile).

Episode 10

Tyler has a new place to live. He moves with Tracie to John's apartment. Tyler sees several toys, books, and markers. He immediately sits down and scribbles. Tracie tells Tyler this is his new home. **[P]**

Episode 11

Tyler has adjusted to the change in his living environment without any difficulty and quickly considers John's apartment his home. Tracie and John have quickly established a consistent routine for him, and he thrives on this routine. He sees his father, grandmother, and grandfather every day. His favorite stuffed animal "Yellow Bunny" is always nearby. **[P]**

Episode 12

No news this week.

Episode 13

Tyler sees his Daddy every afternoon or evening at his grandmother's house. He wonders why his father always lies in bed. He can tell his Daddy is sad because he doesn't say very much and doesn't want to play.

Episode 14

When he goes to see his father, Tyler actually tends to spend most of his time interacting with his great-grandmother Mary or his grandfather Gil. He especially likes to spend time with his grandfather. Gil takes him to the park to play on the playground equipment, plays ball with him in the yard at their home, and lets Tyler sit on a tall stool to watch as he works in his workshop.

Episode 15

Tyler sees his Daddy move from the bed to the wheelchair and watches with curiosity as everybody in the family cheers when he does this. Tyler sits in his father's lap with delight as Mark navigates about the house in a wheelchair.

OCAMPO HOUSEHOLD

OCAMPO FAMILY STORY OVERVIEW

Character	Season 1	Season 2	Season 3
DANILO OCAMPO	Dr. Ocampo has class II heart failure and is a full-time caregiver to his wife Lydia. This story depicts the day-to-day life of disease management and the caregiver role. Danilo does not want any outside help. He maintains a very consistent schedule for Lydia, and they get along quite well. When Lydia falls and breaks her hip, he spends all of his time at the hospital at her bedside because he is not confident she will get good care without him.	Danilo reluctantly agrees to Lydia's transfer to a rehabilitation hospital. Danilo's perception is that Lydia is receiving poor care at the facility. Eventually she is discharged home. He initially has the help of a niece, but after she leaves, he is unable to care for Lydia. He tires easily and is fatigued. He develops acute exacerbation of heart failure, has a myocardial infarction, and dies.	
LYDIA OCAMPO	Lydia has moderate dementia. Her husband cares for her in the home, and she rarely goes out in public. The consistent routine at home that Danilo provides helps Lydia function at an optimal level. Lydia falls and breaks her hip in episode 10 and is admitted to the hospital for an ORIF. Confusion escalates at the hospital. Issues managing her post-op pain, nausea, infection, and anemia also present.	Lydia is transferred to a rehabilitation hospital for continued care. She receives appropriate care, yet she continues to be more confused than she was prior to her fall. A niece comes to help with her care when she is discharged home. After Danilo dies, she is placed in a nursing home.	Lydia continues to live in a nursing home. She has no visitors. She gradually declines, due to lack of mobility and poor nutrition. She becomes confined to bed, does not eat, becomes incontinent, and develops a decubitus ulcer. Lydia eventually dies.

CONCEPTS   *Cognitive Impairment, Coping, Elimination, End of Life, Fatigue, Infection, Mobility, Nutrition, Oxygenation, Perfusion, Role Performance, Sleep, Stress, Tissue Integrity*

DANILO OCAMPO
Season 1

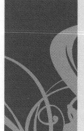

Biographical Information

Dr. Danilo Ocampo is a 74-year-old retired pathologist. He lives in his home with Lydia, his wife of 51 years. Their only child, a son, was killed at age 22 in an automobile accident. Danilo was born and raised in the Philippines and came to the United States when he was 23. He is the last living member of his immediate family. He has a few nephews and a niece in the Philippines, but no relatives live nearby.

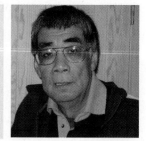

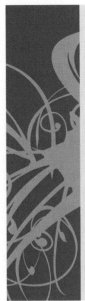

Dr. Ocampo's health has been declining for the past few years. He has a medical history that includes hypertension, myocardial infarction, angina, and class II heart failure. Because of these cardiovascular disorders, he takes multiple medications, including metoprolol, lisinopril, Aldactone, furosemide off and on, potassium (K+) when taking furosemide, aspirin, isosorbide dinitrate, and nitroglycerin. He has a good understanding of the pharmaceutical properties of the medications. At times, he is not sure he gets good health care because of all the medications he takes. He often does not believe they are helpful, because he experiences many side effects and has required multiple admissions to the hospital. He usually feels better after a few days in the hospital, but typically checks himself out of the hospital before his physicians are ready to discharge him.

Because Lydia has dementia, most of Danilo's time and energy are spent managing their household and taking care of her. He has been resistant to outside help, believing he can care for her better than anyone else. He maintains a very consistent schedule, and they get along quite well. Although at one time in their lives they were very socially active, at this point, they rarely go out.

Episode 1
No news this week.

Episode 2
No news this week.

Episode 3
Danilo has a typical week at home and is feeling pretty good. On one day this week, he goes to the bank, grocery store, and home super center for some basic items. He does not leave Lydia for more than 1 hour at a time when running errands. While out, he calls her to be sure she is fine. **[P]**

Episode 4
Danilo cooks dinner and encourages Lydia to help. He recognizes her mental decline and hopes his efforts will keep her as functional as possible. He also recognizes that she is past the point at which she could live by herself and decides he probably needs to meet with an attorney to discuss care for Lydia, should he precede her in death. He has never formalized any such documents in the past.

Episode 5
No news this week.

Episode 6
Dr. Ocampo has an appointment with his attorney, Mr. Wolf, to discuss planning for Lydia, should he die. He is encouraged to write a living will and durable power of attorney. He also discusses in general terms how to best manage her health care. He is encouraged to explore life care communities, board and care homes, and assisted living facilities. Although he does not make any immediate decisions, he knows he needs to get serious about doing something for Lydia. **[P]**

Episode 7
No news this week.

Episode 8
Because the weather is beautiful, Danilo goes through the drive-through of a fast-food restaurant to pick up some chicken and then takes Lydia to a park for a picnic. Lydia does not say much, but he enjoys spending a quiet afternoon with her out of the house.

Episode 9
No news this week.

Episode 10
Danilo wakes up in the middle of the night to the screams of his wife. He finds her on the floor in the bathroom and recognizes from the position of her leg that she has broken her hip. He calls for an ambulance to take her to the emergency department. The day of her surgery, Danilo spends the entire day at the hospital. He is concerned that nobody will know how to best care for his wife. She is confused, and he can see that she is scared. He tries to calm her as best he can. Eventually, late that evening, he goes home exhausted and not feeling well himself.

The next morning, Danilo arrives at the hospital at about 10 a.m. He finds Lydia in restraints, yelling for help.

Her breakfast tray is untouched. Danilo is frantic and calls for the nurse. Lydia's primary nurse is Bobby. Danilo complains to him about the current condition of his wife and the poor care she is receiving. Bobby tries to explain that there had been an emergency on the floor that morning and that the restraints were necessary to keep Lydia safe. Danilo removes the restraints, cleans Lydia up, and feeds her breakfast. A nursing technician comes by the room and tells Danilo she had not fed Lydia or bathed her yet today because she knew Danilo would come to the hospital this morning, and figured he would prefer to feed and bath his wife. Danilo feels angry and decides he cannot trust the hospital staff to care for Lydia. **[VC]**

Episode 11

Danilo has had a frustrating and exhausting week. Lydia remains in the hospital with complications stemming from her surgery. He becomes very anxious about Lydia's care and has ongoing arguments with the nursing and medical staff. He asks many individuals the same questions about her condition, care, and plans for discharge, but he gets different answers from everyone. He feels he must be at the hospital during meal times, or Lydia will not eat. It is Danilo's perception that her complications have resulted from inappropriate care and that he needs to get her out of the hospital and back home if she is to survive.

Danilo spends as much time at the hospital as he can; as a result, he quits attending to his own self-care management. He has become increasingly short of breath and is very fatigued. He notices his legs have become edematous. Danilo goes to the drugstore to use the "self-serve" blood pressure machine and finds his blood pressure is elevated (152/106 mm Hg). Still, he resists the idea of seeing his physician or going to the emergency department, for fear of being admitted. Instead, he increases his dose of furosemide and lisinopril by one-half tablet each per day and tries to get a bit more rest. **[P]**

Episode 12

Danilo continues to be short of breath and fatigued, but the swelling in his legs has lessened. He also checks his blood pressure at a drugstore and finds that it has dropped to 142/98 mm Hg, which he finds acceptable. He reduces his medication doses to normal levels.

The discharge planner makes arrangements for Lydia to be transferred to a rehabilitation hospital as soon as a bed is available. Danilo argues with the discharge coordinator and Bobby (Lydia's primary nurse), about taking her home so that he can take care of her properly. They convince him that the care she will receive at the rehabilitation hospital will be excellent, will facilitate her recovery, and will allow him needed rest. Danilo reluctantly agrees, knowing he has pushed his limits the past few weeks. **[VC]**

Episode 13

Danilo continues to spend most of his time at the hospital. He talks to Bobby regularly about every aspect of Lydia's care.

A bed finally becomes available at the rehabilitation hospital, and Lydia is transferred there. Danilo notices she has become more confused again. Because of the experiences at the other hospital, Danilo is not trusting of the care Lydia will receive. He spends most of his time at the rehabilitation hospital and talks with the staff frequently about Lydia's needs and care. **[P]**

Episode 14

Danilo is unhappy with the lack of progress he has seen during the week Lydia has been at the rehabilitation hospital. She is still confused. The hospital staff gets her out of bed frequently, and she yells and cries. He wishes they would leave her alone so she could rest and wonders if they remember that she is an old woman with a broken hip.

Danilo continues to go back and forth between the hospital and his home. He feels exhausted and frequently short of breath from trying to take care of his wife at the hospital and still manage to keep the house in order at home. He does not take his medications consistently, has a hard time sleeping, and gets little rest. Danilo experiences several episodes of angina, which he manages successfully with nitroglycerin.

He goes to the physician's office without an appointment and is seen by a nurse practitioner. He makes it clear that he will not agree to being admitted, but he feels as though he'd better check in, given his ongoing symptoms. The nurse practitioner auscultates his heart and lungs, noting fine crackles in the lower bases bilaterally; no extra heart sounds are noted. She also observes pitting 3+ edema in the lower extremities. The nurse practitioner makes several suggestions that would offer social support, such as Meals on Wheels and a housecleaning service, to help minimize the stress of keeping up his home. After checking his potassium level (3.9 mEq/L), she increases his furosemide and lisinopril to the maximum dose levels and asks Danilo to come back and see her the following week. **[P]**

Episode 15

Danilo continues to feel tired and frequently experiences angina. He believes if he could take Lydia home he would feel better, because he wouldn't have to do all of the running around he does. He also believes he can take better care of her than the people at the rehabilitation hospital and continues to argue with the nursing and medical staff about the care she receives. The discharge coordinator meets with him and tries to help him understand the progress that Lydia is making. Danilo does not believe that she is progressing all that much. **[VC]**

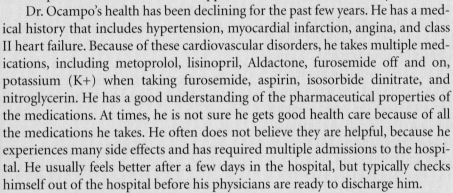

DANILO OCAMPO
Season 2

Biographical Information

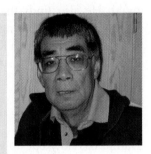

Dr. Danilo Ocampo is a 74-year-old retired pathologist. He lives in his home with Lydia, his wife of 51 years. Their only child, a son, was killed at age 22 in an automobile accident. Danilo was born and raised in the Philippines and came to the United States when he was 23. He is the last living member of his immediate family. He has a few nephews and a niece in the Philippines, but no relatives live nearby.

Dr. Ocampo's health has been declining for the past few years. He has a medical history that includes hypertension, myocardial infarction, angina, and class II heart failure. Because of these cardiovascular disorders, he takes multiple medications, including metoprolol, lisinopril, Aldactone, furosemide off and on, potassium (K+) when taking furosemide, aspirin, isosorbide dinitrate, and nitroglycerin. He has a good understanding of the pharmaceutical properties of the medications. At times, he is not sure he gets good health care because of all the medications he takes. He often does not believe they are helpful, because he experiences many side effects and has required multiple admissions to the hospital. He usually feels better after a few days in the hospital, but typically checks himself out of the hospital before his physicians are ready to discharge him.

Dr. Ocampo's wife has dementia, and she recently has suffered a hip fracture. She spent several weeks at Neighborhood Hospital and more recently was admitted to the rehabilitation hospital. Danilo has been very distressed about the care Lydia has received and her increased level of confusion. It is his opinion that she has not been well cared for, and he wants to bring her home to take care of her himself. Because of his own health issues, Dr. Ocampo's niece, Kristina, has agreed to come from the Philippines to stay with them to help care for her aunt when Lydia is discharged.

Episode 1

Danilo speaks with the medical staff about discharging Lydia and tells them that his niece is coming to stay with them to help care for Lydia. They agree to a discharge next week. **[P]**

Episode 2

Danilo's grandniece, Kristina, has arrived to stay with them. She is the granddaughter of his late brother. She is a college student and is in between semesters. Danilo is very happy to bring Lydia home and feels sure that, once she is back home, she will improve. **[P]**

Episode 3

Danilo is happy to have Kristina at their home to help him. She has not only been caring for Lydia, but has been taking care of many things around the home. Danilo is feeling more rested than he has for the past couple months.

Episode 4

No news this week.

Episode 5

Danilo continues to feel good. He has energy, and the swelling in his legs has subsided. He is aware that Kristina's school break is coming to an end. She offers to take a semester off from school to stay with them longer. Although he likes having Kristina around to help, he believes he can take care of Lydia independently and does not want to keep Kristina from attending school. He encourages her to go back home. **[VC] [P]**

Episode 6

Danilo is somewhat surprised at how much work it takes to care for Lydia. Since Kristina left, Danilo has not been able to sleep very well, because Lydia is often awake at night. He also finds that keeping up with the laundry, shopping, and preparing meals is tiring. He did not appreciate just how much Kristina was helping until she left. Despite this, Danilo is sure they will manage just fine. **[P]**

Episode 7

No news this week.

Episode 8

Danilo has not kept up with optimal management of his own health—for example, he has not consistently taken his medications and is not getting adequate rest. During the middle of the night this week, Lydia attempted to leave the house. Because of situations such as this, Danilo is unable to sleep well. He attributes his poor sleeping patterns to caring for Lydia, but also is not sleeping well because of orthopnea. He also experiences shortness of breath frequently while awake and has noticed an increase in edema in his legs over the past couple of weeks.

Episode 9

Danilo has been feeling progressively more fatigued. He is unable to sleep more than a few hours at a time. Twice this week he has had episodes of angina, which he promptly treats with nitroglycerin. He knows he should make an appointment with his cardiologist, but he becomes concerned that, if he is admitted to the hospital, Lydia could be sent away from their home for care. He decides to self-manage by increasing his dose of furosemide (Lasix). He feels better the following day. **[P]**

Episode 10

Danilo ran out of his lisinopril medication last week. Although he called in for a refill, he has been too tired to drive to the drugstore to pick up his prescription. He is feeling increasingly fatigued and short of breath. The leg edema has increased significantly over the past couple of days, and he again self-medicates with furosemide (Lasix). Following a sleepless night, Danilo continues to feel even more fatigued. He is too tired to help Lydia with anything. He begins to cough and experiences slight pressure in his chest. This is relieved, but the sensation soon returns. Within a few hours, he is coughing up blood-tinged, frothy sputum and realizes he is in trouble. Danilo calls 9-1-1.

Paramedics respond to the Ocampo home about 15 minutes after the call. By this point, Danilo is extremely anxious and somewhat confused. The paramedics note his vital signs (respiratory rate, 36 breaths/minute; heart rate, 132 beats/minute; blood pressure, 100/60 mm Hg; oxygen saturation, 85%) and immediately placed him on oxygen and a cardiac monitor. They note that he is in sinus tachycardia. An intravenous line is started, and 4 mg of morphine sulfate and 80 mg of Lasix are administered.

The paramedics transport Danilo to the emergency department (ED). In the ED, Dr. Gordon quickly makes a diagnosis of acute heart failure and myocardial infarction. Danilo's condition further deteriorates shortly after arriving in the ED. He goes into ventricular fibrillation and, despite exceptional emergency care and resuscitative efforts, Dr. Danilo Ocampo dies. **[MR] [VC]**

LYDIA OCAMPO
Season 1

Biographical Information

Lydia Ocampo is a 69-year-old female who has been married to Danilo for 51 years. Their only child, Emillo, was killed at age 22 in an automobile accident. His death devastated Lydia, but over time she adequately adjusted and coped with the loss. Lydia was born and raised in the Philippines and came to the United States with Danilo when she was 18. All of Lydia's brothers and sisters have passed away, but she has a niece and a few nephews who still live in the Philippines. She and Danilo have no relatives nearby.

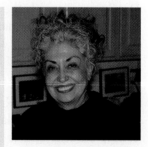

Continued

Lydia's overall physical health is good, and her only known condition is Alzheimer disease. She has had dementia for several years. Her husband is her caregiver, and she benefits from the consistent routine that he provides. Lydia rarely socializes and spends most of her time at home. She is fully ambulatory and feeds, dresses, and toilets herself. She gets confused at times and is easily distracted.

Episode 1
No news this week.

Episode 2
No news this week.

Episode 3
Danilo leaves Lydia at home for about an hour while he runs errands. He assures her that he will only be gone for a little while. She spends time crocheting a scarf, but cannot remember who the scarf is for when she finishes. While he is out, Danilo calls Lydia and tells her he will be home soon. Although Lydia had forgotten he had left the house, she tells him she is doing just fine. **[P]**

Episode 4
Lydia helps Danilo make dinner. She is still able to do many routine things in the kitchen herself, but with assistance. Unassisted, Lydia may do such things as place food to be baked in the refrigerator instead of in the oven, leave burners on, or place food items in the dishwasher. With verbal cues, she is better able to stay on track. While in the kitchen preparing dinner, Lydia is getting ready to heat soup on the stove and places a plastic container on the burners. Danilo reminds her to use a saucepan instead of a plastic bowl. She comments on how silly she is. After dinner is over, Lydia begins to empty the dishwasher (before it ran) and puts dirty dishes away in the cupboards. Danilo stops her and tells her the dishwasher has not yet cleaned the dishes. **[VC]**

Episode 5
No news this week.

Episode 6
Lydia goes into the den to watch television. Several of her favorite television shows come on in the middle of the day, yet she cannot remember the names of any of them. She becomes frustrated because she can't figure out how to turn on the television; Danilo turns on the television and, noting her frustration, tells her he finds remote controls confusing, too. **[P]**

Episode 7
No news this week.

Episode 8
Lydia goes with Danilo for a picnic. She enjoys being outside and watching the animals. She sees a playground and thinks about her son Emillo. She wonders aloud if he has come home from school yet. Danilo reminds her that he died many years ago. She then remembers he died and feels sad—but still wants to go home to be sure he is not home alone.

Episode 9
No news this week.

Episode 10
During the middle of the night, Lydia gets out of bed to urinate. While rushing to the bathroom, she experiences urinary leakage. Her foot slips on the floor, causing her to fall on the ceramic tile floor, hitting the toilet and edge of the tub on the way down. She screams in pain, awakening Danilo. An ambulance takes her to the emergency department, where she is diagnosed with a left hip fracture. She is sent to the operating room for an open reduction internal fixation (ORIF) of the left hip. She is admitted to the medical-surgical floor following surgery.

When Lydia wakes up, she finds that there is a dramatic change in her surroundings and is extremely confused. She does not know where she is or what is happening to her. She is in a strange room, in a strange bed. There are strange sounds and smells all around her. She is in pain. She feels nauseous and vomits several times immediately after surgery. She has uncomfortable tubes in her arms. She attempts to resolve this by pulling them away from her body, but they are quickly replaced. A large object is placed between her legs, making it difficult for her to change positions and get comfortable. Strangers come into her room and do things to her regularly. She tries to fight them off to protect herself. She yells frequently for somebody to help her and speaks in Tagalog, her native language. She tries to get out of bed to escape the situation, only to be scolded. Although she is fairly calm when Danilo is with her, she is often restrained when he is not present. When Lydia is tied up, she becomes terrified and cries for help. She refuses to eat unless Danilo feeds her, because she is afraid the strangers are trying to poison her. **[MR]**

Episode 11

Lydia remains at the hospital because she has developed an infection in her incision and needs intravenous antibiotics and dressing changes. She is pale, and her hemoglobin and hematocrit dropped to 7 g/dL and 30%, respectively; thus, she requires a transfusion of 2 units of packed red blood cells for anemia. Her oral intake has been inadequate, but she has been well hydrated by the intravenous fluids. She has been incontinent ever since the Foley catheter was removed. Attempts at physical therapy have been unproductive. The physical therapists are successful at transferring her from the bed to a chair, but this requires nearly full assistance.

She continues to be more confused than she was when at home, but is calmer than she was immediately after surgery. However, the nursing staff finds her to frequently be uncooperative. Danilo is with her much of the time, and she finds his presence and the sound of his voice comforting. **[P]**

Episode 12

Lydia remains at Neighborhood Hospital. She is still confused, but is beginning to recognize some of the nurses and is becoming familiar with the routine on the floor.

She no longer has an IV, but she still is getting wet-to-damp dressing changes to the incisional wound. The wound is no longer infected and is beginning to heal. Lydia's hemoglobin and hematocrit levels are still low (10 g/dL and 36%), but within an acceptable range. She still has not progressed with physical therapy, but is more cooperative when they come to work with her than she was last week. Her nutritional intake improves, particularly when Danilo is present to feed her. She remains incontinent. **[P]**

Episode 13

Some strangers come into Lydia's room, place her on a hard cart, and put her in the back of a van. She is sure she is being kidnapped. She yells and tells the intruders to leave her alone. She is wheeled into another building and placed in another room and a different bed. Her confusion increases for several days after her transfer to the rehabilitation hospital. **[P]**

Episode 14

Lydia remains in the rehabilitation hospital, where she is receiving excellent care from the nursing staff. She is placed on a very consistent routine, which has resulted in improvements in her nutritional intake. She is also beginning to make progress with physical therapy by getting out of bed regularly and using the toilet. Although she is still more confused than she had been at home, her level of confusion has decreased dramatically. **[P]**

Episode 15

Lydia continues to progress well at the rehabilitation hospital.

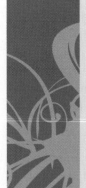

LYDIA OCAMPO
Season 2

Biographical Information

Lydia Ocampo is a 69-year-old female who has been married to Danilo for 51 years. Their only child, Emillo, was killed at age 22 in an automobile accident. His death devastated Lydia, but over time she adequately adjusted and coped with the loss. Lydia was born and raised in the Philippines and came to the United States with Danilo when she was 18. All of Lydia's brothers and sisters have passed away, but she has a niece and a few nephews who still live in the Philippines. She and Danilo have no relatives nearby.

Lydia has Alzheimer disease and, until recently, she experienced relatively good health. A few months ago, she fell and broke her hip. She spent several weeks at Neighborhood Hospital. Her recovery was slow due to a number of

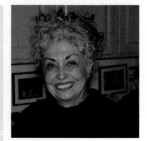

Continued

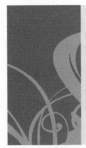

postoperative complications that included anemia, nutritional deficits, a wound infection, and a high level of confusion. In recent weeks, she was admitted to a rehabilitation hospital, where she is making progress, both nutritionally and from a mobility standpoint. At this time, she remains confused. She needs assistance ambulating, bathing, toileting, and getting dressed. Her appetite has improved, but she requires verbal cues and encouragement to eat.

Episode 1

Lydia remains at the rehabilitation hospital. Danilo comes to see her every day. **[P]**

Episode 2

Lydia is discharged home. She recognizes her surroundings, but remains confused and requires full care. A girl is in the home caring for her, but she does not know who she is. She asks the girl if she knows her son Emillo. **[P]**

Episode 3

Under Kristina's care, Lydia makes great progress in her recovery. Lydia is beginning to eat well. She likes the food prepared by Kristina. She is also gradually becoming more independent, although she still requires help with mobility. **[P]**

Episode 4

No news this week.

Episode 5

Although Lydia continues to require assistance with ambulation, she is using a walker and is eating independently now. Kristina has enjoyed caring for Lydia and has been pleased with her progress. She leaves this week to go back to school. Lydia does not understand why she left, but she misses her. She believes Kristina may have been her sister. She usually recognizes Danilo, but sometimes forgets who he is. **[P]**

Episode 6

Lydia is missing the ongoing activity and stimulation she received with her niece. Danilo gets her out of bed, but she ends up sitting in a chair most of the day. **[P]**

Episode 7

No news this week.

Episode 8

During one night this week, Lydia gets out of bed, walks through the house completely naked, and attempts to go out the front door. Danilo hears her attempting to open the door and directs her back to bed. Fearing that she might do this again, Danilo sleeps very little the rest of the night. The next day, Lydia thinks she hears her son Emillo and attempts to go out the front door to find him. **[VC]**

Episode 9

Lydia has not slept at night for a week now. Her confusion has increased to the point at which she is unaware of the time of day—although she is aware she is at home. She attempts to get up out of bed, and Danilo either puts her back in bed or helps her up and sits with her until she is ready to sleep. She frequently calls Danilo "Emillo." Danilo patiently reminds her that Emillo died a long time ago.

Episode 10

This past week, Lydia has only been out of bed to use the restroom. Danilo has been too tired to help her, and she has not independently made the effort to get up. She also has not eaten very much. When paramedics respond to the 9-1-1 call, they find Lydia curled up in bed. She asks them who they are and begins to yell when they put her on a cold, hard cart. She is sure the men are going to kill her. At the emergency department, the nurse tells Lydia her husband has died and attempts to elicit information regarding next of kin. Lydia is unable to answer the questions.

Because there is no medical need for hospital admission, Lydia remains in the emergency department for 30 hours while the hospital social workers work with local authorities to get an emergency placement into a nursing home. **[P]**

Episode 11

Lydia remains at the nursing home. She is persistently confused and alternates between being passive and uncooperative. During the past few weeks, a case manager has been working on Lydia's case. She is able to locate paperwork in the home and in a safety deposit box. She also finds the name of Danilo's attorney, Mr. Frank Wolf, and contacts him. **[P]**

Episode 12

In the several weeks she has been in the nursing home, Lydia has become progressively dependent on her caregivers and accuses them of being her kidnappers.

Danilo's attorney, Mr. Wolf, is contacted this week by the case manager. Although Danilo never made any decisions regarding care for Lydia, he did give Mr. Wolf power of attorney in the event he or Lydia were unable to make decisions independently. Because of the discussion he had with Danilo in the months preceding his death, Mr. Wolf elects to keep Lydia in the nursing home facility and proceeds with trust-related activities. **[P]**

Episode 13

Lydia remains in the nursing home.

Episode 14

Lydia remains in the nursing home. She is placed in a wheelchair and taken to the dining hall for each meal. After her meal, she either sits in a wheelchair in the hall or lies in bed in her room. Lydia has become progressively less responsive; her nutritional status has gradually declined. **[P]**

Episode 15

Lydia remains in the nursing home.

LYDIA OCAMPO
Season 3

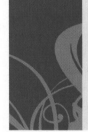

Biographical Information

Lydia is a 70-year-old widow who currently lives at a nursing home. She has Alzheimer disease, and her health has steadily declined in the past year. She has been in the nursing home for several months now and has become completely dependent. Her attorney, Mr. Wolf, has proceeded with the process of selling the family home; the money will be placed in a trust to care for Lydia until she dies.

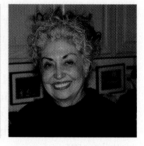

Episode 1

No news this week.

Episode 2

Lydia remains in the nursing home. She has become fairly unresponsive to her caregivers. She sleeps more often and only gets up out of bed when the nursing assistants get her up. She has developed a decubitus ulcer over her sacrum.

Episode 3

An estate sale was held at Danilo and Lydia's home last week. The home was listed for sale and purchased by a middle-aged couple who are in the process of relocating to the community. Proceeds from the sale of the home have been placed in a trust for Lydia's ongoing medical care.

Episode 4

No news this week.

Episode 5

Lydia sleeps most of time. She does not get out of bed very often. When she is placed in a wheelchair, she often falls asleep. She is not interested in eating or communicating. She talks very infrequently and has become completely dependent for all aspects of her care. Despite efforts to turn

her, Lydia's ulcer has increased in size; a wound care nurse comes to see her for ulcer management. **[P]**

Episode 6

No news this week.

Episode 7

No news this week.

Episode 8

Lydia has very poor nutritional intake, and the decubitus ulcer has not responded well to treatment. She is completely incontinent of urine and stool and now does not get out of bed at all. Despite attempts to feed her, she eats very little. Mr. Wolf, Lydia's attorney, is informed of her declining condition, and a do-not-resuscitate order is obtained.

Episode 9

No news this week.

Episode 10

A nursing assistant taking morning vital signs walks into Lydia's room and finds that Lydia has died during the night. Mr. Wolf is contacted, and he prepares a letter notifying Lydia's niece, Kristina, of her passing. **[P]**

REYES HOUSEHOLD

REYES FAMILY STORY OVERVIEW

Character	Season 1	Season 2	Season 3
ANGELO REYES	Angelo is a healthy male with well-controlled type 1 diabetes mellitus. He and his wife go through infertility work-ups. The story also addresses his daily management of DM. He has an episode of vitreous hemorrhage with the threat of retinal detachment and undergoes an outpatient vitrectomy procedure.	The story follows his experiences associated with his wife having a high-risk pregnancy. In addition, Angelo gets the flu and develops ketoacidosis. He is treated in the ED and does not require hospitalization.	Angelo is supportive of his wife during her difficult pregnancy, but is frustrated that she won't slow down at the advice of her physician. His babies are born during this season, and the story depicts the stress associated with being a parent of infants in the NICU.
RACHEL REYES	Rachel is trying to pregnant. She begins infertility work-ups and becomes obsessed with getting pregnant. The story describes the stress associated with this process, not only for Rachel, but also for her husband.	Rachel completes her infertility work-ups and begins taking Clomid. She finally becomes pregnant (with twins). This story follows her pregnancy. She represents a high-risk pregnancy.	As the pregnancy progresses, Rachel develops preeclampsia. She is told to slow down her work activities After developing HELLP syndrome, Rachel is taken for an emergency cesarean section, and her infants are delivered prematurely. She feels a great deal of regret, but is relieved when she is able to take them home.
PETER AND MARISSA REYES	Not born yet	Not born yet	Peter and Marissa are born prematurely, due to their mother's preeclampsia. There are initial problems with thermoregulation, glucose regulation, and respiratory status. Infant care for healthy premature newborns is emphasized in this story.

CONCEPTS   *Acid-Base, Family Dynamics, Fluid and Electrolytes, Immunity, Interpersonal Relationships, Metabolism, Nutrition, Oxygenation, Perfusion, Reproduction, Role Performance, Sensory Perceptual, Stress, Sexuality, Thermoregulation*

ANGELO REYES
Season 1

Biographical Information

Angelo Reyes is a 40-year-old Hispanic architect who has been married to Rachel for the past 3 years. Angelo considers himself to be healthy, but has had diabetes mellitus (DM) type 1 since the age of 13. The only ongoing problem Angelo has is diabetic retinopathy which has caused retinal hemorrhage in the past. He is very compliant with diabetes management and considers it to be

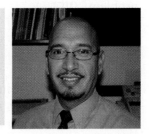

Continued

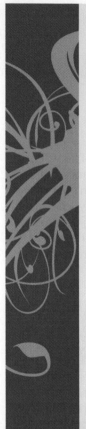

more of an annoyance than a real problem in his life. He attributes his successful disease management to a very structured lifestyle. His daily routine is as follows:

- Wakes up at 5:30 a.m. and checks his blood sugar. If within a normal range, he gives himself an insulin injection (22 units Regular/12 units NPH), takes a shower, and gets dressed. He eats a bowl of cereal and a banana each morning for breakfast and leaves the house about 6:30 a.m., arriving at work by 7 a.m.
- At 10 a.m., he eats a snack (usually an apple or raisins).
- At noon, he checks his blood sugar; if it is within normal range, he eats a sandwich and fruit.
- Between 12:30 and 1 p.m., he walks at a park close to his office.
- At 2:30 p.m., he eats another snack (such as a granola bar or soda).
- Leaves the office at 5:30.
- Arrives home by 6 p.m., checks his blood sugar, and administers his evening dose of insulin (16 units Regular/8 units NPH).
- Eats dinner at 6:30 p.m
- Three nights a week, Angelo goes to the gym at 7:30 p.m. to work out. On these evenings, he may slightly decrease the dose of insulin to compensate for the exercise.
- Checks his blood sugar at 9:30 p.m., has a snack of peanut butter and crackers, and goes to bed immediately after the evening news at 10:30.

Since getting married, Angelo's wife has been very anxious to get pregnant and start a family. Rachel has extensively researched infertility on the Internet and has, in his opinion, become obsessed with getting pregnant. Although he would like to have a child, he has not been enthusiastic about infertility work-ups, partially because of the huge expense involved. However, after 3 years without a pregnancy, he agrees to begin the process because he knows how important it is to her.

Episode 1
No news this week.

Episode 2
Rachel has an initial work-up with her gynecologist today. She comes home after the appointment and tells Angelo that he needs to have an examination by an urologist, because (in her words) he may be "the problem." **[VC]**

Episode 3
No news this week.

Episode 4
Angelo has an appointment with the urologist and needs to take off from work during the morning to go. He does not tell his coworkers why he is gone that morning, because he finds the process a major invasion

of his privacy. He dreads going to the examination. Because the appointment is at 9:30 a.m., Angelo takes his morning snack with him and ends up eating a box of raisins on the exam table while waiting for the physician to come into the examination room.

The urologist takes a history and learns that Angelo has had type 1 diabetes mellitus (DM) since age 13. Further, it is revealed that Angelo has a positive family history for type 1DM (his uncle). Angelo's medical history reveals no past exposure to chemicals, no past trauma to his genitalia, no history of sexually transmitted infections, and no history of impotence. A physical examination reveals no abnormalities of his reproductive organs or testes. The urologist gives Angelo lab requisitions for a blood test to assess hormonal levels and a semen analysis. He is instructed to obtain a semen sample following 48-72 hours

e of days. He is scheduled to see his ophthal-
he following week. **[P]**

13

elects to take a week off from work following his
y. He sees the ophthalmologist, who tells Angelo
rgery was a success, and there was no evidence of
al detachment. Angelo is relieved.

He goes with Rachel for her biopsy and is glad
rything goes smoothly. She is not feeling well after

the procedure, so he spends the afternoon with her. He worries a little bit about the amount of work he has missed lately due to his eye surgery and all of Rachel's tests.

Episode 14

Angelo's vision is gradually improving, and he goes back to work this week.

Episode 15

No news this week.

ANGELO REYES
Season 2

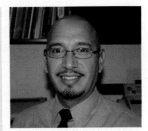

Biographical Information

Angelo Reyes is a 40-year-old Hispanic architect who has been married to Rachel for the past 3 years. Angelo considers himself to be healthy, but has had diabetes mellitus (DM) type 1 since the age of 13. He is very compliant with diabetes management and considers it to be more of an annoyance than a real problem in his life. He attributes his successful disease management to a very structured lifestyle. His daily routine is as follows:

- Wakes up at 5:30 a.m. and checks his blood sugar. If within a normal range, he gives himself an insulin injection (22 units Regular/12 units NPH), takes a shower, and gets dressed. He eats a bowl of cereal and a banana each morning for breakfast and leaves the house about 6:30 a.m., arriving at work by 7 a.m.
- At 10 a.m., he eats a snack (usually an apple or raisins).
- At noon, he checks his blood sugar; if it is within normal range, he eats a sandwich and fruit.
- Between 12:30 and 1 p.m., he walks at a park close to his office.
- At 2:30 p.m., he eats another snack (such as a granola bar or soda).
- Leaves the office at 5:30.
- Arrives home by 6 p.m., checks his blood sugar, and administers his evening dose of insulin (16 units Regular/8 units NPH).
- Eats dinner at 6:30 p.m
- Three nights a week, Angelo goes to the gym at 7:30 p.m. to work out. On these evenings, he may slightly decrease the dose of insulin to compensate for the exercise.
- Checks his blood sugar at 9:30 p.m., has a snack of peanut butter and crackers, and goes to bed immediately after the evening news at 10:30.

The only ongoing problem Angelo has had is diabetic retinopathy. Recently, he underwent a vitrectomy following a retinal hemorrhage. His surgery was successful.

Since getting married, Angelo's wife has been very anxious to get pregnant and start a family. Because they were unsuccessful at getting pregnant, Rachel has undergone an extensive infertility work-up and testing. He has found the process to be very stressful, and it has created tension between the two of them. Angelo is also somewhat concerned about the amount of work he has recently missed.

of abstinence of ejaculation within the next couple of weeks. Angelo is very embarrassed about this entire process and leaves the physician's office feeling humiliated. **[P]**

Episode 5

Angelo is notified by the urologist that all of his lab results are normal. He feels relieved that the "problem" does not lie with him. Rachel expresses surprise that his results were normal. Angelo gets an A_{1C} test done this week; his level is 5.8%. **[P]**

Episode 6

Rachel has her first appointment with the infertility specialist this week, and she shares with Angelo every detail about the visit, including all the tests and the general game plan. Angelo wonders just how much this is all going to cost and hopes that, if they are successful, there will be money left over to raise the baby. **[P]**

Episode 7

No news this week.

Episode 8

This is the week Rachel has her postcoital exam. Angelo is very embarrassed about the idea that he has to leave work to have sex with his wife, knowing she is going to be examined shortly thereafter. He goes along with this because he knows how important it is to Rachel, but he finds the process very humiliating. On the day of the test, he tells his coworkers that he's not feeling well due to his diabetes and thinks he should just go home.

Angelo finds that having sex on demand for a test is not at all enjoyable and is in fact stressful. Additionally, he has to eat lunch earlier than normal and is unable to take his lunchtime walk. Because he is not planning to go back to work, Rachel asks Angelo to go with her to the appointment. He feels embarrassed, knowing the physician is examining his wife right after they had sex. At 2 p.m. Angelo eats his mid-afternoon granola bar snack while in the waiting room and wonders if eating lunch too early will cause problems for him later that day. At 6 p.m. that same evening, Angelo's glucose levels are much higher than normal, and he adjusts his insulin dose. He decides to skip working out at the gym that evening. **[P]**

Episode 9

Angelo thinks his wife is acting very moody this week. She learns her hormonal levels are the probable cause of the infertility and that she needs to have a hysterosalpingogram. This creates a great deal of tension between the two of them, and Angelo finds the situation very stressful. Angelo also notices that his glucose levels are running consistently higher this week and has
ments with his diet a

Episode 10

No news this week.

Episode 11

Angelo has an A_{1C} test done aga
7.5%, which is higher than he typic
Angelo about her experience getting
gogram, and he is glad he was not there w
He thinks she is taking this whole pregnan
too far, but says nothing. **[P]**

Episode 12

While at work one morning this week, Angelo no
"glob" appear in the visual field of his left eye. He calls
ophthalmologist immediately and is told to come into th
office.

At the ophthalmologist's office, Angelo describes t
vision in his left eye as "patchy"—he sees multiple da
reddish-black spots. Although he is generally still able
see, he can't focus on small detail easily. Reading, fo
example, is difficult. The physician tells Angelo that he is
having another vitreous hemorrhage; however, at this
time, he is at risk for experiencing retinal detachment. H
is advised to have a vitrectomy and is scheduled for
procedure the following day as an outpatient at the h
tal. Because he will undergo general anesthesia f
procedure, he may not eat or drink anything aft
night. The procedure is scheduled for 8 a.m.

The next morning, Angelo gets up at 6
checks his blood sugar; because it is 124 mg
is not able to have breakfast before the p
decides to administer one-half of his no
dose of insulin. Angelo arrives at the h
and is taken to the outpatient surger
prepare for the procedure. At 8:30 a
waiting to go to surgery. Rachel as
the delay and is told they are waiti
it shouldn't be much longer. At
waiting in the preoperative hol
get anxious about the effect
sugar. At his request, the nur
level, and it is 108 mg/dL.

By 9:20 a.m., Angelo is
procedure is performed
12:15 p.m., Angelo is rea
scriptions for moxiflox
lution (Vigamox) and
(Pred Forte) and to

Episode 1

Angelo realizes that he and his wife have been through a great deal of stress during the past several months. With all of the work-ups and eye surgery, he believes they deserve a really nice, long vacation. He also thinks it might be good to give her something else to think about besides getting pregnant. He books a 2-week trip to Europe with a travel agent as a surprise for Rachel. The trip is nearly a year away, but he plans to have it paid off by the time they go. He decides to wait until her birthday to tell her about the trip.

Episode 2

No news this week.

Episode 3

Angelo feels badly for his wife when she has her menstrual period. He has come to believe that having a baby is just not in the cards for them. Although this disappoints him, he can envision a long and happy life without children. He wishes there was something he could do to relieve his wife of the ongoing disappointments that she experiences and wishes she could be more accepting of the situation.

Episode 4

Angelo has the A_{1C} test done this week, and his level is 6.7%. He is pleased that he continues to have excellent glycemic control. **[P]**

Episode 5

Angelo has a terrible time at the company picnic because of the smoky air conditions caused by the nearby forest fires. One of his coworkers has asthma and did not come, he suspects, because of the conditions. He is surprised that the picnic was not cancelled.

Episode 6

Angelo is shocked and very excited about Rachel finally getting pregnant. At the same time, he remains cautious, because he knows things might not work out. Angelo also quickly realizes that the 2-week vacation he secretly planned will fall around Rachel's due date, so it will have to be cancelled. He is glad he did not tell Rachel about it, or she would have felt badly. **[P]**

Episode 7

Rachel asks Angelo to go with her for her first prenatal visit. He hates to miss work, but wants to support her in every way that he can. He is excited to see the baby on the ultrasound, but then is shocked when the technician points out to them the presence of two babies. Twins! Angelo does not know what to think or say.

Episode 8

The flu has been going around the office for the past few weeks. Angelo thinks he has been spared until he wakes up in the morning on Monday feeling achy and tired. Still, he does not feel all that bad, so he decides to go to work. Throughout the day, he feels progressively worse. He leaves work in the mid-afternoon so that he can go home to lie down. Because he is not particularly hungry at dinner, he eats a small meal and accordingly gives himself a reduced dose of insulin.

By late in the evening, Angelo is vomiting and begins to run a fever. He continues to vomit well into the next day (Tuesday). His entire body aches, and he feels so tired that it's an effort to get off the bed. He sleeps off and on the entire day, only getting up to go to the bathroom to vomit and urinate. Despite not eating, his glucose level is elevated, however, he is reluctant to give himself insulin, fearing his glucose levels will plummet. By Wednesday morning, the vomiting subsides. Angelo believes he is on the road to recovery, but remains very nauseated. He begins urinating frequently, but is also drinking a large volume of fluids because he is exceedingly thirsty. Angelo knows he has some catching up to do because of the amount of fluids lost the previous day. He continues to sleep off and on.

When Rachel comes home, she takes Angelo to the Neighborhood Hospital emergency department (ED). By this time, Angelo is in no position to protest. He is treated by Dr. Gordon for acute diabetic ketoacidosis and dehydration. He is treated with fluids and insulin, and then sent home after 7 $^1/_2$ hours in the ED. **[MR] [P]**

Episode 9

Angelo is very sympathetic to the nausea and fatigue Rachel has been experiencing, particularly after his recent experience with the flu and subsequent of ketoacidosis. This impacts him somewhat, because he is used to coming home and having dinner prepared for him to eat at exactly 6 p.m. On many nights this week, Rachel has been asleep on the couch when he arrives home, and he has had to prepare dinner. This causes him to eat later than he would like (6:30 or 7 p.m.) and thus affects his workout routine on nights he goes to the gym. Angelo knows that Rachel's fatigue and nausea are temporary, and he doesn't mind making the adjustments. **[P]**

Episode 10

No news this week.

Episode 11

Angelo is happy to see that Rachel is back to her usual self. He is pleased that the pregnancy is progressing well and starts to think about how they might arrange the spare bedroom into a nursery.

Episode 12

This week is Rachel's birthday. Angelo buys her a diamond bracelet in honor her motherhood. The bracelet is expensive, but he figures this may be one of the last opportunities he has to buy his wife a nice gift. After the babies are born, assuming Rachel stays at home to care for them, they will have to make adjustments to their budget. **[P]**

Episode 13

Angelo has been busier than usual at work this past week. He has a new project that is very time consuming. To accommodate the need to increase his work hours and yet maintain his schedule, two evenings a week (after coming home and taking his insulin and eating dinner), he goes back to the office from 6:30–9:30 p.m. He is still able to have his evening snack and be in bed by 10:30 p.m. He also decides to go to his office for a few hours over the weekend. He does not like to go back to the office, but recognizes the need to stay on his regimen.

Episode 14

No news this week.

Episode 15

Rachel talks with Angelo about taking childbirth education classes in the evening next month at the Neighborhood Patient Education Center. He has heard all about such classes from his friends who have become fathers. He is interested in going, but is not so sure about the process. He is somewhat concerned that the classes will interfere with his evening dinner, insulin, and exercise regimen. He hates the thought of having to make changes when he has established a routine that works so well for him. **[P]**

ANGELO REYES
Season 3

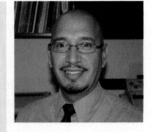

Biographical Information

Angelo Reyes is a 41-year-old Hispanic architect who has been married to Rachel for the past 4 years. Angelo considers himself to be healthy, but he has had diabetes mellitus (DM) type 1 since the age of 13. He is very compliant with diabetes management and considers it to be more of an annoyance than a real problem in his life, although he recently had an episode of diabetic ketoacidosis. He attributes his successful disease management to a very structured lifestyle. Angelo and his wife are expecting twins soon. He is anxious to become a father, but also apprehensive about the changes that are likely to take place in their lives.

Episode 1

Angelo has been going with Rachel to childbirth classes during the past couple of weeks. He has been able to adjust his schedule so that it does not interfere with his diabetes management too much. He finds the classes very informative, and they make him feel much more a part of the pregnancy. He is excited when Rachel tells him they are going to have a boy and a girl.

Angelo meets with his physician about the possibility of getting an insulin pump. He worries that, after the babies are born, he won't be able to stay on the strict schedule he has been following for all these years. After talking with the physician, he decides not to rush into anything and instead will think about it for awhile.

Episode 2

Rachel tells Angelo about the babies being in a breech position and that Dr. Tito told her to "slow down." Rachel tells Angelo that Dr. Tito obviously does not know about the real estate business. Angelo reminds Rachel that Dr. Tito does know the pregnancy business, and he encourages her to reduce her workload and cut back to part-time until the babies are born. Angelo senses that this is not what Rachel wanted to hear. **[P]**

Episode 3
No news this week.

Episode 4
Angelo gets a phone call from Rachel. She tells him that Dr. Tito wants to put her in the hospital because of some swelling and a headache, but she doesn't have time for this. Angelo becomes angry with Rachel for putting her career before her well-being and potentially the well-being of the babies. He tells her that refusing hospitalization is not an option, and she needs to do exactly what Dr. Tito suggests. **[P]**

Episode 5
Angelo can see that Rachel continues to look swollen, especially around her face. When she tells him her headaches have returned, he insists she call Dr. Tito immediately. He leaves work to take her to Dr. Tito's office. Shortly thereafter, he is on his way to the hospital with her, worried that Rachel and the babies are in danger.

Angelo is told that Rachel will have a cesarean section later in the evening. Angelo immediately begins to plan how he will manage his diabetes around the change in his schedule for the day. He is nervous all day as they wait for her surgery, as he knows the babies will be premature and is worried about their survival. He finds the hospital chapel and spends time praying for Rachel and his unborn children. He has never felt such a sense of fear and desperation in his entire life, but he knows he needs to be strong for Rachel.

Angelo is present during the delivery of his children. He is thrilled and scared at the same time. They are so tiny! They are taken to the Neonatal Intensive Care Unit shortly after birth. Angelo stays with Rachel as they complete the procedure, relieved that she is safe. **[P]**

Episode 6
Angelo is relieved that the babies seem to be doing better. The first few days were very difficult for him, because he felt as though he had no control over the situation. He also felt somewhat helpless in providing emotional comfort to Rachel. He goes with Rachel after work each evening to spend time with the babies.

Episode 7
Angelo continues to go to the hospital each evening after work to see the babies. He can see the gradual improvement in their conditions and is amazed to see how quickly they are growing.

Episode 8
No news this week.

Episode 9
Angelo is excited to know that the babies are coming home next week. His mother wants to visit at their home when the babies leave the hospital, but he is reluctant to allow her to come because she is a heavy smoker.

Episode 10
The babies are home at last. Angelo is more than willing to help Rachel, but he is just not sure how to help. He cannot believe the amount of work that goes into taking care of two tiny babies.

Angelo convinces his mother to delay her visit until the babies get a little bigger, when they will be at lower risk for an infection. Angelo's mother is offended at his request, reminding Angelo that she raised him and his brother, and did not seem to make her children sick. **[P]**

Episode 11
Angelo and Rachel continue to adjust to life with two tiny babies. Angelo feels tired from the frequent nighttime feedings and at times wishes he could just get a good night's sleep. He often feels guilty leaving the house to go to work, because Rachel is alone at home caring for the babies.

Episode 12
Rachel's mother is visiting this week. Angelo gets along well with his mother-in-law, but is hopeful she does not decide to stay for an extended visit.

Episode 13
Angelo has an A_{1C} test this week and is pleased to learn that his results are 5.4%. **[P]**

Episode 14
No news this week.

Episode 15
Angelo encourages Rachel to stay at home, rather than go back to work. He admits that finances will be tight, but feels it is the only answer; he is completely against putting Peter and Marissa in day care due to the risk of their getting sick, and he really does not want anybody else coming into their home to care for the babies.

RACHEL REYES
Season 1

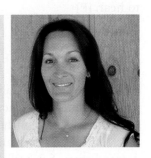

Biographical Information

Rachel is a healthy, happily married 38-year-old woman. She and her husband Angelo have been married for 3 years. It is a first marriage for both, and they have been attempting to conceive a child ever since. Rachel and Angelo have both been heavily focused on their careers all of their adult lives. Rachel works as a realtor in a large real estate company. She is physically active, tries to eat a healthy diet, only drinks alcohol occasionally, and does not use any tobacco products.

Since getting married, Rachel has been very anxious to get pregnant and start a family. She stopped taking oral contraceptives (after taking them for the previous 18 years) shortly after getting married. After one year of failing to conceive, Rachel began searching the Internet for sites related to pregnancy and infertility. Rachel's research also made her very aware of the huge expense associated with infertility work-ups and treatment, as well as the lack of insurance coverage for this expense. So, she and Angelo have been hopeful that she would get pregnant without intervention, if they just give it enough time. She learned to monitor ovulation by measuring her body temperature and has been faithfully recording these patterns, along with dates of intercourse, for the past year in a spiral notebook kept next to her bed. She also read that men who wear brief underwear may have a reduction in fertility. Despite his initial protests, Rachel was able to get Angelo to begin wearing boxer-style underwear during this past year. Although she considers adoption a potential alternative, Angelo is against this idea, citing that he is not interested in raising someone else's child.

Being acutely aware that her biological clock is ticking, Rachel has become increasingly obsessed with having a child over the past few months and has convinced Angelo that they should consult infertility specialists to help them conceive. She makes an appointment with her women's health physician for an initial infertility work-up.

Episode 1
No news this week.

Episode 2
Rachel has her first appointment with her gynecologist to discuss her concerns regarding her inability to get pregnant. During this work-up, a medical history is taken, which includes age at menarche and a description of menstrual cycles. Rachel shares with the gynecologist the notebook documenting her temperatures for the past year. The physician notes the lack of a biphasic temperature curve, suggesting inadequate hormonal function and ovulation. Rachel's history also includes evidence of rubella immunity. The doctor performs an examination, which includes a pelvic exam, Pap smear, and a culture for Chlamydia. The gynecologist refers Rachel to an infertility specialist and suggests that her husband be examined by an urologist. Despite the information about her temperature pattern suggesting hormonal dysfunction and/or a problem with ovulation, Rachel is quite sure the problem lies with Angelo, because he has type 1 diabetes mellitus. **[P]**

Episode 3
Rachel sells two homes this week and is thrilled! **[P]**

Episode 4
Angelo sees the urologist this week. Rachel wants to know everything that happened at the visit and what he learned. She is disappointed to learn that Angelo has no answers for her, and she will have to wait for the semen analysis to be completed before she knows more. Rachel learns from her gynecologist that the Pap

smear a few weeks ago was normal, and the culture was negative.

Episode 5

No news this week.

Episode 6

Rachel has her first appointment with the infertility specialist. During this initial visit, a through history is taken. Rachel shares with the physician the ovulation charts she has maintained and the results of Angelo's semen analysis. The physician outlines the general plan for the infertility work-up and explains that the process is not only expensive, but very long and drawn out, which can be very frustrating. The diagnostic process could take several months and require time away from work to complete the exams. The following blood tests will be run at one time: thyroid and androgen levels; daily blood samples for follicle stimulating hormone (FSH), luteinizing hormone (LH), and progesterone; and prolactin levels for 1 month to evaluate hormonal production and regulation. The physician suggests that Rachel begin these tests within a couple days of starting her next menstrual cycle. Other planned tests include a postcoital exam, hysterosalpingogram, endometrial biopsy, and laparoscopy. Rachel assures the physician that she and Angelo want to proceed. **[P]**

Episode 7

No news this week.

Episode 8

Rachel has scheduled a postcoital exam this week, because she is expected to ovulate within the next few days. The test will assess the quality of the cervical mucus and characteristics of the sperm. Rachel and Angelo were instructed to abstain from intercourse for several days prior to the exam. Because the sample of cervical mucus must be obtained within a few hours of intercourse, Angelo needs to come home during the middle of the work day to accommodate Rachel's 1 p.m. appointment.

Episode 9

Rachel has a follow-up visit with the infertility specialist to discuss the lab results. Her thyroid and androgen levels are within normal range. Her follicle stimulating hormone (FSH) level failed to rise early in the cycle, the luteinizing hormone (LH) level failed to rise mid-cycle, and the progesterone level failed to rise at end of the cycle. The prolactin level is normal. The results from the postcoital exam show that the sperm are

mobile, and the cervical mucus is thicker than expected. The physician tells Rachel that these results point to a probable imbalance in hormonal regulation as the cause of the infertility. She wants to complete the other diagnostic tests, however, to rule out other coexisting problems. **[P]**

Episode 10

No news this week.

Episode 11

Rachel is scheduled for a hysterosalpingogram to visualize her uterus and fallopian tubes. This test needs to be done within one week following menses. Although Rachel wanted to do this test last month, but she was out of town at a realtor continuing education program. Rachel's test is scheduled for 9 a.m. She plans on taking the early part of the morning off from work, with the intention of being in the office by late morning.

On the day of the test, there are scheduling problems at the radiology office, because one of the technicians called in sick. Rachel is furious at the suggestion that her appointment be rescheduled for the following month. She yells at the receptionist, telling her that she MUST have this test today. The receptionist tells Rachel that, if she is willing to wait, they could probably work her in, but it would likely be in the afternoon. Rachel agrees to wait. She calls work and tells them she is not sure when she will be in, but that she will come as soon as she can. Rachel's test is finally done at 3 p.m.; following the test, Rachel just goes home. **[VC]**

Episode 12

Angelo has a problem with his eye, requiring outpatient surgery. Rachel takes a day off from work to take him to his procedure and then take care of him at home afterward. Angelo is scheduled to have his procedure at 8 a.m. At 8:30 a.m., he is still in the pre-op holding area. Rachel asks the nurses what they are waiting for and is told they are just waiting for the doctor to arrive. At 9 a.m., they are still waiting in pre-op holding, and Rachel can see that Angelo is getting a bit anxious about his blood sugar. She goes to the nurses' desk and begins yelling at the staff, telling them that her husband is a diabetic and can't lie there all day without eating. The nurses attempt to apologize, but Rachel isn't interested in hearing their excuses. When the operating room technician comes to take Angelo into surgery, Rachel lets her know the delay in the surgery is unacceptable. The technician is annoyed with Rachel and could care less what she thinks.

Later in the day, after they are home from the hospital, Rachel gets a phone call from her physician, informing her that the results of her hysterosalpingogram are normal. **[P]**

Episode 13
Rachel has an endometrial biopsy performed to evaluate the quality of her uterine lining. Rachel experiences pain and cramping during and after the procedure, so she takes the rest of the day off from work. **[P]**

Episode 14
Rachel receives a follow-up report from the endometrial biopsy that the results are normal. This week, she has her laparoscopy procedure, which she hopes will be the last diagnostic test. The laparoscopy shows no evidence of endometriosis.

Episode 15
No news this week.

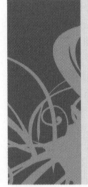

RACHEL REYES
Season 2

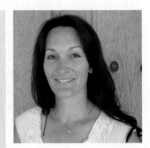

Biographical Information

Rachel is a healthy, happily married 38-year-old woman. She and her husband Angelo have been married for 3 years, and they have been attempting to conceive a child ever since. She has been working with an infertility specialist during the past several months. It has been a very exhausting and expensive experience, but Rachel remains hopeful that she will be able to conceive.

Rachel and Angelo have both been heavily focused on their careers all of their adult lives. Rachel works as a realtor in a large real estate company. She is physically active, tries to eat a healthy diet, only drinks alcohol occasionally, and does not use any tobacco products.

Episode 1
This week, Rachel has another appointment with her infertility specialist. The physician reviews the tests performed and the results, and explains the next steps to take. The decision is made to start Rachel on a prescription of clomiphene citrate (Clomid). She is told that, because this drug stimulates ovarian activity, there is an increased risk of multiple pregnancies. Rachel has already read about Clomid and is anxious to get started. The physician tells her that, with luck, she might become pregnant in the next few months. Rachel purchases several home ovulation test kits on the way home from her appointment so that she can plan intercourse to coincide with ovulation cycles.

Episode 2
No news this week.

Episode 3
It has been 4 weeks since Rachel's last period. She has been performing a home pregnancy test every day to see if she has become pregnant. When she starts her period this week, Rachel is devastated and misses work. She attributes the failure to get pregnant this month to working too many hours. **[P]**

Episode 4
Rachel continues to feel sad that she did not get pregnant. She wants the medication to work, but is also aware that, if she does not get pregnant after 4–6 cycles, it is not likely to work. She thinks about getting pregnant nearly all the time and worries about what to do next if the medication is not successful.

Episode 5
Rachel and Angelo go to a picnic with Angelo's architectural firm this week. However, the nearby forest fire causes the air conditions to be very bad, so they leave early. Almost everyone at the picnic is feeling the effects of the air. Rachel has a mild cough after being out in the smoky air all day. She worries that inhaling the smoky air might be a reason the Clomid is not effective.

Episode 6
This week, Rachel tests positive for pregnancy with one of her home tests. She runs the test a second time to be sure it is positive. She is so excited that she calls Angelo at work to tell him the news and also calls the physician's office. She is asked to come in the following day to confirm the pregnancy. The following morning, Rachel runs another

home pregnancy test as soon as she wakes up to be sure she is still pregnant. At the infertility specialist's office, Rachel's pregnancy is confirmed with yet another pregnancy test. She is referred to Dr. Gayle Tito at Neighborhood Women's Health Specialists for prenatal care, because of her expertise in working with older pregnant women. It is suggested that Rachel schedule a prenatal visit within a few weeks. **[P]**

Episode 7

Rachel has her first prenatal visit with Dr. Tito. She asks Angelo to go with her for moral support. During the visit, a comprehensive history and examination are completed. Rachel is shocked when she is told that it appears as though they will have twins. She knew that was a possibility, but really did not believe that it would happen. **[MR]**

Episode 8

Angelo stays home sick with the flu for a couple of days. On Wednesday, Rachel has a home showing that lasts until late afternoon; when she finally gets home at 6 p.m., she is shocked at how Angelo looks. He is lethargic, very flushed, and breathing very fast. Rachel knows he is in trouble and needs to take him to the Neighborhood Hospital emergency department.

Rachel spends the entire evening into the early hours the following morning with Angelo while he is treated for ketoacidosis. It scares her to think about what might have happened if she had not come home when she did. It also makes her realize how fragile Angelo is when he becomes ill.

Episode 9

Rachel has begun to adjust to the idea of having twins. She knows that she is not the first person in the world to have the experience, but worries that it will be difficult. She has been feeling very tired and nauseated. She knew to expect this, but did not realize just how nauseated and fatigued one might get with a pregnancy. She suspects that having twins and the busy schedule she keeps contribute to her symptoms all the more. She has another prenatal visit with Dr. Tito this week. **[P] [MR]**

Episode 10

No news this week.

Episode 11

At long last, the nausea that Rachel has been experiencing has begun to subside. She has another prenatal visit and is pleased that her pregnancy seems to be progressing well. **[P] [MR]**

Episode 12

Rachel celebrates her 39th birthday this week. She thinks the bracelet Angelo bought for her is beautiful, but worries about how much he might have spent on it. Rachel is enjoying a very busy and successful month as a realtor. She has been able to sell five homes—an all-time record for her. She is pleased that her client base and number of referrals are growing; at the same time, she is beginning to realize that much of the work that has gone into her business will be for nothing after she has the babies. She is thrilled about being pregnant, but also aware of what she will lose. **[P]**

Episode 13

Rachel regularly feels her babies move. She finds the sensation strange, yet pleasant. She does not have any nausea at this point, but she has been experiencing constipation and continues to feel tired. Rachel has her 18-week prenatal visit. **[P] [MR]**

Episode 14

No news this week.

Episode 15

It has been a very busy week for Rachel. She picks up two new clients and is working hard to arrange to show them homes. She has been frustrated with one client to whom she has now shown over 40 homes in the past 3 weeks; still, he cannot seem to make up his mind. At this point, she is not sure she will ever find him something he is willing to buy. Fortunately, Rachel has had more energy than she has had in weeks.

Rachel sees Dr. Tito again this week for a prenatal visit. She talks with Angelo about getting signed up for childbirth education classes at the Neighborhood Patient Education Center. **[MR]**

RACHEL REYES
Season 3

Biographical Information

Rachel is a healthy, happily married 39-year-old woman. She and her husband Angelo have been married for 4 years (a first marriage for both). Rachel and Angelo are pregnant with twins after years of unsuccessful attempts. Rachel is very excited about becoming a mother. Rachel and Angelo have both been heavily focused on their careers all of their adult lives. Rachel works as a realtor in a large real estate company. She has been trying to decide what to do about her career once the babies are born. She is looking into the possibility of working part-time so that she can spend time with her babies, without completely giving up her career.

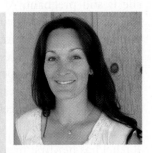

Episode 1

Rachel's pregnancy continues to progress, and she continues to maintain a busy work schedule. Overall she has been feeling well, except that she has noticed swelling in her hands and feet at the end of the day and has been having intermittent contractions. She and Angelo have been going to childbirth classes, and Rachel has decided that she will breastfeed her infants, although she isn't sure how one does this with twins. She sees Dr. Tito this week for her 28-week prenatal visit. An ultrasound shows that the babies are growing—and that she is going to have a boy and a girl. **[MR] [P]**

Episode 2

Dr. Tito has asked Rachel to come in every 2 weeks for prenatal visits at this point in her pregnancy. During this visit, Rachel shares with Dr. Tito that the swelling in her hands and feet has increased. She also tells Dr. Tito that the babies are very active and admits to occasional uterine contractions. During the examination, Dr. Tito determines that Rachel's babies are in a breech position.

Dr. Tito talks with Rachel about her work schedule and learns that she has been as busy as ever as her real estate business has grown. She tells Rachel that she really should reduce her work schedule, or at least slow down and find time during the day for rest. Rachel wonders how she will be able to cut back her hours at this point without giving her clients to other realtors. **[MR] [VC]**

Episode 3

No news this week.

Episode 4

Rachel has done little to cut back on her work schedule. She has built in two 30-minute periods during the day when she lies down on a couch in her real estate office, however, she finds this to be a huge inconvenience.

Rachel has her 32-week appointment with Dr. Tito this week. She reports that the swelling in her hands and feet has not improved (despite resting like the doctor advised), that her face feels puffy, and that she has had a headache for the past couple of days. She also admits to continued intermittent contractions. Dr. Tito, concerned about the symptoms, the observed edema, the elevated blood pressure, and the protein in her urine, strongly recommends that Rachel be admitted to the hospital to rule out preeclampsia. Rachel tells Dr. Tito she has a couple of closings later in the day, but perhaps she could be admitted the following day. After Rachel talks with Angelo, she agrees to the admission.

Rachel stays in the hospital for 48 hours. During this brief hospitalization, the headaches go away, and the edema decreases. Rachel's liver enzymes are found to be elevated, she has protein in her urine, and she continues to have edema in her feet. She is given steroids (betamethasone 12 mg intramuscularly once a day for 2 days) to help the babies' lungs develop, in case they are born prematurely. Rachel is told that the babies are still in a breech position and that she must rest to avoid serious complications. She arranges to begin her maternity leave immediately, deciding selling homes is not worth the risk of having further problems with this pregnancy. **[MR] [VC]**

Episode 5

The headaches and facial puffiness that Rachel experienced last week have returned. She takes a couple of Tylenol tablets, but they are not effective. Rachel is evaluated by Dr. Tito, who immediately admits her to the hospital. Upon admission, a few blood tests are run. Her blood pressure is in the 160/100 mm Hg range. After the test results come back, she is told her liver enzymes are worsening (the fibrinogen and platelet count has dropped). Dr. Tito explains that

Rachel has developed HELLP syndrome (*h*emolysis, *e*levated *l*iver enzyme *l*evels and a *l*ow *p*latelet count) and needs to have a cesarean section delivery in the early evening. She is told she may not eat or drink anything until after the surgery. Rachel is glad she saw a video about this in the prenatal class so that she had an idea of what to expect.

A magnesium sulfate drip is started, causing Rachel to feel hot and panicky. She is assured by the nurse that these symptoms will subside after the initial bolus is in. A neonatal nurse practitioner visits Rachel and Angelo to inform them about what to expect after delivery. They are told the babies will be in the neonatal intensive care unit (NICU), and the couple will be allowed to visit them and ask questions. The nurse encourages breastfeeding the babies and discusses the use of a breast pump.

Rachel cries off and on all day, blaming herself for putting the babies in this position. If they do not survive, she would never forgive herself, and she is sure Angelo would never forgive her either. In the early evening, Dr Tito successfully delivers both infants by cesarean section. Rachel sees her babies, briefly noting that they both have black hair, before they are taken to the NICU. She asks if they are okay, but is only told that they will be evaluated immediately. Rachel is glad Angelo is with her. **[MR] [P]**

Episode 6

When Rachel is discharged from the hospital, she feels cheated because she cannot bring the babies home. She goes to the hospital every day in the morning and at night to see them, and Angelo accompanies her every evening. She is using the breast pump every 3 hours. She is happy that she is producing breast milk for her babies and is thrilled when she is allowed to hold them for the first time.

Rachel has a postpartum check-up with Dr. Tito this week. Although she generally feels well, she reports feeling easily fatigued. Her blood pressure is now 128/82 mm Hg, and her incision is healing well. She is reminded not to lift heavy objects or drive for several weeks. Contraception is discussed with Rachel, but she doesn't think she will need it, because she needed Clomid to get pregnant to begin with. **[P]**

Episode 7

Rachel is pleased that Peter and Marissa are doing so well and learns that they should be able to go home in a few weeks. She continues to make trips to the hospital every day, spending as much time as she can with them. With the help of a lactation consultant, she begins to breastfeed the babies. She comes to know the nurses very well and has developed an interest in the work they do. Rachel considers her job as a realtor; although she has always enjoyed it and has been successful at it, she begins to think about the possibility of going to nursing school in the future. As she watches the nurses interact with the parents and care for the infants, she perceives this to be a much more fulfilling career than selling homes. **[P]**

Episode 8

No news this week.

Episode 9

Peter and Marissa remain at the hospital, but have made steady progress. Rachel is told by the nurses that she can expect to take them home in the next week or so.

Episode 10

Rachel and Angelo are finally able to bring Peter and Marissa home. Rachel is instructed to feed them every 2–4 hours, alternating between breast and bottle feedings, until they are breastfeeding well. Rachel and Angelo quickly learn about the fatigue associated with infants; with twins, it seems at times to be overwhelming. They are told to keep the infants home as much as possible, to keep them away from smoking, to keep them away from anybody who is sick, and to practice good hand washing. They are given information about car safety seats as well. Two days after the babies' discharge, Rachel takes them to see Carolyn Marquette, the pediatric nurse practitioner at Neighborhood Pediatrics for a follow-up visit. **[VC]**

Episode 11

Rachel has another follow-up visit with Dr. Tito this week. Her blood pressure is now 122/72 mm Hg, and her incision has completely healed. A Pap smear is done, and she is told she does not have to return for another visit for a year, unless problems arise. She admits to Dr. Tito that she feels pretty tired; now that the babies are home, she is not getting much sleep. **[P]**

Episode 12

Rachel takes the babies to see Carolyn Marquette, the pediatric nurse practitioner at Neighborhood Pediatrics, for another appointment. She is pleased to learn that the babies continue to gain weight. Her mother comes from out of town to spend the week at their home to help her. Rachel is glad to have the help, because she feels so tired, but at the same time she feels the need to constantly watch her mother to be sure she washes her hands before touching the babies. **[P]**

Episode 13

Rachel takes the babies to Neighborhood Pediatrics for their 2-month immunizations this week. Carolyn Marquette, the pediatric nurse practitioner, tells Rachel about the need to give the babies palivizumab (Synagis), an immunization to prevent RSV, the following month. They will need to have this immunization every month for five doses. The shot, she is told, is very expensive, so Rachel needs to check with her insurance company to ensure coverage. **[VC]**

Episode 14

No news this week.

Episode 15

Rachel's maternity leave is up at the end of next week. Her boss at the real estate office has left a message on her phone, telling her they are all looking forward to her return to work. Deep down, Rachel believes that she should give up her career to care for her babies. Although she loves her career, she feels strongly that Peter and Marissa are now her top priority. She explores the possibility of not going back to work and adjusting to one income.

Rachel and Angelo get a letter from the insurance company, denying coverage for the $3,500.00 Synagis immunizations; they are told they will have to cover this expense on their own. Rachel makes a call to the nurse practitioner to inquire about this situation.

PETER AND MARISSA REYES
Season 3

Biographical Information

Peter and Marissa Reyes were born at 33 weeks' gestation to Rachel and Angelo Reyes. Peter weighed 1,600 grams, and Marissa weighed 1,750 grams. Peter was 42 cm long, with a head circumference of 31 cm; Marissa was 42.5 cm, with a head circumference of 31.5 cm. They were born prematurely as a result of their mother's preeclampsia.

Episode 5

Peter and Marissa Reyes come into the world this week at 6:52 p.m. on Thursday at 33 weeks' gestation. At birth, Peter and Marissa have Apgar scores of 6 and 7 at 1 minute, respectively; at 5 minutes, their scores are 7 and 7. They are briefly introduced to their mother and father before being taken to the NICU for evaluation and stabilization.

In the NICU, they are dried off, weighed, placed under a warmer, and examined by the neonatal nurse practitioner, who notes that the findings are consistent with 33 weeks' gestation. Because the infants become slightly dusky during the exam, blow-by oxygen is administered, and their color pinks up. Over the next 15 minutes, however, Peter begins to exhibit grunting and nasal flaring, and his oxygen saturation level drops to 84%. Respiratory therapy is called, and the technician initiates continuous positive airway pressure (CPAP). Blood gasses and chest x-ray reveal that Peter is developing respiratory distress syndrome. The neonatal nurse practitioner intubates him and administers surfactant down the endotracheal (ET) tube, followed by bagging. Additional surfactant is administered for a few minutes, and the ET tube is removed.

Oxygen is administered at $^1/_4$ liter by nasal cannula, and his symptoms resolve. Peter's oxygen saturation improves to 92%. Marissa's oxygen saturation remains stable at 94% on nasal cannula oxygen. Both of their body temperatures remain stable.

In addition to temperature and respiratory support, Peter and Marissa require nutrition and fluid support. Screening glucose levels are drawn; Marissa's glucose is 55 mg/dL, whereas Peter's is only 24 mg/dL. A bolus of D10W intravenous solution is administered to Peter, followed by a continuous infusion. An hour later, Peter's glucose is 44 mg/dL. Both infants are supported on peripheral parental nutrition (D12.5% with 2% amino acids) for several days.

The infants begin to exhibit yellowing of the face when they are 36 hours old, prompting a bilirubin assessment. Marissa and Peter's bilirubin levels are 6.0 mg/dL and 6.8 mg/dL, respectively. The following morning, their bilirubin levels climb to 12 mg/dL and 13 mg/dL, respectively, requiring phototherapy. Their eyes are covered and, wearing only a diaper, they are placed in an isolette for 3 days. Over that time, their bilirubin levels slowly decrease.

Episode 6

Peter and Marissa remain at the hospital. At the beginning of the week, their weights are 1,550 and 1,600 grams, respectively. They remain on peripheral parental nutrition (PPN) for several days and then graduate to feedings fortified with breast milk through a feeding tube. Both babies average intake is about 150 mL/kg/day. They also both have an ultrasound to rule out intraventricular hemorrhage; the findings are negative.

Episode 7

Peter and Marissa gain steady weight this week. Peter now weighs 1,625 grams, and Marissa weighs 1,700 grams. They have improved with their feedings and are now taking approximately 250 mL/day.

Episode 8

No news this week.

Episode 9

Peter and Marissa continue to do well in the hospital. Peter's weight is up to 1,800 grams, and Marissa's weight is 1,900 grams.

Episode 10

Peter and Marissa come home from the hospital this week. They are seen 2 days after discharge by the pediatric nurse practitioner. Their weights are 2 kg and 2.1 kg, respectively.

Episode 11

No news this week.

Episode 12

Peter and Marissa remain healthy and both are making good progress in weight and doing well with breastfeeding.

Episode 13

Peter and Marissa are now 2 months old. During an office visit, Peter weighs in at 2.8 kg, and Marissa weighs 3.0 kg. They receive their immunizations (HBV, DTaP, Hib, IPV, and PCV).

Episode 14

No news this week.

Episode 15

No news this week.

EVELYN RILEY HOUSEHOLD

EVELYN RILEY FAMILY STORY OVERVIEW

Character	Season 1	Season 2	Season 3
EVELYN RILEY	This story focuses on the experiences of a mother struggling to help her children. She is very concerned about the welfare of her grandson Ryan and does what she can to help care for him whenever Jessica will allow her to. She also experiences frustration trying to get help for her son Jason. She knows he has academic and social problems, but can't seem to get help.	Evelyn increases the amount of time she cares for her grandson and has a growing concern for the welfare of her pregnant daughter Jessica. Evelyn also continues to try to get help for Jason. She is finally able to get a neuropsychologist referral, and he validates her concerns and is willing treat Jason. Evelyn is also concerned about her other daughter Jenna's weight gain.	Evelyn continues to support Jessica by caring for both of her grandchildren (Ryan and Carrie). Jessica eventually gets out of her relationship with Casey, reconciles with Evelyn, and moves back home. Evelyn's other concerns continue to focus on her son Jason and daughter Jenna, who has a new diagnosis of type 2 diabetes mellitus.
JENNA RILEY	Jenna is a healthy but overweight and self-conscious teenager. Although she has many friends, she experiences rejection by them at times. She excels in academics. This story focuses on her experiences related to being an overweight 14-year-old.	Jenna continues to have problems with her weight and is affected by the problems her sister and brother experience. She reacts to stress by eating, causing her to continue to gain weight. Her mother has quit buying junk food, but Jenna gets the food she craves at school.	The school nurse notices Jenna's weight gain. Jenna has a medical evaluation and is diagnosed with type 2 DM. The rest of the story in this season depicts issues related to diabetic management of an adolescent.
JASON RILEY	Jason has a history of academic and behavioral problems at school. His mother has been trying to get help for him for some time, but with no luck. It is determined that he needs glasses, but these don't resolve the problems at school.	Jason's problems at school continue. He gets into fights frequently and does poor academically. He is finally referred to a neuropsychologist, who diagnoses Jason with ADHD. Jason starts taking Ritalin, and an IEP is developed at school.	After adjusting to new medication and the IEP, Jason slowing begins to make academic progress, and his social skills improve. He begins to make a couple of friends.

CONCEPTS   *Body Image, Cognition, Family Dynamics, Interpersonal Relationships, Intrapersonal Violence, Metabolism, Nutrition, Pain, Role Performance, Sensory/Perceptual*

EVELYN RILEY
Season 1

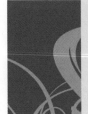

Biographical Information

Evelyn is a 38-year-old single mother in good health. Her ex-husband left Evelyn and her children about 10 years ago. She has never remarried and is not currently involved in a romantic relationship. Although she receives a small amount of child support from her ex-husband on a regular basis, he has had very little contact with her or the children in the past 10 years; in fact, he has not

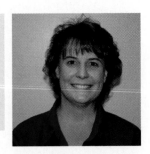

Continued

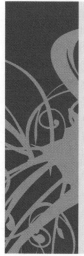

seen his children for over 8 years. Evelyn works out of her home as a medical transcriptionist. She supplements her income by working at a retail store at the mall in the evenings a few nights each week.

Evelyn has three children. Her oldest, Jessica Riley, is 17 and a new mother. Evelyn's relationship with Jessica was good until Jessica became an adolescent. Since that time, it has been very strained, especially after Jessica became pregnant. Jessica moved out of the house when she was 6 months pregnant to an apartment a short distance away. At this point, Evelyn tries to help her daughter by taking care of her baby Ryan when Jessica goes to school and sometimes in the evening. Evelyn's other children, Jenna (14) and Jason (11), live in the home with her. Evelyn has been frustrated by the ongoing school and social problems that Jason has been experiencing. For the past year, she has been attempting to get an appropriate referral to help him, but feels she has been going in circles within the system.

Episode 1
No news this week.

Episode 2
Evelyn is asked by Jessica to babysit Ryan for a few hours in the evening so that she can go to her friend's house for a party. Evelyn begins to become concerned when Jessica fails to pick up the baby by midnight. Jessica finally calls about 1:30 a.m. and tells her mother that she will just pick up Ryan in the morning. Evelyn is angry with Jessica because of her lack of responsibility.

Jason is involved in another fight at school this week. Evelyn is asked to come in for a counseling session with the teacher, principal, and counselor. The counselor suggests that Jason's behavioral issues are related to poor or inconsistent discipline in the home. Evelyn verbalizes that she disagrees and believes that he has some sort of learning problem. She requests that Jason be tested. **[P]**

Episode 3
Evelyn goes with Jessica to take Ryan for his 2-month well-baby visit. Jessica tells her mother that her new boyfriend Casey is going to move in with her, so Evelyn will only need to watch Ryan during the daytime. Evelyn expresses concern and says she's happy to continue caring for Ryan. Jessica tells her mother that she can raise her own baby. **[P]**

Episode 4
Jason comes home with a note from his teacher that he failed to complete his volcano project and that Evelyn needs to ensure that he completes his homework. Evelyn was not aware that Jason even had a volcano project—this was the first she had heard of it. Evelyn also gets a phone call from the school nurse, Violet Brinkworth, telling her that Jason's vision is only 20/100 in both eyes. The nurse suggests that she take Jason for an eye examination.

Episode 5
Evelyn takes Jason to an optometrist this week, who determines that he needs glasses. Evelyn hopes that the glasses will help Jason do better in school. Despite her optimism, she knows deep down that Jason has some kind of learning problem and wishes she could get him some help. Evelyn makes sure Jason gets his homework completed each night this week, but it is a major task. **[P]**

Episode 6
Evelyn is concerned about her grandson Ryan. She voices her concerns to Jessica, including the facts that Ryan does not seem to be gaining much weight and that he often looks dirty —specifically, he has dried milk on his neck, and his clothes are not clean. Evelyn also questions whether living with Casey is in Jessica and Ryan's best interest. Jessica gets very defensive and angry, accusing her mother of disliking Casey and trying to make her feel dumb. Jessica tells her mother that, if she continues to criticize her, she won't let her take care of the baby anymore. Evelyn decides it is best to back off, fearing that she won't be allowed to take care of Ryan. **[P]**

Episode 7
No news this week.

Episode 8
Evelyn arranges a party for Jason and several of his classmates in an attempt to help him make friends. Only a few kids show up at the party, and Evelyn notices that few interact directly with Jason. She continues to feel frustrated with Jason over the ongoing homework battles. She notices that his complaints of headaches have stopped, but the problems with schoolwork remain. The assistant scoutmaster, Pat Richman, tells her that Jason had a "meltdown" at the Boy Scout meeting this week. **[P]**

Episode 9
No news this week.

Episode 10
Ryan is 6 months old this week. Evelyn gets Jessica's permission to take Ryan to his well-baby check-up and to get immunizations. The pediatrician tells Evelyn that Ryan is falling a bit behind on his weight and to feed him more. Evelyn again tries to talk to Jessica about Ryan's care, but Jessica tells her mother to shut up and mind her own business.

Evelyn receives a phone call from the principal's office at Jason's school, because Jason was involved in another fight. She feels at her wit's end with her son; she just can't seem to control him at times. She talks with the school counselor again about getting a referral to a neuropsychologist. The counselor continues to suggest that the problems seem to be the result of inadequate discipline, but agrees that a medical problem might explain some things. Evelyn is advised to start with her family physician. Evelyn schedules an appointment with Dr. Rowe to see if she can be of any help in Jason's situation. **[VC]**

Episode 11
Evelyn learns this week that Jessica is pregnant again and has quit school. Evelyn tells Jessica that the last thing she needs right now is another baby. She has another fight with Jessica about the fact that she is going nowhere in life and needs to get her act together.

Evelyn takes Jason to Dr. Rowe, the family physician, to see if she can offer any help with Jason's ongoing problems. Dr. Rowe's initial response to Evelyn as she discusses the problems is one of skepticism. She tells Evelyn that most 10-year-old boys are hard to control, and Jason will outgrow the problems, but she needs to discipline him more. Evelyn is furious with the accusation and frustrated by the lack of response she is experiencing. She specifically requests a referral to a neuropsychologist, but Dr. Rowe does not feel it is indicated at this time.

Episode 12
This week, Jason's Boy Scout leader tells Evelyn that Jason is no longer welcome to participate in the troop because he bit one of the other scouts during a meeting. **[VC]**

Episode 13
No news this week.

Episode 14
Evelyn, Jenna, and Jason go out of town to visit Evelyn's mother and are gone all week. Evelyn does not find out about Ryan's illness until they return.

Episode 15
Jessica tells her mother that she has found a new preschool for Ryan to attend during the daytime, and wonders if Evelyn can babysit Ryan in the evenings. Despite the fact that this would cut into her hours working at the mall, Evelyn agrees to do this, knowing it will be in Ryan's best interest.

EVELYN RILEY
Season 2

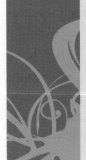

Biographical Information
Evelyn is a 39-year-old single mother in good health. Her ex-husband left Evelyn and her children about 10 years ago. She has never remarried and is not currently involved in a romantic relationship. Although she receives a small amount of child support from her ex-husband on a regular basis, he has had very little contact with her or the children in the past 10 years; in fact, he has not seen his children for over 8 years. Evelyn works out of her home as a medical transcriptionist. She supplements her income by working at a retail store at the mall in the evenings a few nights each week.

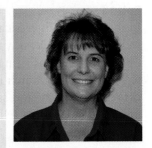

Continued

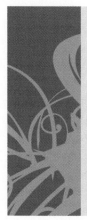

Evelyn has three children. Her oldest, Jessica Riley (18), is the mother of a 10-month-old son and is expecting another baby. Evelyn's relationship with Jessica was good until Jessica became an adolescent. Since that time, it has been very strained. Jessica lives in a one-bedroom apartment with her son Ryan and boyfriend Casey. Evelyn does not like Casey and fears for her daughter and grandson's safety. She helps Jessica as much as possible by taking care of Ryan when Jessica works in the evenings. Evelyn's other children, Jenna and Jason, live in the home with her. Evelyn has been frustrated by the ongoing school and social problems that Jason has been experiencing. For the past year, she has been attempting to get an appropriate referral to help him, but feels she has been going in circles within the system.

Episode 1

No news this week.

Episode 2

Evelyn spends most of her day catching up with medical transcription work. She works 3 evenings at the mall and takes care of Ryan two evenings this week. She feels exhausted!

Episode 3

Evelyn receives a call from the school, informing her that Jason has been involved in another fight. The school administrators request that she come to the school immediately for a meeting. At the meeting, the principal and counselor suggest that they might need to expel Jason because of his ongoing behavioral issues. Evelyn becomes very angry and recaps the effort she has made, pointing out that she has been attempting to get help for her son for the past couple of years, but has met resistance every step of the way—both from the school and in the community. Evelyn suggests that, before the school decides to expel her son, perhaps they should pay attention to the needs of the students and actually try to facilitate a solution to the problem.

The school counselor looks back over the Jason's file, considers what Evelyn has said, and admits that perhaps they have not been as helpful as they could have been. The counselor vows to help Evelyn with a referral to a neuropsychologist.

Episode 4

Evelyn notices the weight Jenna has been gaining and suggests to her that she stop eating so many snacks and try to get some exercise after school. Evelyn tells Jenna that she will only buy two bags of chips a week at the store, so she needs to make them last. She also decides to start making Jenna her lunches to ensure that she eats healthy foods at lunch. Jenna tells her mother that she is too tired after a long day of school to feel much like exercising. Evelyn hopes that Jenna passes this "teenage laziness phase" soon. **[P]**

Episode 5

No news this week.

Episode 6

Evelyn takes Jason to his first appointment with the neuropsychologist. Jason meets with the psychologist independently first and then with Evelyn. The psychologist asks for Evelyn's permission to obtain copies of Jason's school records, which would provide a history from the school system's perspective about his behavioral issues. The neuropsychologist also obtains permission from Evelyn and Jason to talk with his current and former teachers. **[P]**

Episode 7

Evelyn invites Jessica to the house for a family get-together. She is relieved when Jessica and Ryan arrive at the house without Casey.

Episode 8

Jessica asks Evelyn if she can watch Ryan each night this week, explaining that she needs to get more hours in to pay some bills, because Casey is out of work again. Evelyn agrees to do this and arranges for Jenna to watch Ryan while she works her shifts at the mall. Although she is angry that Jessica must work more hours, she is glad that Casey is not taking care of Ryan.

Evelyn takes Jason for his second visit to the neuropsychologist, who interviews Evelyn regarding Jason's behavior at home. Evelyn tells him that Jason is impulsive, can't attend to homework for more than 15 minutes at a time, has a hard time getting organized, and frequently forgets books and homework. The psychologist shares with Evelyn what he learned from the school records. She is angry to hear that there is repeated documentation of references to her child as obstinate and mean-spirited. One entry even implies that the school might consider investigating his home situation. **[VC]**

Episode 9

No news this week.

Episode 10

This week Evelyn takes Jason to another appointment with the neuropsychologist. After meeting with Jason, the psychologist shares with Evelyn that he has contacted Jason's previous and current teachers. He tells Evelyn that he is impressed by the consistency of the descriptions from the past three teachers regarding what they perceive to be Jason's challenges: unable to attend to tasks, distracted, can only attend to a task for 5–10 minutes, does best in very structured situation (especially if they remove distractions and provide frequent prompts), and seems to do best in a consistent routine. These symptoms suggest attention deficit hyperactivity disorder (ADHD).

Evelyn agrees with this analysis, because it is consistent with what she sees at home. She is relieved that somebody finally believes her and that there really is a problem other than a lack of discipline. The psychologist suggests medication and environmental modifications in the classroom. He also suggests family counseling—primarily to benefit Evelyn, because it is hard to be a single mother of a child with ADHD. Evelyn agrees to talk with the school to see what kinds of modifications can be made available for her son. She is not so sure about having Jason take medication, because she has heard many negative things about methylphenidate (Ritalin). **[VC]**

Episode 11

Evelyn takes her grandson Ryan to the pediatrician's office because of poor eating, fever, and congestion. She does not want to take the chance of Ryan becoming severely ill again.

This week, Evelyn tells the principal about the ADHD diagnosis made by the neuropsychologist and the need for classroom accommodations. The principal and counselor are relieved to hear that there may be a way to help Jason. They request additional testing in the district office.

Episode 12

Evelyn takes Jason down to the school district offices for additional testing. She is so glad to finally be getting the cooperation she felt she should have had two years ago. **[P]**

Episode 13

Evelyn gets a phone call from Jessica, who is crying. Jessica tells her mother that she is going to the hospital in an ambulance and needs her to pick up Ryan from her apartment. Evelyn later learns that Casey has been arrested and is suspected of injuring Jessica. She is relieved when she learns that Jessica's baby is born healthy. Evelyn hopes Jessica will get away from that creep now. **[P]**

Episode 14

Evelyn is thrilled to see and hold her new granddaughter Carrie, but is disappointed when Jessica tells her that she and Casey have worked things out. She wants to shake sense into her daughter, but at the same time feels helpless. She worries about the safety of her daughter and her two grandchildren and is glad Social Service is following up on the situation.

Evelyn attends a meeting with the school nurse, counselor, principal, teacher, and neuropsychologist to set forth an individualized educational plan (IEP) for Jason. In this plan, recommendations are made by the professionals and the school system to structure the classroom and assignments. The purpose of the IEP is to establish specific goals for Jason during the academic year. Because he has poor reading skills, one goal that everyone agrees to is for Jason to read at his grade level. Another goal is to improve his social skills and to become more accepted by his peers. Finally, it is suggested that he focus on self-management skills, such as remembering to bring home and turn in homework. The neuropsychologist suggests that Jason's desk be placed in the classroom away from the window and that he be given two sets of textbooks—one for home and one for school. Furthermore, additional hands-on activities to increase Jason's academic engagement are recommended, as is a quiet environment for testing. It is also again suggested that Jason start taking methylphenidate (Ritalin), which the psychologist strongly believes is necessary for Jason to make progress. **[P]**

Episode 15

Jason is started on Ritalin this week. Evelyn has reluctantly agreed to this, but is still somewhat concerned. She has read that Ritalin is "overused" and has become a way for society to control energetic children. Although she knows deep down that her son needs help, she wonders if drug therapy is the right answer.

EVELYN RILEY
Season 3

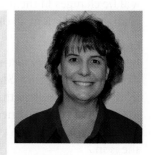

Biographical Information

Evelyn is a 39-year-old single mother in good health. Her ex-husband left Evelyn and her children about 11 years ago. She has never remarried and is not currently involved in a romantic relationship. Although she receives a small amount of child support from her ex-husband on a regular basis, he has had very little contact with her or the children. Evelyn works out of her home as a medical transcriptionist. She supplements her income by working at a retail store at the mall in the evenings a few nights each week.

Evelyn has three children. Her oldest, Jessica Riley (18), is the mother of an 18-month-old son Ryan and a 6-week-old daughter Carrie. Evelyn's relationship with Jessica is strained. Jessica lives in a one-bedroom apartment with her two children and boyfriend Casey. Because of his abusiveness, Evelyn does not like Casey and fears for her daughter and grandchildren's safety. Evelyn's other children, Jenna and Jason, live in the home with her. After several frustrating years, Evelyn has recently been able to get Jason help with his ongoing school and social problems. He has recently started taking methylphenidate (Ritalin) and receiving special accommodations at school to facilitate his learning. Evelyn has noticed that Jenna has gained weight. Knowing it is a sensitive topic, Evelyn attempts to gently suggest that she watch her weight.

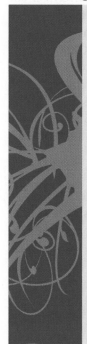

Episode 1

While talking with Jessica on the phone this week, Evelyn is suddenly cut off. When she calls back a few minutes later, Casey answers the phone and tells her that Jessica suddenly had to go the bathroom. Evelyn thinks this is odd. A few days later, Evelyn sees a bruise on Jessica's face. Jessica explains that she ran into a door, and specifically answers "no" when asked if Casey hit her. Evelyn does not believe Jessica's explanation. **[P]**

Episode 2

Evelyn receives a phone call from the school nurse, Violet Brinkworth, about Jenna. The nurse tells Evelyn that she is concerned about Jenna's weight gain and suggests that she have a medical evaluation to determine if there is a condition that might explain it. Evelyn confirms with the nurse that she has noticed the weight gain and is concerned, but it never occurred to her to take her to see a physician. **[P]**

Episode 3

Evelyn takes Jenna to see Dr. Rowe, as suggested by the school nurse. She is glad that Dr. Rowe listens to her when she shares her concerns—unlike her previous experiences when trying to get help for Jason. Evelyn is surprised at the number of lab tests ordered and is worried. She has problems sleeping because of all of her concerns.

Episode 4

No news this week.

Episode 5

This is an overwhelming week for Evelyn. She learns that her daughter Jenna has diabetes, Jason is an emotional wreck after being involved in another fight at school, and she notices bruises on Jessica's face again. She wonders about the effect that all of this stress is having on her own sanity and which of the problems she should be most concerned about. How can she manage it all? Evelyn is relieved to know that Carrie and Ryan have not been harmed. She tells Jessica that she knows Casey is beating her and pleads with her to get away from him. Evelyn sleeps very poorly all week because of all the worry about her three children. **[VC]**

Episode 6

Evelyn takes Jenna to an appointment with Dr. Yin, the pediatric endocrinologist. Dr. Yin talks with Evelyn and Jenna about diabetes and outlines the major components of treatment. She writes a prescription for Jenna and asks them both to work with Marjorie, the certified diabetic educator (CDE). She talks with Evelyn privately about typical psychosocial issues and adherence issues associated with teens who have type 2 diabetes.

Evelyn announces to both Jenna and Jason that there will be changes in the foods they eat and explains that the changes will benefit all of them. **[P]**

Episode 7

Evelyn is again very disturbed by the obvious beatings her daughter is enduring. She pleads with Jessica to get away from Casey—or, if nothing else, to let her keep the children so they are not near him. Evelyn does not understand why Jessica won't talk with her about the trouble she is in.

Evelyn and Jenna have additional meetings with Marjorie, the diabetic nurse educator, this week. Evelyn had heard of diabetes, but did not realize the complexity and seriousness of the disease.

Jason invites a classmate to spend the night this weekend. It has been many years since Jason has had a friend to their home for a sleepover. Evelyn is pleased to see that her son has a friend.

Episode 8

No news this week.

Episode 9

At 4 a.m., Evelyn gets a phone call from her oldest daughter. Jessica tells her mother that she left Casey, but is in hiding because she is fearful that he will come looking for her and her children. Jessica does not reveal her location, but asks her mother to call her employer to let them know she will be gone for a few weeks.

Evelyn feels so helpless, knowing the trouble her daughter is in, yet she is thankful that Jessica and the grandchildren are away from Casey. She wonders how many more problems she will have to deal with. Evelyn sees Casey driving by her home several times this week and worries what he might do.

Evelyn does not tell Jenna and Jason about Jessica. She figures they have enough on their minds, and she does not need to burden them with Jessica's problems.

Episode 10

Casey knocks on the front door and asks Evelyn if she would help him find Jessica and the kids. He tells Evelyn that they have had some problems, but he is ready to work things out. Evelyn is glad she doesn't know where Jessica is. She does not share any information with Casey, but worries that he will find Jessica and the children.

This week, Evelyn meets with members from Jason's school and learns that he is doing better since he began taking the medication and following the educational plan. Evelyn is pleased with this news. **[P]**

Episode 11

Evelyn is relieved to learn that Casey has been arrested and is in jail. She is also relieved that Jessica is able to come out of hiding and return to her apartment. She worries, however, that Casey will find a way to post bail and harm Jessica.

Episode 12

No news this week.

Episode 13

No news this week.

Episode 14

Over the past few weeks, Jessica has spent a great deal of time at home with Evelyn. Evelyn talks with Jessica about the need to let go of past anger and move forward. For the first time in several years, Evelyn feels as if she and Jessica really understand each other. Evelyn suggests that Jessica and the kids move back home until she can get back on her own two feet. When Jessica agrees to this, Evelyn is overjoyed. **[P]**

Episode 15

Evelyn, Jason, and Jenna help Jessica and her kids move back home this week. Evelyn knows the transition may be hard at first, but is relieved to know that her daughter and grandchildren are safe.

JENNA RILEY
Season 1

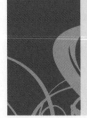

Biographical Information

Jenna is a healthy but overweight 14-year-old girl who lives with her mother Evelyn and brother Jason. Her older sister Jessica lives a short distance away in her own apartment with her infant son Ryan. Jenna misses having her older sister around and looks up to Jessica. Jenna has had minimal contact with her father and does not really even know him.

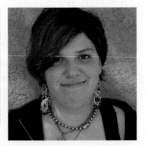

Continued

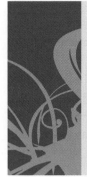

Because her mother works a few evenings each week, Jenna is responsible for her younger brother Jason. She gets along okay with her brother, but thinks he is such a weirdo. She is a good student in the eighth grade at the local middle school. She has many friends and spends a great deal of time on the phone or in computer chat rooms talking with friends in the evening. Jenna is self-conscious about her weight. She knows she should try to lose weight, but just doesn't really know how and doesn't have much discipline when it comes to resisting snacks. She finds it very hard to not join in with her friends when they eat.

Episode 1

No news this week.

Episode 2

Jessica's baby spends time at the house several times in the evening this week. Jenna likes it when Ryan is there and fantasizes about the day she will have a baby of her own. She hears her mother wondering out loud when her sister is going to pick up Ryan and take him home. **[P]**

Episode 3

No news this week.

Episode 4

Jenna attends a slumber party at her friend's house. They stay up all night and eat popcorn and pizza, and drink soda while watching movies. The girls also practice applying make-up, painting their fingernails and toenails, and doing each other's hair. One of the girls asks Jenna about a dark streak across the back of her neck near her hair line; Jenna looks in the mirror and sees the streak, but doesn't know what it is. She unsuccessfully tries to wash it off. Because it does not hurt and is hidden by her hair, she doesn't think much more about it. The following day, Jenna sleeps the entire afternoon and does none of her chores. **[P]**

Episode 5

Jenna's brother comes home with new glasses this week. Jenna is quick to tell him the glasses make him look weirder than he already looks.

Episode 6

Jenna is aware that her mother and sister are fighting about Jessica's boyfriend and about the baby. She finds this upsetting and eats one-half a package of cookies after school. Jenna's mother becomes angry when she learns this and tells Jenna that she needs to start watching what she eats. **[P]**

Episode 7

Jenna has her first menstrual period this week. She recognizes what it is because of classes she had at school and because of things her friends told her. Evelyn buys Jessica some tampons and feminine napkins.

Episode 8

Jenna is teased at school by several of the boys in her class about being a "piggy." This hurts Jenna's feelings tremendously. Jenna and her friends make a pact to not talk to the boys until they apologize. Jenna eats three pieces of cake at Jason's party. **[P]**

Episode 9

No news this week.

Episode 10

Jenna gets her report card at school this week and is pleased that she has all A's again. She likes the fact that people consider her smart. Jenna is aware that her brother has been in a fight at school again. She does not understand why he fights all the time and why he just can't sit down and do his homework the way she does. She is angry at him for making their mother upset. Jenna also knows that her mother is very worried about Ryan and Jessica. She spends each evening in a computer chat room with her friends while eating chips and drinking soda. **[P]**

Episode 11

Jenna knows that Jessica is pregnant, but still does not have a good understanding of how that all works. Her mother is so wrapped up in that situation and with Jason that Jenna feels almost invisible. She has gained several pounds over the past few months, but does not feel she has any control over her eating. She sometimes hates the way she looks and feels. **[P]**

Episode 12

Jenna goes to a slumber party with several girls. The girls talk about their boyfriends at school. Jenna does not have a boyfriend, and she suspects the reason is because she is fat. Although she remains friends with the girls, she begins to feel like somewhat of an outsider because of her weight. She wonders why she can't be skinny like her sister Jessica.

Jenna's brother was kicked out of Boy Scouts this week. She wonders why he can't control himself. **[P]**

Episode 13

There is an announcement at school that try-outs for the school Spirit Squad will be held in a couple of weeks. Jenna's friends talk about the try-outs and ask Jenna if she plans to try out. The girls on the Spirit Squad tend to be the popular girls at school. Jenna would love to be on the squad, thinking it could help her to become popular. However, she is becoming increasingly self-conscious about her weight and worries that people might laugh at her. She tells her friends that her mother doesn't have enough money for the uniforms and other expenses associated with Spirit Squad, because all their money goes to help her pregnant sister. **[P]**

Episode 14

Jenna goes out of town with her mother and Jason to visit her grandmother. Jenna loves to spend time with her grandmother, but knows she has been sick lately with thyroid problems. **[P]**

Episode 15

No news this week.

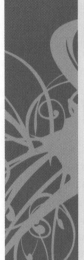

JENNA RILEY
Season 2

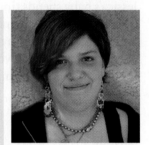

Biographical Information

Jenna is a healthy but overweight 14-year-old girl who lives with her mother Evelyn and brother Jason. Her older sister Jessica lives a short distance away in her own apartment with her son Ryan and boyfriend Casey. Jenna misses having her older sister around and looks up to Jessica.

Because her mother works a few evenings each week, Jenna is responsible for her younger brother Jason. She also often watches her nephew Ryan when he spends time in their home. She gets along okay with her brother, but thinks he is such a weirdo. She is a good student in the eighth grade at the local middle school. She has many friends and spends a great deal of time on the phone or in computer chat rooms talking with friends in the evening. Jenna is self-conscious about her weight. She knows she should try to lose weight, but just doesn't really know how and doesn't have much discipline when it comes to resisting snacks; she always feels hungry! She finds it very hard to not join in with her friends when they eat.

Episode 1

No news this week.

Episode 2

Jenna learns that all of her friends have made the Spirit Squad. She wishes she had tried out, but did not want to face the possible embarrassment of not making the squad because of her weight. She had hoped to hang out with her friends after school this week, but they now have Spirit Squad practice. Feeling hurt and left out, Jenna goes home and eats cookies. She hides the box of remaining cookies under her bed. **[P]**

Episode 3

Jenna wakes up one morning this week with a huge pimple. She has been noticing little pimples lately, but this one, she believes, can be seen from a mile away. Her mother does not even comment on the pimple. Jenna realizes her mother has been very distracted between worrying about her brother Jason and her sister Jessica.

Jenna frequently stays after school to watch her friends at Spirit Squad practice. On one day after school this week, the Spirit Squad girls were making posters for the assembly. When Jenna offered to help, she was told that only Spirit Squad members could make the posters. **[P]**

Episode 4

Jenna is irritated with her mother for commenting on her weight and is further annoyed when she is unable to find her favorite chips or cookies after school. Using her allowance, she buys candy from the store and hides it in her room so her mother won't know she has it. Jenna feels very tired in the afternoon and evening—too tired to get into an exercise routine. **[VC]**

Episode 5
No news this week.

Episode 6
Jenna recognizes that her clothes are fitting tightly. She asks her mom if they could go shopping sometime soon, but does not explain why. She is relieved when her mother does not comment about her weight gain. Jenna has more pimples on her face and is beginning to really hate the way she looks.

Episode 7
Jenna helps her mother make a cake for their family get-together. She secretly eats four pieces of cake over the course of the day and is glad that her mother doesn't notice. She feels very tired and spends the entire evening lying on the couch and watching TV.

Episode 8
Jenna takes care of her nephew Ryan twice this week while Evelyn works at the mall. Jenna and Jason absolutely love taking care of Ryan. They find many games to play with him during the evenings.

Jenna hates the fact that she has more pimples. She washes her face three times a day, but the pimples continue to develop. **[P]**

Episode 9
No news this week.

Episode 10
Jenna hates the fact that there is (in her opinion) nothing good to eat at their house anymore and hates the lunches her mother makes for her. She usually trades most of her lunch away to other kids for foods that she likes. She constantly wants to drink soda pop and often drinks five cans in a day. She frequently needs to get up in the middle of the night to urinate. Jenna thinks this is causing her to be even more tired and vows to quit drinking sodas after 9 p.m.

Jenna sets up a Web page on YourZone.com this week. On the site, Jenna describes herself as a cheerleader and says that she is 19 years old. The picture she posts is not of herself, but rather one of a thin girl without pimples that she found on the Internet. **[P]**

Episode 11
Jenna is pleased with the number of responses to her Web site. Several guys have written to her, and she enjoys the attention. Jenna tells her friends that she has a new boyfriend. **[P]**

Episode 12
No news this week.

Episode 13
Jenna's sister has her baby this week. Jenna loves holding the new baby. She also found out that Casey hit Jessica and had to go to jail. Jenna wonders why her sister has such a jerky boyfriend. **[P]**

Episode 14
Jenna is deeply disappointed that none of the boys ask her to the roller skating party. All of her friends on the Spirit Squad were asked to go with boys from school. Jenna decides to go to the party anyway. Her friends on the Spirit Squad practically ignore her at the party, so Jenna spends time with some of the other girls. Jenna takes comfort in the fact that she regularly communicates with several guys on the Internet. Even though she makes up a lot of stuff about herself, she likes the idea that boys are interested in her.

Jenna wants to lose weight, but doesn't know how. Even though her mom has tried to force her to change her eating habits, Jenna can't stay away from soda and can't stop eating junk foods at school. She also feels too tired after school to exercise. **[P]**

Episode 15
No news this week.

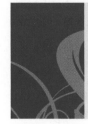

JENNA RILEY
Season 3

Biographical Information
Jenna is a healthy but overweight 15-year-old girl who lives with her mother Evelyn and brother Jason. Her older sister Jessica lives a short distance away in her own apartment with her boyfriend Casey and her children Ryan and Carrie. Jenna has had minimal contact with her father and does not really even know him.

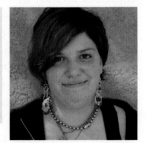

Continued

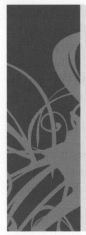

Because her mother works a few evenings each week, Jenna is responsible for her younger brother Jason. She also often watches Ryan and Carrie when they spend time in their home. She gets along okay with her brother, but thinks he is such a weirdo. Jenna is a good student in the ninth grade at the local middle school. She has many friends and spends a great deal of time on the phone or in computer chat rooms talking with friends in the evening.

Jenna has recently gained a lot of weight. She is very self-conscious about her weight and believes her friends sometimes avoid her because she is fat. She knows she should try to lose weight, but just doesn't really know how and does not have much discipline when it comes to resisting snacks; she always feels hungry! She frequently hides the foods that she eats so that her mother will not make comments about what she is eating.

Episode 1
No news this week.

Episode 2
During a gym class activity, Jenna goes to the school nurse, Violet Brinkworth, complaining of a twisted ankle. After examining the ankle, Violet talks with Jenna about other things that might be bothering her. Jenna tells the nurse that nobody wanted her on their team because she is too slow and that one of the boys told her she had a body like a penguin.

As the nurse talks with her more, Jenna shares that she has gained a lot of weight and is not happy about the fact that she is so heavy. She does not understand why she cannot be skinny like her sister. The nurse notices a dark pigmentation on the back of Jenna's neck and suggests to her that perhaps she might need to see a doctor to determine why she is gaining so much weight. Violet gets Jenna's permission to contact her mother about this matter. **[VC]**

Episode 3
Jenna continues to feel rejected by her friends on the Spirit Squad. She tries to join them at lunch, but is frequently told that the table is already full. She goes to the practices to watch, but the girls ignore her presence. She is no longer invited to join them in any activities. Although they don't come out and say it, she is sure they don't want to hang around with her anymore because she is fat. Jenna begins hanging around with a different group of girls.

She has an appointment with Dr. Rowe, the family physician, this week. Dr. Rowe takes a history and completes a physical exam. During the family history, Jenna is surprised to hear her mother report that obesity and diabetes run in her father's side of the family; specifically, both her father and paternal grandmother have the disease.

Jenna's blood pressure is 120/78 mm Hg, and her body mass index (BMI) is 24.8, which places her at the 90% percentile for girls aged 14. A capillary blood glucose test done in the office is 158, and a urine dipstick shows a trace of glucose. Dr. Rowe also notices acanthosis nigricans on the back of Jenna's neck.

Based on the history and clinical findings, Dr. Rowe recognizes the need to test Jenna for diabetes. She orders an outpatient thyroid stimulating hormone blood test and a fasting blood glucose test to be performed on two different days. A follow-up appointment is scheduled for 2 weeks later. In the meantime, Jenna is encouraged to try to lose some weight by changing her dietary patterns and exercising.

Episode 4
Jenna goes to the outpatient lab for blood tests on two different days this week. She hates the fact that she is unable to have breakfast until after her blood is drawn. After getting to school on both mornings, Jenna eats some donuts purchased from the snack machine.

Jenna continues to communicate with many people on YourZone.com. She particularly likes a 20-year-old guy named Tom. Jenna has told Tom that she is also 20. In several messages, he tells her that he has fallen in love with her and wants to meet her in person. He asks Jenna where she lives. Jenna wants to meet Tom, but she is afraid that, when he realizes she is really 14 and fat, he won't love her anymore. **[P]**

Episode 5
Jenna returns to Dr. Rowe's office this week for a follow-up visit. Dr. Rowe tells Jenna and Evelyn that, based on the history, lab results, and other clinical findings, Jenna has type 2 diabetes. She recommends that a pediatric

endocrinologist manage Jenna's diabetes and provides her mother with a referral. Jenna has heard of diabetes before, but doesn't know much about it. She doesn't think it is too big of a deal, because she feels fine, but she is hopeful she will lose weight.

Tom, Jenna's Internet friend, continues to ask her to meet him. Jenna finally admits to Tom that she is really 14 and a little overweight, and that the picture she posted is not really her. Tom tells Jenna that it doesn't matter—that he loves her and wants to meet her. Jenna is pleased with the fact that Tom still loves her, but wonders if she should be dating a 20-year-old guy. Jenna tells her friends at school about Tom; they warn her not to tell him anything else and suggest that she stop communicating with him. Jenna thinks her friends are just jealous. **[VC]**

Episode 6

It is report card time and, once again, Jenna has made straight A's. The recent teasing from her peers has been difficult, but she feels very proud to see her name near the top of the honor roll list.

Jenna has an appointment with Dr. Rena Yin, a pediatric endocrinologist, this week. Another history, work-up, and blood tests are completed. Dr. Yin elects to start Jenna on metformin, 500 mg twice daily, to be taken with meals.

Jenna and Evelyn also meet with Marjorie, a nurse who is a certified diabetic educator (CDE), to begin the process of learning about diabetes self-management. Marjorie outlines the four major components of self-management: nutrition therapy, an increase in physical activity, self-monitoring of blood glucose, and drug therapy. Jenna immediately likes Marjorie, because she doesn't make her feel uncomfortable about the fact that she is fat. She seems to accept her just the way she is. **[VC] [P]**

Episode 7

Jenna continues to meet with Marjorie, the CDE. The primary focus of initial education efforts is on self-monitoring of blood glucose. Marjorie teaches Jenna how to perform a finger stick and measure her glucose level. She is instructed to do this twice a day for a few weeks to see how the new medication is working. Jenna hates poking her finger.

Over the course of meeting with Marjorie, Jenna opens up to her and tells her about the teasing at school and about her boyfriend Tom, whom she met on the Internet. Concerned about what Jenna might be telling this man, Marjorie talks with Jenna further about the situation and points out that it could be a very dangerous

situation for her. It never occurred to Jenna that Tom might not be who he says he is. Marjorie shares a brochure on Internet safety for teens and asks her to read it so they can discuss it on their next visit. She also suggests that Jenna talk with her mother about this. **[P]**

Episode 8

No news this week.

Episode 9

Jenna has completed most of the initial diabetic education. She feels like she learned a lot, but does not perceive her disease to be really all that bad. Marjorie suggests to Jenna that she attend diabetes camp to be held in a few months. Jenna likes the idea of going to a camp with other girls who have the same problem.

Although she adheres to the finger pokes and medication regimen, Jenna does not stick to her diet or attempt to increase her activity. The new diet leads to many fights with her mother. She feels there are so many limitations to what she can eat that she often feels left out among her friends at school. She does not want to tell her friends that she has diabetes, because she doesn't want to be perceived as different.

Episode 10

Jenna has no interest in following a diet. She finds herself thinking about food all the time and ends up eating compulsively at school. Jenna quickly figures out that, if she doesn't stick to her diet, the elevated glucose level is stored in the memory of the glucose monitor. She tries to erase the higher numbers so that Marjorie and her mother will not see them, but is afraid she might break the meter and get into trouble. Instead, she figures out she can use her friend's blood to register good blood glucose measurements on the monitor. **[P]**

Episode 11

Jenna learns that Casey is in jail and sees his picture in the Neighborhood Newspaper. She learns that he has been beating up Jessica, and Jessica has been trying to get away from him. Jenna is afraid of Casey and hopes she never sees him again.

Jenna continues to eat whatever she pleases at school. She frequently feels very tired and grouchy. Jenna has noticed that, if her blood glucose levels are high, she can lose weight more easily. She does not understand how this works, but likes the idea of losing weight. She continues to use her friend's blood for the glucose measurements. **[P]**

Episode 12

No news this week.

Episode 13

Darren, one of Jenna's friends, figures out how to alter the memory on the blood glucose device. Jenna tells him what numbers to program into the monitor and figures out that this frees her from having to follow a diet (except when at home). She is quite sure nobody will ever know the difference. **[P]**

Episode 14

It has been a couple of months since Jenna began a treatment plan for diabetes management. She has a follow-up visit with Dr. Yin (the pediatric endocrinologist) and Marjorie, the CDE. She proudly shows her record of blood glucose levels from her blood glucose monitor, which reflects excellent glycemic control. She claims to have been following the diet, exercising, and taking her medication. Dr. Yin and Marjorie note that she has lost 4 pounds since her last visit and that her HbA_{1C} level is 13.1%. Dr. Yin and Marjorie recognize the need for additional education with Jenna and confront her about the measurements recorded on the glucometer. **[VC]**

Episode 15

Jenna is excited about the fact that Jessica is moving back home with them. She has missed her older sister and loves her children. Despite some of her recent disappointments with the diabetes and excessive weight gain, Jenna takes comfort in the close relationships she experiences within her family.

JASON RILEY
Season 1

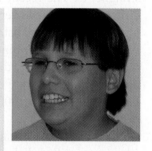

Biographical Information

Jason is an active, healthy 11-year-old boy. He is currently in fifth grade at the public grade school near his home. He lives with his mother Evelyn and his 14-year-old sister Jenna. He has never had much contact with his father. Jason's home life has been somewhat stressful the past year or so because of ongoing fights between his mother and oldest sister Jessica; the conflict resulted in Jessica moving out of the house. Jason gets along well with his mother, but he has typical sibling conflicts with Jenna.

Jason has had problems in school for the past 3 years. Teachers report that he has difficulty staying on task and won't follow directions. Although he made some progress last year with his fourth-grade teacher, his grades have been consistently poor. His mother tries to help him with homework after school or in the evenings, but these sessions frequently turn into battlegrounds. It takes Jason hours to complete fairly simple assignments, resulting in a great deal of frustration for him and his mother. The fact that he frequently comes home from school with headaches further aggravates the situation. In addition to problems with academics, Jason has problems with social interactions. His teachers at school find him to be disruptive in the classroom. During the past year, he has been frequently sent to the principal's office for misbehaving. He is frequently teased at school. Most of his time at home is spent playing video and computer games and watching TV.

Episode 1

No news this week.

Episode 2

Jason gets in a fight at school this week when another classmate does not give him the green paint during an art activity. Jason is sent to the principal's office because he is perceived to be the instigator by the teacher. Jason explains to the principal that he wanted the green paint, but nobody would give it to him, so he punched his classmate to get it. He tells his mother he had a headache all day at school. **[P]**

Episode 3

Jason comes home from school with a headache twice this week. His mother suggests that he join the Boy Scout

Troop associated with his school, hoping he'll get interested in something besides video games and make some friends. Jason is not thrilled about the idea, but agrees to try it. **[P]**

Episode 4

Violet Brinkworth, the school nurse, performs vision screening tests at Jason's school this week. Violet tells Jason he may need glasses. He attends his first Boy Scout meeting and finds that some of the boys in the troop are the same ones who often tease him at school. Still, he likes the Scoutmasters and decides to go again next week. Jason fails to complete a volcano project at school, and his teacher sends a note home to inform his mother. His mother grounds him for a week, which he thinks is "just dumb." **[P]**

Episode 5

Jason's mother takes him to the optometrist's office this week to get fitted for glasses. Jason hates the fact that he has to wear glasses, but the eye doctor says they might help his headaches go away. The following day Jason is teased at school for wearing glasses, and Jenna tells him he looks like a nerd. **[P] [VC]**

Episode 6

No news this week.

Episode 7

At school, Jason continues to be teased about being weird and for wearing glasses. He was given a permission slip to take home for an upcoming field trip, but he completely forgot about it and lost it. He is still going to Boy Scout meetings—he likes the meetings because the leaders do not tolerate teasing among the boys. His favorite Boy Scout leader is Pat Richman. He is looking forward to going on a hike over the weekend with his troop. **[P]**

Episode 8

Jason has a party at his house this week. Only some of the kids he invited come to the party. He also has a bad meeting at Boy Scouts this week. He gets confused listening to directions while working on a badge and becomes disruptive. When he is disciplined by the head Scoutmaster, he becomes angry and has a temper tantrum. The assistant scoutmaster, Pat Richman, helps him to settle down and talks with his mother briefly after the meeting. **[P]**

Episode 9

No news this week.

Episode 10

Report cards come out this week. Jason has a 'C' and two 'D's, and a F. On the playground at recess, he gets into a fight with another kid because he is teased for being dumb. Jason is unable to concentrate long enough to complete his homework assignments that evening, leading to another fight with his mother. She tells him he can't watch TV for two days. This makes him angry, and he gets on his bike and rides away, despite Evelyn's demands that he stay home. He goes to the nearby park, finds a stick, and hits the playground equipment.

One of the kids that Jason invited to his party several weeks ago is having a birthday party. All of the kids at school are talking about it, but Jason does not get invited. He does not understand why he doesn't get an invitation and is hurt, but he is too embarrassed to ask his friend about it. **[VC]**

Episode 11

Jason is taken to a doctor's appointment to get some help with all the problems he is experiencing. He finds the discussion between his mother and Dr. Rowe very embarrassing. He also knows Mom is really mad at Jessica, but does not know why.

Episode 12

This week, Jason becomes angry at the Boy Scout meeting during a game. In his frustration, he bites one of the other scouts. The Scoutmaster takes Jason home and tells his mother that he can no longer come to the meetings. Jenna teases her brother about being so dumb that he can't even be a Boy Scout. After getting home from scouts, his mother sends him to his room, where he spends the rest of the evening. He feels like such a failure. He wishes he could just kill the boys in the Scout troop. **[P]**

Episode 13

No news this week.

Episode 14

Jason goes to his grandmother's house this week with his mother and sister, Jenna. He enjoys being away from school, but is miserable that he does not have a computer or video game to play while there. His sister annoys him, and they frequently argue. He spends most of his time watching TV until his mother tells him to go out and play. He goes outside and throws rocks at cars from behind a hedge. **[P]**

Episode 15

No news this week.

JASON RILEY
Season 2

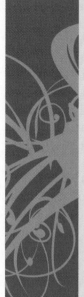

Biographical Information

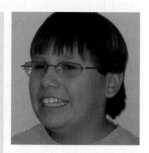

Jason is an active, healthy 12-year-old boy. He is currently in fifth grade at the public grade school near his home. He lives with his mother Evelyn and his 14-year-old sister Jenna. He has never had much contact with his father. Jason's home life has been somewhat stressful the past year or so because of ongoing fights between his mother and oldest sister Jessica.

Jason has ongoing problems in school. Teachers report that he has difficulty staying on task and does not follow directions. His grades have also been consistently poor. His mother tries to help him with homework after school or in the evenings, but these sessions frequently turn into battlegrounds. It takes Jason hours to complete fairly simple assignments, resulting in a great deal of frustration for him and his mother. In addition to problems with academics, Jason has problems with social interactions. His teachers at school find him to be disruptive in the classroom. During the past year, he has been frequently sent to the principal's office for misbehaving and was kicked out of Boy Scouts. He is frequently teased at school. Most of his time at home is spent playing video and computer games and watching TV.

Episode 1
No news this week.

Episode 2
Jason is the target of teasing at school in gym class. His mother suggests that he resolve the problems by talking to his teachers instead of getting into fights. He tells the gym teacher about the teasing in the locker room, but doesn't think the teacher listens or even cares. The boys in the class call him a "girly-boy" and make fun of him for telling the teacher. After school, Jason tries to share this experience with his mother, but she is busy taking care of his nephew Ryan. This makes him angry, and he runs into his room and tears up one of his school books.

Episode 3
Jason is involved in another fight at school this week with the kids in his gym class. He tells the boys that next time he will bring a knife to school and stab them. Even though they instigated the fight, Jason was the one who threw the first punch. Because of his ongoing problems and his verbal knife threat, the school administrators threaten to expel him. **[P]**

Episode 4
Jason does his best to ignore the ongoing teasing at school and resists the temptation to get into a fight. He is forced to do group work and can't seem to sit still. He hates the kids in his group and is disruptive. When redirected by the teacher, he thinks he is being picked on. It has reached the point at which he really hates going to school. He wishes he could go to a different school where the kids are nice.

Episode 5
No news this week.

Episode 6
Jason's mother takes him to the neuropsychologist for an evaluation this week. The psychologist talks with Jason in an attempt to get to know him. He asks Jason what he likes to do, what he finds fun, and what school is like for him. Jason tells him that he doesn't like school because the other kids are dumb and they pick on him. Jason also shares that the teachers do not like him. He undergoes psychometric testing. **[VC]**

Episode 7
Jason enjoys the family get-together that his mother has planned. He likes it when his oldest sister Jessica is at home and they are all together. Jason also is glad to see his mother happy for a change.

Episode 8
Jason has another visit with the psychologist this week. He talks more with Jason about school and what his life is like in his home. Jason tells the psychologist about Jessica and her baby, and the fact that she is going to

have another baby. He also tells the psychologist about mean kids at school and that he gets blamed for everything. He tells him that he wishes some of the other kids at school were dead. He admits that he has a hard time remembering what he needs to do for school once he gets home. **[P]**

Episode 9
No news this week.

Episode 10
The psychologist tells Jason that he believes the reason he has trouble at school is because of a problem known as attention deficit hyperactivity disorder (better known as ADHD). He asks Jason if he would be willing to take some medication and maybe make some changes at school to help him feel better. Jason agrees to try the medications and changes at school, but he is sure the kids will still tease him.

Episode 11
Jason's mother has a meeting with the principal and counselor. He is embarrassed by the fact that they are talking about him. He wonders if they will make fun of him.

Episode 12
Jason takes tests this week at the school district offices. He is told that the tests will help his teachers help him learn better.

Episode 13
Jason's sister, Jessica, has her baby this week. He knows his mother has been very upset and knows she does not like Jessica's boyfriend. He overhears his mother tell a friend that Casey was arrested. Jason wonders what it is like to go to jail and is excited to see the new baby.

Episode 14
The neuropsychologist meets with Jason and Evelyn again this week to discuss positive reinforcement and time management strategies. Specifically, he suggests that Jason spend more time interacting with others and less time playing video games at home. He also talks to Jason about taking the medication.

Episode 15
Based on the reports from the school counselor and neuropsychologist, Dr. Rowe (the family practice physician) agrees to write a prescription of methylphenidate (Ritalin) for Jason.

JASON RILEY
Season 3

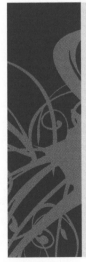

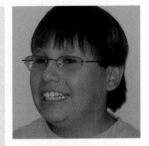

Biographical Information

Jason is an active, healthy 12-year-old boy. He lives with his mother Evelyn and his 15-year-old sister Jenna. He has never had much contact with his father. Jason's home life has been somewhat stressful during the past year or so because of his mother and oldest sister Jessica fighting, and the fact that Jessica just had another baby.

Jason has had problems in school (both academically and socially) for the past several years. He is frequently the target of teasing and often gets into fights. During the past year, his mother has taken him to several meetings and appointments to try to help him. Recently, he was diagnosed with attention deficit hyperactivity disorder (ADHD) and began taking methylphenidate (Ritalin), 10 mg twice a day (before breakfast and lunch). At school, an individualized educational plan and special accommodations have been developed.

Episode 1
Jason takes methylphenidate (Ritalin) before school every morning and again at lunch time, requiring a trip to the nurse's office. Jason feels a bit nervous and less hungry ever since he started to take the medication. He does not want any of the kids to know he takes medication. Likewise, he doesn't want the other kids to know he has a "special plan," because he is afraid of being teased. At home, Jason is not

happy about having limits placed on playing video games. He is not interested in reading books or doing other activities and feels angry about the changes expected of him. **[P]**

Episode 2
No news this week.

Episode 3
Jason has been taking methylphenidate (Ritalin) for a month now. He feels less agitated and has a calmer presence. He has not been in any fights for several weeks and has been able to understand the teacher's instructions in class. Despite this, he gets teased for going to a resource room and for being dumb and weird. The fact that he has no friends makes him feel sad and angry. No matter how hard he tries, nobody likes him. But at least the school work doesn't seem as hard as before. Jason does not like the restrictions placed on video games at home. Sometimes, he plays them late at night after his mother goes to bed, but then he is very tired during school the following day. **[P]**

Episode 4
No news this week.

Episode 5
Jason has a fight at school this week. One of the boys sees him in the nurse's office when he is there to take his medication at lunch and tells all the other kids that Jason takes pills because he is crazy. The kids start calling him "Crazy Jazy." Jason tries to ignore the teasing, but finally punches one of the boys in the stomach and tells him, "I'm going to kill you." He is sent to the principal's office, and his mother is called when he is unable to settle down. He feels out of control and screams, yells, and shouts obscenities at the top of his voice. The school principal tells Evelyn to keep him home from school for the rest of the week.

Episode 6
Report cards are distributed this week. Jason is disappointed because he got all 'C's and a 'D.' He is surprised (and relieved) that his mother signs the report card and does not even comment on the grades. Jason has a better week at school. The boys who teased him previously keep their distance and make no comments to him. One boy in his class, Brian, talks with Jason about a video game they both have.

Jason learns that his sister, Jenna, has diabetes. His mother announces that there are going to be big changes in the way the whole family eats. She will not have any junk food in the house, and everybody is going to eat breakfast every morning. Jason hates having his sister's problems impact the food he has to eat.

Episode 7
Jason's new friend, Brian, spends the night this weekend. They spend most of their time playing video games. Jason is very happy to have a new friend.

Episode 8
No news this week.

Episode 9
Jason has been gradually doing better in school. He has been keeping up with assignments and is better able to follow instructions. He has not been involved in any fights recently. Jason and Brian have another friend named Mike, and Jason is very happy to have two friends at school. Jason is somewhat aware of Jessica's problems with Casey and overhears his mother mentioning to Jenna that Jessica is hiding from him. He does not fully understand where she might hide and pictures Jessica and her kids hiding in a closet or under a bed.

Episode 10
A meeting is held this week with Jason, his mother, his teacher, the principal, and the school counselor. Jason is thrilled when his teacher shares with everyone the progress that he has made over the past month. Jason can tell that his mother is happy with the news, but she does not seem as excited as he thought she might be. He feels a bit disappointed with her response. **[P]**

Episode 11
Jason learns that Casey killed somebody in a car accident and is in jail. He wonders why Casey did that and why he is so mean to his sister, Jessica.

Episode 12
No news this week.

Episode 13
Brian invites Jason and Mike to go on a fishing and camping trip over the weekend. Jason is thrilled to catch his first fish. Brian's father teaches the boys how to clean fish with a knife. They later cook fish over the campfire for supper. Not once during the trip does Jason think about video games. **[P]**

Episode 14
No news this week.

Episode 15
Jason is glad that his oldest sister is moving back home. Although he is not too interested in the baby, Jason loves to play with his nephew Ryan. Ryan breaks Jason's head set, but instead of becoming angry, Jason remains calm. **[P]**

RILEY AND HOLMES HOUSEHOLD

RILEY AND HOLMES FAMILY STORY OVERVIEW

Character	Season 1	Season 2	Season 3
JESSICA RILEY	Because of a difficult relationship with her mother, Evelyn Riley, Jessica recently moved into her own apartment. She has a new infant son and is trying to go to school, work, and take care of her baby. She is struggling financially. Early on in this season, she meets Casey. He moves in with her and she gets pregnant again.	During this season, the focus is on Jessica's prenatal care. During the pregnancy, she becomes the victim of domestic violence. Near term (38 weeks), she is kicked in the abdomen by Casey, causing her to go into labor. She delivers a healthy infant daughter.	The domestic violence continues to escalate. Jessica continues to defend Casey, believing that he will eventually become a good father. Eventually she seeks refuge in a shelter. Jessica and her kids move back home with Evelyn, and she plans to go back to school and finish a degree so that she can support herself.
CASEY HOLMES	Casey meets Jessica at a party and shortly thereafter moves in with her. He agrees to care for baby Ryan when Jessica is at work. Little does she know, he neglects Ryan. Casey parties heavily; he is a substance abuser and has difficulty holding jobs.	Casey becomes physically and verbally abusive to Jessica while she is pregnant. When she is near term he kicks her in the abdomen during a fight, causing her to go into labor. Because of all the commotion, neighbors call police. He is arrested for drug possession.	Casey continues a pattern of domestic violence and substance abuse. He gets arrested again and sent to jail. During this period of time, Jessica breaks off their relationship.
RYAN RILEY	Ryan is 1 month old at the beginning of the story. Although he is healthy, he has colic and cries a lot. He receives good care at his grandmother's house, but is poorly cared for and neglected at his own home. He has a serious episode of RSV and dehydration, requiring hospitalization. Failure to thrive is diagnosed during hospitalization, and social services intervenes.	Ryan turns 1 year of age during this season. He spends less time around Casey and is mandated to go to a social services preschool. He spends an increasing amount of time in his grandmother's (Evelyn Riley) care. Ryan flourishes physically and mentally in this environment.	Ryan stays at his grandmother Evelyn's house more than with Jessica at this point. He is very happy to be with his grandmother, where he stays healthy and safe.
CARRIE HOLMES	Not born yet.	Carrie is born at end of Season 2. She is healthy, despite the traumatic onset of labor. She is overall healthy and well cared for by her grandmother.	Carrie is a healthy infant. She has an episode of otitis media.

CONCEPTS   *Elimination, Family Dynamics, Fatigue, Fluid/Electrolyte Balance, Immunity, Infection, Interpersonal Relationships, Interpersonal Violence, Nausea & Vomiting, Nutrition, Oxygenation, Reproduction, Sleep, Substance Abuse, Thermoregulation, Tissue Integrity*

JESSICA RILEY
Season 1

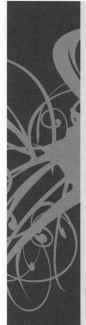

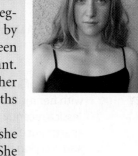

Biographical Information

Jessica Riley is a 17-year-old single mother of a 1-month-old infant, Ryan. Ryan's father ended his relationship with Jessica when she was 4 months pregnant. She has not seen or heard from him since that time, but has been told by friends that he left the state. Her relationship with her mother Evelyn has been strained for the past several years and worsened when she became pregnant. Because she was constantly fighting with her mother, Jessica moved out of her mother's home into a small, one-bedroom apartment when she was 6 months pregnant.

Jessica grew up in a single-parent home. Her father left the family when she was 7. She is the oldest child and has two younger siblings, Jenna and Jason. She recently completed her GED and is now trying to go to school part-time for an associate's degree in cosmetology at the local community college. She also works nearly full-time as a waitress at a restaurant, but because she has been supporting herself and her baby, she struggles financially. Her mother Evelyn helps by watching her baby a few hours each day. Additionally, Jessica receives government assistance in the form of WIC coupons and Medicaid. Jessica does not exercise and eats mostly fast food. She smokes about one-half pack of cigarettes a day and drinks alcohol socially when she parties.

Episode 1

Jessica often feels overwhelmed while trying to care for her infant, work, and go to school. Ryan experiences colic almost every night, spits up frequently, and cries constantly. She is so tired of listening to Ryan cry! Jessica has made several visits to the emergency department (ED) during the past couple of weeks, but the doctors (in her opinion) don't do anything. She tried to breastfeed her baby, but concluded that she did not have enough milk, so she switched to formula. She believes this may be causing Ryan's colic. Jessica is not getting enough sleep and feels frazzled. She misses being able to go out with her friends whenever she feels like it. **[P]**

Episode 2

Jessica's friend, Amy, invites her to a party at her home. Jessica believes she deserves a break from Ryan and asks her mother to watch him for a few hours. Jessica is thrilled to go out! At the party, she meets a guy named Casey, and they spend the rest of the evening together. Jessica calls her mother and tells her she will just pick up Ryan in the morning. Casey goes with Jessica back to her apartment and spends the night with her. **[P]**

Episode 3

Jessica and her mother Evelyn take Ryan for his 2-month well-baby visit at the pediatrician's office. Jessica met the pediatrician at the hospital when Ryan was born. She tells the pediatrician about her ongoing problems with Ryan's colic and that she has a hard time getting enough sleep. The pediatrician assures her that this stage will pass and praises her for the weight Ryan has gained since birth.

Jessica has been with Casey almost constantly since meeting him at the party a few weeks ago, and they decide to live together. Casey moves in with Jessica and Ryan, and agrees to watch the baby in the evenings so that Jessica can work more hours. Jessica is thrilled to have someone to take care of her and Ryan. She tells her mother that she only needs Evelyn to watch Ryan during the daytime. Evelyn expresses concern about the live-in boyfriend and offers to keep Ryan, but Jessica tells her mother she can raise her own baby.

Episode 4

No news this week.

Episode 5

Casey criticizes Jessica for holding the baby too much. He tells her that she has turned Ryan into a spoiled brat, and the reason he cries so much is because he always wants attention. Jessica decides Casey is right and holds Ryan less often.

Jessica is working many evenings and likes the fact that she is starting to have a little more money to spend.

However, she sometimes wonders if Ryan is being fed when Casey takes care of him; she finds a nearly full bottle of milk with him in the crib, and he always needs his diaper changed when she comes home. Casey sometimes yells at Jessica when she returns home about her "damn baby" that won't quit crying and says he has better things to do with his time. Although she has some concerns, she doesn't say anything, for fear that Casey might leave her; she loves and needs Casey. **[P]**

Episode 6

Jessica has another fight with her mother. Evelyn voices her concerns about Ryan not gaining enough weight, and says that he often looks dirty—he has dried milk on his neck, and his clothes are dirty. She also questions whether living with Casey is in Jessica's or Ryan's best interest. Jessica gets very defensive and angry, accusing her mother of not liking Casey and trying to make her feel dumb. Jessica tells her mother that, if she continues to criticize her, she won't let her take care of the baby anymore. **[P]**

Episode 7

Jessica has her 18th birthday this week. She and Casey celebrate by going out for pizza. Jessica hopes that Casey gets another job soon. Ryan is due for his 4-month well-baby check-up and immunizations. Because she has a test at school, Jessica cancels the appointment. Casey convinces her that immunizations are not that important anyway. **[P]**

Episode 8

No news this week.

Episode 9

No news this week.

Episode 10

Jessica experiences nausea and fatigue 4 days this week. She also notices breast tenderness. She recalls that these symptoms are similar to how she felt shortly after she became pregnant with Ryan. Although she thinks it is possible that she is pregnant, she is pretty sure she is not because she just had a baby, and her menstrual cycles have been irregular. She cannot recall when her last period was, but decides to just wait to see when she gets her next period.

Jessica allows her mother to take Ryan for his 6-month check-up and immunizations this week. Following the physician visit, Evelyn tells Jessica that, according to the pediatrician, Ryan is falling a bit behind on his weight and needs to be fed more. Evelyn again voices her concerns about Ryan's care. Jessica tells her mother to shut up and mind her own business. **[P]**

Episode 11

Jessica continues to be nauseated and has a hard time keeping anything down. While at work, she becomes dizzy and faints. Her coworkers urge Jessica to go to a doctor to get checked out. She goes to the Neighborhood Hospital emergency department and, following a workup, is told that she is pregnant. Jessica is instructed to follow up with her health-care provider for prenatal care. Jessica quits going to school because she recognizes that, with another baby on the way, she will need to work more hours to make ends meet. **[VC]**

Episode 12

Jessica goes for her first prenatal visit at the same women's health care practice where she went when she was pregnant with Ryan. On this visit, Jessica meets Carol Ramsey, a nurse midwife, and immediately likes her. An ultrasound scan shows her pregnancy to be about 16 weeks' gestation.

Jessica is advised to decrease or stop smoking, avoid alcohol, eat a nutritious diet, and take prenatal vitamins. She is instructed to go to the outpatient lab within a couple of days for a multiple marker screen (MMS). **[MR]**

Episode 13

Over the past few weeks, Jessica notices that Casey has become increasingly possessive. He frequently questions her about men she works with at the restaurant and discourages her from hanging out with her friends. On one evening this week, he accuses her of having an affair with a male colleague from work after he calls to ask her to cover a shift for him. When she denies having an affair, Casey pushes her down to the floor and threatens to harm her if she ever leaves him. **[VC]**

Episode 14

Ryan has had a cold all week. Because Evelyn is out of town, Jessica's friend, Carol, agrees to babysit during the day while Jessica is at work. When she picks up Ryan, Carol tells Jessica that he did not eat anything, and she thinks he has a fever. Jessica knows he has been sick all week and observes that Ryan is sleeping. She is glad he is finally not crying. When she drops off Ryan at home on her way back to work for the evening shift, she asks Casey to keep an eye on him because he might have a fever.

When Jessica gets home from work later in the evening, she finds Casey asleep on the couch. She picks up Ryan and feels how hot he is. He is also limp, like a rag doll. Jessica notices that he is making funny noises when he breaths. She is frightened and immediately takes him to the Neighborhood Hospital emergency department, where Ryan is admitted with dehydration. While at the hospital, he is also diagnosed with respiratory syncytial virus and failure to thrive.

Episode 15
A few days after Ryan is discharged from the hospital, a social worker makes a home visit, meeting with Jessica alone while Casey is at work. A detailed history is taken, and issues regarding child care, feeding practices, and Casey come to light. Based on the visit, the social worker advises Jessica to take Ryan to Kangaroo Junction Preschool, a special school for children at risk for domestic abuse or neglect, during the daytime and to Jessica's mother in the evenings. Specifically, the social worker recommends that Casey not care for Ryan. Fearing Casey's

reaction to the situation, Jessica tells Casey that the lady from the hospital made her aware of a free day-care service for kids, and that her mother wants to watch the baby more frequently during the evenings. She is relieved that Casey does not question her further on this.

Jessica also goes for her 20-week prenatal visit. When Carol Ramsey, the nurse midwife, asks her how things are going, Jessica admits to fatigue, but confirms that she is taking the prenatal vitamins. When asked about her smoking and alcohol intake, Jessica reports that she is still smoking, but not as much. She tells Carol, "Casey smokes, so it is hard not to smoke, and I've only had a few beers since last visit." Jessica does not tell Carol about Ryan's recent illness or the social worker's visit. **[MR] [P]**

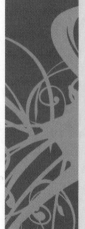

JESSICA RILEY
Season 2

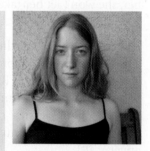

Biographical Information
Jessica Riley is an 18-year-old single mother with a 1-year-old son, Ryan. She has had no contact with Ryan's father since before he was born. Jessica and Ryan live in a small, one-bedroom apartment with Jessica's boyfriend Casey. She is now 6 months pregnant with Casey's child. Although Jessica works full-time at a restaurant, she struggles financially. She is glad Casey contributes to paying the bills and is not sure how she could financially make it without him. Although she was successful at completing her GED, Jessica dropped out of the community college she was attending when she learned she was pregnant with a second child. She didn't think she could afford to go to school with another baby and wanted to focus on working as much as possible.

Jessica grew up in a single-parent home. Her father left the family when she was 7. She is the oldest child and has two younger siblings, Jenna and Jason. Her mother Evelyn helps by watching her baby in the evenings. Additionally, Jessica receives government assistance in the form of WIC coupons and Medicaid, and Ryan attends a government-assisted day-care program. Jessica does not exercise and eats mostly fast food. She smokes about one-half pack of cigarettes a day and drinks alcohol socially when she parties.

Episode 1
Jessica has her 24-week prenatal visit. She continues to see Carol Ramsey, the nurse midwife, and likes her a lot, because she makes her feel comfortable. She tells Carol that she tried to stop smoking, but hasn't been able to. When asked about her alcohol intake, Jessica tells her that she is no longer drinking. She adds that Casey was giving her a hard time about not drinking, so she has been pretending to drink to keep him happy. **[MR] [P]**

Episode 2
No news this week.

Episode 3
After work one evening this week, Jessica picks up Ryan from her mother's home and visits with her for about 20 minutes. When she arrives back at her apartment, Casey yells at her for being late and demands to know where she was. When she tries to explain, he pushes her down, causing her to fall to the floor, and accuses her of

lying to him. Shortly thereafter, he tells her he is sorry and treats her nicely for the next couple of days.

Episode 4
Jessica sees Carol, the nurse midwife, for her 28-week prenatal visit. Jessica tells the nurse that her major complaint at this point is ongoing constipation. When asked about the types of fluids she consumes, Jessica replies that she mostly drinks Cokes. The midwife suggests that Jessica reduce the number of soft drinks she consumes each day and increase her fluid and fiber intake. She also encourages Jessica to consider signing up for childbirth classes, even though she has recently had a baby. An ultrasound is done during the visit, and Jessica is thrilled when she learns that her baby is a girl. Jessica tells Carol, "I love the clothes for baby girls and cannot wait to dress her up."

Later that same day, Jessica is surprised at Casey's reaction when she tells him they are having a baby girl. She thought he would be pleased, but in fact, it is just the opposite. Jessica wonders what she can do to make him love her more. **[MR] [P]**

Episode 5
Jessica wins free tickets to the Neighborhood Zoo in a drawing at work. During the weekend, Jessica and Casey use the tickets to take Ryan to the zoo. On this particular day, Jessica enjoys the attention she receives from Casey. She loves it when they are able to spend time together like a real family. It makes her sad when she thinks about Casey's comments regarding having a girl, but she is sure that he will love their daughter once she is born.

Episode 6
Jessica invites a friend from work over to the apartment for lunch and to visit. After her friend leaves, Casey begins to yell at Jessica and accuses her of sharing secrets about him. Jessica denies this, telling Casey that she and her friend were just visiting. Casey grabs Jessica by the hair and threatens her. He tells Jessica that she is not to bring friends or her stupid mother to their apartment anymore. He also comments that Jessica is becoming a "fat whale."

Jessica has begun to experience leg cramps and heartburn. She does not recall having these symptoms when she was pregnant with Ryan and wonders if the stress of working, caring for Ryan, being pregnant, and trying to keep Casey happy is causing this. She frequently worries about making Casey angry and that he might leave her. **[VC]**

Episode 7
Jessica is very upset to learn that Casey lost his job. She worries about paying bills without his income and arranges to pick up additional shifts. She wishes he would not spend their money on beer.

Jessica is surprised when Casey tells her that he is going with her to her prenatal appointment. During the visit, Casey is very attentive and caring toward her. He dominates the conversation and tells Carol, the nurse midwife, that he just wants to be sure everything is perfect. Jessica is pleased with his level of interest in her pregnancy, but recognizes that his presence makes it difficult to talk with the midwife. Casey tells Carol that everything is fine, and Jessica doesn't really have a chance to tell the midwife about the heartburn and leg cramps she has been experiencing. **[MR] [P]**

Episode 8
Jessica comes home from a long day of work to find Casey drinking and smoking pot. She asks Casey if he has been able to find a job yet, because she is worried about making the rent payment. Jessica is surprised when Casey stands up and hits her on the left side of her abdomen, yelling that she is stupid and fat, and has no right to tell him what to do. Jessica knows that she is not seriously hurt, yet she lies in bed all night crying. The next morning, she goes to work, hoping to have a good day in tips. **[P]**

Episode 9
Jessica is confused by Casey's behavior. One day he is such a sweet guy, full of compliments and very apologetic about his occasional bad behavior—and then the next day he hits her. She tries to figure out what she is doing wrong that causes him to yell at her and hit her. She is relieved that Casey leaves Ryan alone.

Jessica has her 34-week prenatal visit. Carol talks with Jessica about fetal development and begins describing the birth process. During the exam, Jessica is scared when Carol asks her about the bruises on the side of her abdomen where Casey struck her. She tells the nurse that she bumped into a table, but Jessica can tell the midwife does not believe her story. She tells Jessica that sometimes she sees bruises like this on women who have been hit and asks her if that is what happened to her. Jessica denies being hit and again says she bumped into a table. **[MR] [P]**

Episode 10
No news this week.

Episode 11
Jessica goes in for her 36-week prenatal visit, accompanied by Casey. The nurse midwife asks Jessica and Casey about more visible bruises on her abdomen. Jessica becomes scared about what Casey might say or do and is relieved

when he tells Carol that Jessica is very clumsy and runs into things. Jessica quickly acknowledges that it's true.

Carol asks Casey to step out of the exam room during the vaginal exam. She says to Jessica, "It has been my experience that many women who have bruises like this have been hit." Jessica again denies that this is the case, telling the nurse midwife that she really is just fat and clumsy. Carol shares with Jessica that shelter information can be found in the women's bathroom, but Jessica tells the midwife she does not need anything like that. **[MR] [VC]**

Episode 12

Jessica sees Carol Ramsey, the nurse midwife, for her 37-week prenatal visit. During the vaginal exam, the midwife tells Jessica that her cervix is thinning and beginning to dilate slightly. Jessica asks her how much longer it will be before the baby comes. She hopes to have the baby soon so she can be thin and look pretty again. Casey has been nice to her this week, although he has made several comments about how fat she looks.

Jessica continues to work full-time, but it has become increasingly difficult, as she is very tired by the end of the day. She is so tired that she doesn't even have the energy to take care of Ryan. Several times this week, she has asked her mother to keep Ryan overnight for her and take him to day care in the morning. Jessica misses Ryan, but is relieved not to have to take care of him. **[MR] [P]**

Episode 13

Jessica takes the evening off from work because she is feeling very tired. She fixes dinner for Casey before going to work. While fixing dinner, Ryan begins crying in the other room, and she interrupts her cooking to attend to his needs.

When they all finally sit down to eat, Casey throws his plate against the wall and screams at Jessica for making a "lousy dinner." He then proceeds to yank her out of her chair and hit her in the back, knocking her down to the floor. She gets up crying, and he hits her in the abdomen, saying, "You care more about that damn brat than me and what I want." She falls to the floor, and he kicks her in the abdomen. Jessica screams in pain. Somehow, she gets off the floor and makes it into the bedroom. The neighbor in the next apartment hears the commotion. Knowing that Jessica is pregnant and in an abusive relationship, the neighbor calls the police.

When the police arrive, they find Casey watching television and smoking a joint. Jessica is doubled over on the bed crying, and Ryan is in his crib crying. The police note that she is pregnant and call for an ambulance. They

ask her if she was hit, and she denies it. The police tell Jessica that they are arresting Casey for drug possession and further questioning. Jessica calls her mother and asks her to come get Ryan and then meet her at the hospital. When the paramedics arrive, they start an IV, place Jessica on oxygen, and transport her to the hospital. At the hospital, the triage nurse sends her directly to the labor and delivery unit.

Jessica delivers a healthy female infant later in the evening. Because she suffered a small abruption to the placenta, the nurse midwife and physician suspect trauma from abuse. In the immediate postpartum period, Carol, the nurse midwife, talks with Jessica privately. Jessica is told that she had a small abruption, and that the placenta had an infarct. Carol explains that, in these situations, trauma is suspected. She also shares with Jessica that sometimes women in abusive relationships get hit or kicked in abdomen. Jessica cries and admits that this is what happened, but insists that Casey didn't mean to do it and will never do it again. Jessica tells Carol that she will not press charges.

Social work is called for a referral before Jessica is discharged. Jessica is told that a social work referral is required because of the risk of intimate partner violence and drug charges against Casey. Jessica worries about this, fearing that Casey will be angry if he finds out. The social worker makes a home visit the day after Jessica and the baby are discharged, and Jessica is relieved that Casey is not home. Jessica tells the social worker everything is fine and that there are really no problems. **[P]**

Episode 14

Casey and Jessica decide to name the baby Carrie. Jessica is happy, because Casey is kind and sweet to her. She notices the efforts he seems to be making to be a good father. He tells her he is so sorry that he hurt her, but is also glad she finally had the baby. Jessica knows how sorry he is and is glad that Casey didn't have to stay in jail. She anticipates that their problems are now in the past.

Jessica takes a few weeks off from work to be home with the baby. She would like to take more time off, but cannot afford to. Casey agrees to pick up extra shifts until she can go back to work. Jessica's mother spends time at the apartment, helping with the baby. Jessica becomes angry with her mother when Evelyn suggests that she leave Casey and move back home with her children. Jessica does not understand why her mother cannot see that Casey has changed.

The social worker makes another visit this week to assess the home situation. Jessica once again tells her that everything is fine and that Casey is an excellent father. **[P]**

Episode 15

Jessica has a postpartum exam with Carol Ramsey, the nurse midwife. Carol tells Jessica that everything is normal, with the exception of a slightly low hematocrit level. She also notes that Jessica's breasts have reduced in size. Jessica explains that she has decided not to breastfeed.

Carol starts Jessica on a contraception patch and explains that she should apply a new patch each week. Carol also explains the need to eat a healthy diet and take vitamins and iron. When asked about the situation at home, Jessica tells the midwife that everything is great and that Casey is a wonderful father. Carol admires how beautiful Carrie is and notes that she has contact dermatitis on her bottom. Carol suggests that Jessica use an ointment and change the brand of diapers she is using. **[P]**

JESSICA RILEY
Season 3

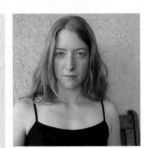

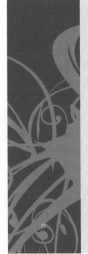

Biographical Information

Jessica Riley is an 18-year-old single mother with a 17-month-old son, Ryan, and a 6-week-old daughter, Carrie. Jessica and her children share a one-bedroom apartment with Carrie's father, Casey. Jessica has not heard from Ryan's father since before he was born.

Jessica works full-time at a restaurant, but struggles financially. She is glad Casey contributes to paying the bills and is not sure how she could financially make it without him. She has earned her GED, but dropped out of the community college after she became pregnant with Carrie.

Jessica grew up in a single-parent home. Her father left the family when she was 7. She is the oldest child and has two younger siblings, Jenna and Jason. Her mother Evelyn helps by watching her baby in the evenings. Additionally, Jessica receives government assistance in the form of WIC coupons and Medicaid, and Ryan and Carrie attend a government-assisted day-care program.

Episode 1

Jessica has a much-needed day off from work. She is very happy to stay at home with Casey and her two children. Because of his night-shift work schedule, Casey lies down for an afternoon nap. Jessica gets a phone call from her mother. While on the phone, Carrie begins to cry. Before Jessica can get off the phone, Casey hangs the phone up on her, hits her on the left side of the face, and screams at her to keep the damn baby quiet. Crying, Jessica runs to get Carrie to protect her. She is thankful that Casey leaves the apartment. During the course of the next several days, Jessica tells her coworkers and mother that she ran into a door. **[P]**

Episode 2

Jessica's bruises are healing. She has a visit with the social worker this week and tells her things have been going well. When the social worker asks Jessica if the marks on her face are bruises, Jessica replies that she bumped her head on a door. Jessica is relieved that Carrie and Ryan look fine.

Episode 3

Jessica is thrilled when Casey tells her he is moving to the day shift. She is sure that, if they can spend their evenings together, Casey will be happier and won't hit her anymore.

Episode 4

No news this week.

Episode 5

When Casey fails to come home one night this week, Jessica stays up all night concerned for his safety. When he finally comes home, Jessica asks him where he has been and why he didn't call. She also points out to him that he is supposed to be at work. She does not expect Casey's reaction. Casey strikes her in the head and throws her against the wall. Jessica hits the back of her head against the wall, causing a large, painful bump. She does not understand what she did wrong to cause him to act this way, but his behavior frightens her.

At work, Jessica again has to explain her facial bruises and swelling to her coworkers. Her mother Evelyn does not believe her explanations and attempts to talk with Jessica about getting away from Casey. Jessica tells her mother that she just sometimes makes him mad, but Casey does not mean to harm her. **[VC]**

Episode 6

When Casey does not come home one night this week, Jessica thinks better than to ask him where he has been. She is afraid that he will hurt her or her children. When at home together, she does everything she can think of to win Casey's approval. Because he is out of work again, Jessica is worried about money and hopes to work more hours at the restaurant.

The social worker makes a home visit to see Jessica, Carrie, and Ryan—partly because of a concern raised by Ryan's teacher, Miss Webb. The social worker again notes old bruises on Jessica's face, but sees that the children appear well fed and unharmed. The social worker talks with Jessica about removing herself from her current situation. Jessica tells the social worker she will think about it, but that things are fine.

Episode 7

Jessica is thrilled to see all the money Casey pulls from his pants pocket. She asks him how he got so much money and wonders if he found a job. Her question is answered with a beating to the head and stomach. He yells at Jessica and asks her when she is going to lose some weight.

The next day, Jessica avoids seeing her mother, but is confronted by several coworkers. They tell her that it is obvious what is going on and plead with her to get away from Casey. One of the girls tells Jessica about the battered women's shelter in town and asks her to go there if things get any worse. Jessica tells them it is all her fault, and Casey is not to blame. There is no way they could ever understand why she can't leave Casey. She loves and needs him, but at the same time, she is afraid of him. Jessica's mother Evelyn also pleads with Jessica to get away from Casey—if not for herself, for the safety of her children. Jessica wants to talk to her mother, but just can't figure out where to start.

Episode 8

It has been a couple of weeks now since Casey hit Jessica. She is beginning to think that things are going to improve. Jessica picks up Carrie and Ryan from day care and is told that Carrie feels hot. Jessica also notes that Carrie feels hot and is very irritable. Because it is after hours, she takes Carrie to the emergency department, where she is treated by Dr. Gordon for an ear infection. **[P]**

Episode 9

At 2:15 a.m., Casey unexpectedly begins pounding on Jessica's head with his fists while she is asleep. She screams in pain and tries to get away. Casey yells at her for not waiting up for him. Jessica can tell Casey has been drinking, and he is acting very strange. She is able to get out of bed, but he catches her and continues to beat her. She finally gets away from him, and he laughs at her, telling her she is fat and ugly. Shortly thereafter, Casey passes out on the couch.

Jessica quickly gathers a few belongings and her two children, and leaves the apartment. She recalls what her friend told her about the battered women's shelter and goes there directly. At the shelter, Jessica is told that she and her children can stay there temporarily until other arrangements can be made. She is assured that it is unlikely Casey will find her. Jessica is told that the most dangerous time for women is when they leave their abuser; for this reason, she must not reveal to Casey where she is.

From the shelter, Jessica calls her mother and explains the situation. Evelyn pleads with Jessica to come home, but Jessica knows that Casey will look for her there. Jessica doesn't even tell her mother exactly where she is, other than to say that she and the children are in a safe place. Jessica promises to get back in touch with Evelyn in a few days. She asks her mother to call her boss at work to let him know that she'll be out for a few weeks, but to tell him nothing else.

Episode 10

Jessica, Ryan, and Carrie spend a long week at the shelter. She meets several other women who have had similar experiences. The shelter staff and professional counselors spend time with Jessica and the other women, talking with them about domestic violence and abusive situations, and helping them consider alternative long-term plans. They talk with Jessica about the possibility of pressing charges against Casey and getting a restraining order. During the week, Jessica experiences a range of emotions, from anger toward Casey for the way he has treated her, to sadness over missing him and wanting to work things out with him.

Jessica is able to spend a little time with her mother during the week. Evelyn is so grateful that Jessica and the kids are safe. Evelyn tells Jessica that Casey came by and demanded to know where she and the kids were. She warns Jessica to stay away from him. **[P]**

Episode 11

Jessica calls Casey this week to talk and let him know that she and the kids are okay. She tells him she hopes they can patch things up. Casey tells Jessica that he loves and misses her, and wants her to come back home. He asks

Jessica where she is (something the shelter staff told her would happen), and when she refuses to answer, he becomes angry and threatens to kill her. Jessica hangs up, knowing now that she can never go back home to Casey.

A couple of days later, Jessica learns that Casey has been arrested and is in jail on armed robbery and vehicular homicide charges. She believes that, as long as he is in jail, she can return to her apartment and try to get back into a regular routine.

Episode 12
No news this week.

Episode 13
Although she has returned to work, Jessica finds herself deeply in debt. Both of her credit cards are at their limits, and she is behind on paying her rent and utilities. She feels overwhelmed with the responsibility of trying to support her two children independently. Jessica figures out that, even if she worked 24 hours a day for the next 2 months, she would still remain in debt. If it were not for her WIC coupons and other government assistance, Jessica knows her kids would be hungry. She finds herself wishing that Casey was not in jail so he could help her pay the bills.

Episode 14
Jessica has been spending most of her free time with her children at her mother's house. She is comforted by the company of her mother and siblings as she continues to work through her feelings. Jessica feels reconnected to her family; in fact, she feels a connection with them that she cannot remember ever experiencing. She has come to appreciate her mother's tireless efforts, not only for Ryan and Carrie, but also for her siblings, Jason and Jenna. She hopes to be as good of a mother as Evelyn.

It is during this week that Jessica makes the decision to move back home in the hopes of having the opportunity for a new start. Evelyn agrees to help her get back into school. Jessica knows this is the best chance she has to support herself and her children in the years to come. **[P]**

Episode 15
Jessica moves back to her mother's home this week. Within a few days of moving, she receives a letter in the mail from Casey. She wonders how he knows that she moved back home with her mother. She feels uneasy and worries about her safety and the safety of her children in the future. **[P]**

CASEY HOLMES
Season 1

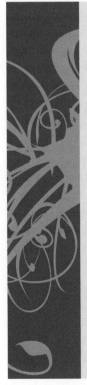

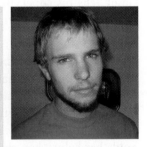

Biographical Information

Casey Holmes is a physically fit 23-year-old male who had a troubled youth. His parents divorced when he was very young, and he bounced back and forth between parents—both of whom remarried. Growing up, he often saw his father hit his stepmother when he was angry. As an adolescent, Casey became involved with a gang and was arrested a few times for petty crimes, such as shoplifting and vandalism. He never finished high school and moved out on his own at the age of 18. Since that time, he has held a number of odd jobs and has made an effort to stay out of trouble.

For the past several months, Casey has been working as a basic laborer for a general construction company, performing tasks such as shoveling, raking, hauling mortar in wheelbarrows, and running a jackhammer to break up concrete. He has not been given an opportunity to learn more advanced skills, because his supervisors and coworkers note that he often shows up late for work and displays little motivation. Casey is paid minimum wage and has health insurance as a job benefit. He feels that he is underpaid for the type of work he does. Casey also has a savings plan option as an additional job benefit, but he does not participate, because he would rather just have the money to spend. On most days after work, Casey shares a 12-pack of beer with his buddies and smokes dope. He also uses other drugs when he can afford to buy them. He sometimes worries about the possibility of getting caught in a random drug screen, but he figures he can always get another job.

Episode 3

Casey has spent nearly every spare moment with Jessica since meeting her a few weeks ago. He has spent very little time around infants or children, so he thinks it is cool. He decides to move in with Jessica and offers to take care of Ryan in the evenings while she works. One day this week he has a hangover in the morning and is late to work. The superintendent emphasizes to Casey the need to get to work on time, but Casey perceives his boss as just giving him a hard time. **[P]**

Episode 4

Casey takes care of Ryan in the evenings. He finds that he does not really like doing it. Because Ryan spits up a lot, he figures the kid must not be too hungry and just quits trying to feed him. He does not often change Ryan's diapers because it is gross, and he knows Jessica will do it when she comes home anyway. The main reason Casey hates taking care of the baby is because Ryan cries a lot. When Ryan cries, Casey feels angry. Often, he copes by putting the baby in his crib, closing the door, and then playing video games or watching a movie with the volume up very loud so that he doesn't have to hear Ryan.

At work, Casey is disciplined by his supervisor for failing to wear ear protection while using a jackhammer. Casey tells his supervisor that he just forgets to wear it, and that it is uncomfortable. **[VC]**

Episode 5

Casey has been busy and tired from working all day and needs to get out and hang with his buddies. Sometimes, Casey leaves the baby alone in the apartment to get away from the crying. He figures that, as long as Ryan is in the crib, he should be okay. He is critical of how often Jessica holds her baby when she is at home. He tells her that she has turned him into a spoiled brat, which is why he cries so much when she is away.

Casey is late to work once this week and is also written up for failing to use protective ear equipment again while using a jackhammer.

Episode 6

Casey has a party several nights in a row at the apartment while Jessica is at work. Casey and his friends use cocaine, smoke pot, and drink beer while they are partying. His friends poke fun at him for "babysitting." He puts Ryan in the bedroom with the door closed so that he doesn't bother them. Casey fails to show up for work 2 days in a row and is fired from his job.

Episode 7

Casey is looking for a job. Jessica has an appointment with the doctor for Ryan to get shots, and she can't get off work. When she asks Casey if he would take Ryan, he tells her that Ryan is healthy, and it would be stupid to give shots to healthy kids unless they were living in a Third World country. **[P]**

Episode 8

Casey is still looking for a job. He borrows money from Jessica to buy beer and gets drunk every day this week. **[P]**

Episode 9

Casey gets a job at with a landscape contractor. He works hard during the day and comes home very tired. He drinks beer and smokes a joint to unwind and continues to take care of Ryan in the evenings. **[P]**

Episode 10

No news this week.

Episode 11

Jessica tells Casey she is pregnant. He is happy with this news, because this now means that Jessica is his. He tells Jessica he hopes it is a boy, and they should name their baby Casey Jr. He celebrates by having his buddies over to drink beer. **[P]**

Episode 12

No news this week.

Episode 13

Casey is suspicious that Jessica is having an affair. After a phone call from a man, Casey pushes her to the floor, telling her that he'll hurt her if she ever leaves him. The next day, Casey feels badly about this and buys Jessica flowers.

Episode 14

On her way out the door for an evening shift, Jessica tells Casey that Ryan has been sick and asks him keep a close eye on him. After Jessica leaves for work, Casey puts Ryan in his crib, goes to the refrigerator, and opens a can of beer. He drinks beer and smokes pot most of the evening and only checks in on Ryan once. Casey is passed out asleep on the couch when Jessica comes home. He does not wake up until the following morning, when Jessica calls him from the hospital to tell him about Ryan. **[P]**

Episode 15

Casey learns that a woman from the hospital came by the apartment. Jessica tells Casey that the woman came from the hospital to see how Ryan was doing. She also tells Casey that the woman told her about free babysitting, so he would no longer have to watch Ryan in the evening. Casey is glad to hear this. **[P]**

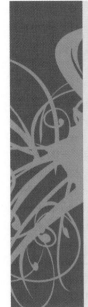

CASEY HOLMES
Season 2

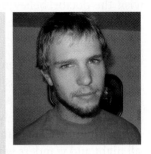

Biographical Information

Casey Holmes is a physically fit 23-year-old male who had a troubled youth. His parents divorced when he was very young, and he bounced back and forth between parents—both of whom remarried. Growing up, he often saw his father hit his stepmother when he was angry. As an adolescent, Casey became involved with a gang and was arrested a few times for petty crimes, such as shoplifting and vandalism. He never finished high school and moved out on his own at the age of 18. Since that time, he has held a number of odd jobs and has made an effort to stay out of trouble.

Casey lives with his pregnant girlfriend Jessica Riley and her son Ryan. He does not particularly like Ryan and thinks Jessica spoils him. He is very proud of the fact that Jessica is pregnant with his baby. He is controlling of Jessica and does not want anybody else looking at her. On most days after work and into the evening, Casey drinks beer and smokes dope with his buddies. He is irritated that Jessica does not party with him as much as she did when they first met. Casey also uses other drugs when he can afford to buy them.

Episode 1

Casey and his buddies are partying in their apartment when Jessica gets off work one evening this week. Casey pops a beer open for Jessica and tells her to drink it, because she has some "catching up" to do. He is happy that she takes the beer he offers her. **[P]**

Episode 2

No news this week.

Episode 3

Casey is pretty angry by the time Jessica arrives home from work nearly one-half hour late one evening this week. He had mental images of someone at work touching her, and he was sure she probably enjoyed it. As soon as she comes in the door, he begins to yell at her, wanting an explanation of where she was and who she was with. He is so angry that he pushes her to the floor. Casey later feels sorry for what he did and vows to make it up to her. He treats her nicely for the next couple of days. **[P]**

Episode 4

Casey is angry when Jessica tells him they are going to have a girl, and he tells her that she should be giving him a son. He says he doesn't even know why anyone would want a girl. **[VC]**

Episode 5

Casey has been late to work several days during the past couple of weeks. His boss tells him that, if he wants to continue to have a job, he needs to be on time. Casey does not like the fact that his boss hassles him so much. Over the weekend, Casey takes Jessica and Ryan to the zoo. He does not particularly like zoos, but he enjoys the outing. While at the concession stand, he notices a girl working behind the counter and thinks she is hot.

Episode 6

Jessica has a girlfriend over to the house for lunch and to visit. Casey does not like the way her friend looks at him. He later overhears them laughing, and he is sure they are talking about him. After she leaves, Casey yells at Jessica, accusing her of sharing secrets about him. He grabs Jessica by the hair and shakes her while he yells at her. He tells her, "Whatever happens between us stays between us, and if you tell anybody anything, I will kill them." Casey also tells Jessica that she is starting to look like a fat whale. He is not sexually attracted to her because of her weight gain.

Episode 7

Casey is fired from his job this week. He failed to check the hydraulic fluid level prior to operating the Bobcat and, because the fluid level was low, the pump burned out and significantly damaged the equipment. Casey buys a 12-pack of beer on the way home.

A few days later, Casey accompanies Jessica to her prenatal visit. He is curious about what goes on during her visits and wants to impress the medical personnel. He is very attentive to Jessica during the visit and asks many questions. He also wants to see if she is really going to visit the doctor, believing it's possible she is meeting another man during these "appointments." **[VC]**

Episode 8

Casey is enjoying listening to music and smoking pot when Jessica starts hassling him about getting a job. He yells at her that she is not going to start bossing him around and telling him what to do. He hits her on the side of her abdomen. He is annoyed with the fact that she cries all night and wonders why she can't just get over it. **[P]**

Episode 9

No news this week.

Episode 10

No news this week.

Episode 11

Casey has found a night job working in a warehouse. The pay is okay, and at least he won't have to work all that hard. The worst part about the job, in Casey's opinion, is that the hours are not great for the party scene. However, he is told that a day position may open up in the near future.

Casey accompanies Jessica to her prenatal visit. Right before the midwife exposes Jessica's abdomen, he tells Carol that Jessica is clumsy and has some bruises on her abdomen from running into things. He steps out of the room during the exam and wonders if they will talk about the bruises. Before they leave the appointment, he asks Carol how long he will have to wait before he can have sex with Jessica after the baby is born, and how long she will be moody.

Episode 12

Casey buys flowers for Jessica this week and tells her she is wonderful. He also tells her he will be glad when she is no longer pregnant.

Casey smokes cocaine with his friend Robert. They run out of cocaine and don't have the money to buy more, so Casey and Robert break into some cars and steal stereo systems, which they sell at a pawn shop for drug money. Casey misses work twice this week. **[P]**

Episode 13

Casey watches Jessica making dinner while he watches TV and thinks to himself that she is getting so fat! Ryan is in the other room crying, so Jessica stops what she is doing to attend to Ryan. When he finally sits down to eat, Casey throws a plate against the wall and screams at her for making a "lousy dinner." He then proceeds to hit her hard in the abdomen, saying, "You care more about the damn brat than me and what I want." She falls to the floor screaming. Ryan is in the other room crying. Casey lights up a joint to relax. When the police arrive, they find Jessica doubled over and crying, Ryan in his crib crying, and Casey watching TV and smoking a joint. The police arrest Casey for drug possession and take him in for further questioning. Casey spends a couple of days in jail before his buddy, Robert, bails him out. He learns that Jessica had their baby and is anxious to get home to see her.

Episode 14

Casey and Jessica agree to name their baby Carrie. Casey wants to be a good father. He helps Jessica with some of the infant care duties, but completely ignores Ryan. Casey does not like seeing the baby sucking on Jessica's breast. He thinks it looks ugly and tells Jessica she should feed the baby with a bottle. Jessica tells Casey that a lady from the hospital will be coming by to see Carrie every once in a while. **[P]**

Episode 15

Casey does not like all the attention Jessica gives the baby. He also wishes the baby was a boy. At the same time, he proudly tells everyone at work about his daughter, because he enjoys the attention it brings him. Casey and Robert break into more cars for drug money this week. Casey considers it easy money, and it pays much better than his warehouse job.

CASEY HOLMES
Season 3

Biographical Information

Casey Holmes is a physically fit 24-year-old male. He lives with his girlfriend Jessica Riley, their 6-week-old infant daughter Carrie, and Jessica's 17-month-old son Ryan. Casey does not particularly like Ryan and thinks Jessica spoils him. He is proud to be a father, but wishes Carrie were a boy. During Jessica's pregnancy, he physically abused her on several occasions.

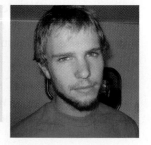

Continued

Each time, he felt badly for hurting her and vowed to make it up to her. He has not injured Jessica since the night she went into labor.

Casey works the night shift at a warehouse as a stocker. He spends a lot of his free time with his buddies drinking beer and smoking dope. Casey and his friend Robert have recently been vandalizing cars for drug money.

Episode 1

After working a night shift, Casey is sleeping during the afternoon while Jessica is home with her children. When Carrie's cry wakes him up, he is angry. He walks out into the living room to find Jessica talking on the phone. He hangs up the phone and strikes her on the left side of her face. He tells her that he is not to be disturbed while he is trying to sleep and to make the damn baby shut up. When Jessica starts to cry, he leaves the apartment for a couple of hours. **[P]**

Episode 2

Casey and Robert spend most of their free time this week partying with friends.

Episode 3

A day-shift position opens up at the warehouse where Casey works, and he applies for the position and gets it. He is happy to be able to get back to working during the day. Casey and Robert break into a home this week. **[P]**

Episode 4

No news this week.

Episode 5

Casey goes to a party with Robert after work. He stays out all night drinking and smoking crack. When he gets home the next morning, Jessica is hysterical; she was worried about where he might have been, whether he was okay, and that he might miss work. Casey hits Jessica in the face, throws her against the wall, and shouts, "You are not my mother, and I can do whatever the hell I want!" He goes to the refrigerator to pop open a beer. Casey is fired from his warehouse job. **[P]**

Episode 6

Casey has been on a partying binge for the entire week. He has been staying out late and, in some cases, all night. At one party this week, he meets a girl by the name of Amber, and they end up having unprotected sex. Casey thinks she is better looking than Jessica. He is glad Jessica has not asked him where he has been. **[P]**

Episode 7

Casey is looking for a job this week. He applies at several places, but is not very enthusiastic about any of the job leads. Casey and Robert steal a car and strip it of its parts to sell at a salvage yard. He becomes angry when Jessica

asks him where he got the money, and to punish her, he kicks her in the stomach and tells her to lose some weight. Casey sees Amber twice this week. **[P]**

Episode 8

No news this week.

Episode 9

Casey comes home after partying and finds Jessica asleep. He wakes her up and begins to beat her because she did not stay up and wait for him. He later falls asleep. When he wakes up the next morning, Jessica and the kids are gone.

Episode 10

Casey has been looking for Jessica all week. He is furious that she has left. He parks in front of Evelyn's house, expecting to find Jessica and the kids there, but sees no sign of them. He asks Evelyn where they are, and she tells Casey she really doesn't know. He frequently checks at the restaurant to see if she is at work, but does not find her there. **[P]**

Episode 11

Jessica calls Casey this week, and he tells her to come back home. She tells him she misses him and loves him, but can't come back right now. Casey promises to never hurt her again and asks Jessica where she is. When Jessica does not tell him, he threatens to kill her.

Later that same evening, Casey and Robert attempt armed robbery at a local business. While attempting to flee, they are involved in an automobile crash that kills two innocent victims. Casey and Robert are booked in the Neighborhood Jail on charges of armed robbery and vehicular homicide.

Episode 12

Casey is in jail.

Episode 13

Casey is in jail.

Episode 14

Casey is in jail.

Episode 15

Casey remains in jail. He finds out from his buddies that Jessica and the kids have moved back to her mother's home. He writes a letter to Jessica, asking her forgiveness and for her to come visit him.

RYAN RILEY
Season 1

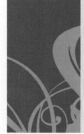

Biographical Information

Ryan Riley is a 1-month-old infant boy who was born to Jessica Riley, a 17-year-old single mother. Although his mother had minimal prenatal care, he was a healthy, 6-pound, 4 -ounce infant at birth, and there were no complications during labor, birth, or immediately following birth. Ryan's grandmother, Evelyn, is his primary caretaker while Jessica is at work or at school, although many other people take care of him as well.

Episode 1

Ryan screams and cries almost nonstop for several hours every night this week. He is inconsolable. No matter what Jessica does, he continues to cry. He is taken to the emergency department (ED) twice this week; both times, he is discharged with a diagnosis of colic.

Episode 2

No news this week.

Episode 3

Jessica and Evelyn take Ryan to the clinic for his 2-month immunizations and well-child visit. He weighs 10 pounds at this visit, and his mother and grandmother are praised for his excellent weight gain. **[MR]**

Episode 4

No news this week.

Episode 5

Ryan isn't seeing his grandmother as much as he used to and begins to experience inconsistent care. During the daytime, he goes to his grandmother's house. While there, his grandmother and Aunt Jenna hold him frequently, talk to him, and play with him. Additionally, he is fed consistently and kept clean. He finds his grandmother's voice comforting.

When Ryan is picked up and taken home, he has a different experience. He is usually put in his crib, and there are many loud noises. This upsets him and makes him cry. When his mother holds him, he finds it comforting, even though it is for only short periods of time. Casey holds him infrequently and is rough. He never looks at him, and he yells a lot. Feedings at home are inconsistent. Often, Ryan is put in his crib with a propped bottle, but the bottle often falls away, and Ryan can't get it. Ryan's diapers are changed infrequently, and he has developed an uncomfortable rash.

Episode 6

No news this week.

Episode 7

Ryan is now 17 weeks old. He is supposed to go for a well-baby check-up this week, but his mother cancels the appointment. He often feels hungry and is cranky. He is being fed about 4 to 5 ounces four times a day. He cries frequently and does not see his grandmother as much as he used to.

Episode 8

No news this week.

Episode 9

No news this week.

Episode 10

Ryan is now 6 months old. With Jessica's permission, Ryan's grandmother takes him to the pediatrician for a well-baby visit. He weighs 14 pounds. The pediatrician notes a change in his weight pattern and asks Evelyn about Ryan's home situation regarding feedings. Evelyn is able to describe her routine when she takes care of Ryan, but admits it is only a few hours a day. She tells the physician that she is unable to describe Ryan's feeding patterns in the evening. **[MR]**

Episode 11

No news this week.

Episode 12

No news this week.

Episode 13

No news this week.

Episode 14

Ryan is now 9 months old. He has been sick off and on for the past week with a cold. Because Evelyn is out of town this week, Jessica's friend, Carol, babysits Ryan for the day while Jessica works the first part of a double shift. Ryan does not feel good at all. He is not interested in eating or playing and has no energy.

Jessica picks up Ryan from Carol's house, takes him home, and leaves him with Casey for the evening while she goes back to work. Ryan is put in his crib and left alone all evening. During the course of the evening, Ryan gets worse and has nothing to drink. When Jessica comes home later that evening, Ryan feels very sick and is having problems breathing. His mother immediately takes him to the hospital.

The emergency department physician, Dr. Gordon, asks Jessica how long Ryan has been sick, how many wet diapers he had in the past day, and when he last ate. Jessica tells Dr. Gordon that Ryan has had a cold for a week or so, but got sick just today. She admits that she doesn't know when he last ate or the number of wet diapers he has had. She tells Dr. Gordon that she has been working a lot of hours during the past several days.

Ryan stabilizes in the emergency department with oxygen and fluid support. After a work-up, he is diagnosed with dehydration and bronchiolitis. He is admitted to the subacute pediatric unit. The admitting orders include an IV fluid infusion of D5 $\frac{1}{4}$ NaCl with 10 mEq KCL; urine bag for output measurement; O_2 by nasal cannula at 2 L/min; suction of nares and nasal pharynx; and Pedialyte to encourage oral fluids while the respiratory distress resolves. **[MR]**

Episode 15

Ryan spends the entire week at the hospital. As his respiratory syncytial virus (RSV) resolves, he starts taking oral fluids and eating baby food. His medical records are obtained from the pediatrician's office, and his weights at birth, 2 months, and 6 months are analyzed. A rapid weight gain is noted during his 7-day hospital admission, and Ryan now weighs 16 pounds. A diagnosis of failure to thrive is confirmed. The social service department is consulted, and a home visit is planned shortly after discharge. Discharge teaching includes the topics of infant feeding and nutrition, general care, developmental milestones, and safety. Ryan is scheduled for a follow-up visit at the pediatrician's office 1 week after discharge.

A few days after discharge, a social worker makes a home visit and takes an extensive history; issues regarding child care, feeding practices, and Casey come to light. Based on the visit, the social worker advises Jessica to take Ryan to Kangaroo Junction Preschool, a center for children at risk for domestic abuse or neglect, during the daytime and to Evelyn's home in the evenings. Specifically, it is recommended that Casey not care for Ryan.

RYAN RILEY
Season 2

Biographical Information

Ryan Riley is Jessica Riley's 1-year-old son. Ryan lives in a one-bedroom apartment with his mother and her boyfriend Casey. Ryan recently was hospitalized with dehydration, respiratory syncytial virus (RSV), and failure to thrive. Because he was found to be underweight and undernourished, Social Services made arrangements for him to attend Kangaroo Junction Preschool during the day and encouraged Jessica to take Ryan to his grandmother's home in the evenings when she is working.

Episode 1

Ryan has been attending the new day care for a couple of months now. He has a very consistent routine and enjoys the social interaction with his caregivers at the center. His grandmother Evelyn takes Ryan in for his 12-month immunizations and well-child exam. On this visit, Ryan weighs 20 pounds; the pediatrician remarks to Evelyn that he is really starting to show some good progress. Evelyn is pleased and shares the good news with Jessica. **[P]**

Episode 2
No news this week.

Episode 3
Ryan is picked up by his mother from Evelyn's home. When they get home, he is put in his crib, and then hears yelling and his mother crying. The noises frighten Ryan, and he begins to cry. Casey comes into the room and yells at him loudly to shut up—and then slams the door. **[P]**

Episode 4

No news this week.

Episode 5

Ryan goes to the zoo with Jessica and Casey. He sits in a stroller nearly the entire time playing with paper. He gets cranky while in the stroller and wants to be held by his mother. Jessica gives him a bottle with Coke in it. Ryan is happy to drink the soda. **[P]**

Episode 6

No news this week.

Episode 7

No news this week.

Episode 8

Ryan has not seen his mother very much during the past week. He has been spending nearly all his time at the day care center or with his grandmother. He loves his grandmother's home because Evelyn, Jenna, and Jason are always there to play with him. Ryan takes his first steps this week.

Episode 9

No news this week.

Episode 10

Because Ryan is now walking, he finds all sorts of things to explore at home. He does not like it when Casey is there, because he yells at him frequently and puts him in his crib. Ryan does not like this because he gets bored in his crib. Although Casey has never hurt him, the yelling frightens him. **[P]**

Episode 11

Fifteen-month-old Ryan has been running a fever and has a great deal of nasal drainage and congestion. He does not feel well at all. Worried about how ill he was the last time he was sick, Evelyn takes him to Neighborhood Pediatrics to be examined. Ryan is diagnosed with an upper respiratory infection. Evelyn is instructed to give him plenty of fluids and children's acetaminophen (Tylenol) for the fever. Ryan's weight on this visit is 21 $1/2$ pounds.

Episode 12

Ryan feels much better this week. He has spent nearly all of his time with his grandmother during the past few weeks because his mother has been working additional hours. He usually sees his mother between the time he is picked up from day care and when she has to go back to work for the evening shift. Often he spends the night with his grandmother. Ryan misses seeing his mother, but he is very happy at his grandmother's house. **[P]**

Episode 13

Ryan is picked up by his mother from day care this week, and she takes him home. As soon as they get home, he is put in his crib. He does not want to be in the crib. Ryan tries to climb over the rails to escape the crib, but is unable to. He cries until his mother comes into the room and spends some time with him. Later, he hears shouting and then hears his mother screaming. He is frightened and begins to cry. He then hears very loud music, and his mother crying. Later, some strange men come into his room, which frightens him further. Ryan is not comforted until his grandmother picks him up and takes him to her home.

Episode 14

Ryan sees there is a baby in the house. His mother tells him this is his sister, and her name is Carrie. Ryan does not understand any of this, but he likes the baby. **[P]**

Episode 15

No news this week.

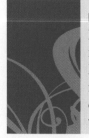

RYAN RILEY
Season 3

Biographical Information

Ryan Riley is Jessica Riley's 17-month-old son. As an infant, Ryan was diagnosed with failure to thrive, but this condition has improved over the past year. Ryan lives in a one-bedroom apartment with his mother, infant sister, and his mother's boyfriend Casey. He attends Kangaroo Junction Preschool during the day and stays with his grandmother Evelyn in the evenings when his mother is working.

Episode 1

Ryan has done well at the Kangaroo Junction Preschool program. He has come to understand a predictable and orderly routine both at day care and at his grandmother's home. At day care, he has social interactions with many other children his age, primarily engaging in parallel play.

His world is not orderly and structured in his mother's home. Because of this, there are no rituals for bedtime, mealtime, or morning routine. This week, Ryan sees Casey hit his mother, making his mother cry. He holds his favorite toy Boo Bear for comfort.

Episode 2

The social worker makes a visit to see Jessica, Carrie, and Ryan. The social worker sees that the living conditions are messy, but the children appear healthy and show no evidence of neglect or abuse. She watches Ryan at play talking to Boo Bear and playing with blocks on the floor, noting these behaviors to be age appropriate.

Episode 3

Ryan's baby sister goes with him to Kangaroo Junction. He watches as they put her in a room with other babies. Ryan goes with the older children to Miss Webb's room. Ryan is delighted to use crayons to draw a picture.

At home, Ryan protests when Jessica takes a marker away from him. He cries until she gives it back to him to keep him quiet. He makes marks on the wall and receives a spanking as punishment.

Episode 4

No news this week.

Episode 5

Ryan cries when he sees Casey hit his mother and throw her against the wall. He is further frightened by the yelling. Casey tells Ryan, "You shut up, or I'll bust your chops." Later in the week, while at Kangaroo Junction, Miss Webb observes Ryan hitting stuffed animals with his hands and telling them to "shut up."

Episode 6

The social worker comes by to see 20-month old Ryan this week. She observes a curious child who is very busy with purposeful behavior. He places his favorite stuffed toy Boo Bear under a pillow so that he can hide and stay safe. He goes into the kitchen and pulls pots and pans out of the cupboards, places various toy objects in the pots, and then puts the lids on the pots. Later he goes back to the kitchen to retrieve a specific toy from the pot. The social worker does not note evidence of physical abuse.

Episode 7

Ryan spends the night with his grandmother four nights this week. He enjoys being there because he sits on her lap before bed and looks at storybooks while she reads to him. When at home, he brings books to his mother for her to read, but is told no. He often gets angry and cries when he does not get his way.

Episode 8

No news this week.

Episode 9

Ryan is very upset that his routine has changed again. He is taken by his mother to a strange home. There are other children there, but they are different from the children at his school. He wants to see his grandmother. He wants to see Miss Webb. He wants to go back home. He clutches Boo Bear for comfort.

Episode 10

Ryan remains at the new house. He has quickly learned a new routine here. He stays in a room with his sister and mother. The people at the house are nice to him. There are many toys to play with. He misses his grandmother and asks Jessica about her.

Episode 11

Ryan is very happy to go back to his home and return to his previous routine. He is also very happy to see his grandmother and Miss Webb. He notices Casey is not at the apartment, but does not ask his mother about him.

Episode 12

No news this week.

Episode 13

No news this week.

Episode 14

Ryan goes with his grandmother to the pediatrician's office so that his sister can get her shots. While there, the nurse weighs Ryan, noting that he now weighs 25 pounds at 21 1/2 months of age. The nurse and Evelyn are pleased with the progress he has made in weight gain, noting he is now just below the 25th percentile.

Episode 15

Ryan is happy to move to his grandmother's house. He watches his grandmother and mother set up a crib in the room for his sister and sees that Boo Bear has been placed on a bed in the same room. He knows they will stay here now. [P]

CARRIE HOLMES
Season 2

Biographical Information

Carrie Holmes is a newborn infant girl, daughter of Jessica Riley and Casey Holmes. She was born at 38 weeks' gestation by vaginal delivery after her mother went into labor following a small placental abruption from abdominal trauma. Carrie's Apgar scores were 7 at 1 minute and 9 at 5 minutes. Her initial assessment measurements were as follows:

- Birth weight: 6 pounds, 4 ounces
- Length: 49 cm
- Head circumference: 33 cm
- Chest circumference: 32 cm
- Ballard Scale: 38 weeks

Episode 13

The delivery occurs without fetal complications, and Carrie is perfectly healthy at birth. She is placed on Jessica's abdomen immediately after birth and covered with a warm blanket to maintain her body temperature. Shortly thereafter, Carrie is cleaned, examined, and has erythromycin ophthalmic ointment placed into her eyes. A dose of phytonadione (Vitamin K) and hepatitis B vaccine are administered intramuscularly.

Prior to discharge, a heel stick is performed to obtain a blood specimen from Carrie for routine newborn metabolic screening. A urine sample is collected for a drug screen, which is negative. By the time of discharge (the day after she was born), she is breastfeeding about 7 times a day. She has 6 wet diapers and passes a large meconium stool. Her umbilical cord is drying, and the clamp is removed. **[MR]**

Episode 14

Carrie is settling into her home life with her mother, father, and brother Ryan. Sometimes she is breastfed, and other times she is given a bottle with formula. Jessica does not make it to the Neighborhood Pediatric office until Carrie is 1 week old. She weighs 6 pounds, 1 ounce. She is examined by the pediatrician and found to be in perfect health.

Episode 15

Carrie experiences a change in feeding; she is now getting a bottle with formula instead of her mother's breast for every feeding. Carrie sometimes experiences uncomfortable gas, and this makes her cry. She has also developed a sore rash on her skin. During Jessica's postpartum exam, the midwife examines Carrie and notes that she has diaper rash. Carrie had a repeat PKU test due this week, but Jessica fails to take her to the outpatient lab for the test.

CARRIE HOLMES
Season 3

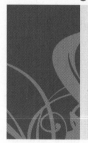

Biographical Information

Carrie Holmes is a 6-week-old infant girl, daughter of Jessica Riley and Casey Holmes. She was born at 38 weeks' gestation by vaginal delivery after her mother suffered a small placental abruption following abdominal trauma. She was perfectly healthy at birth. She is bottle fed and has been in the care of her mother or grandmother Evelyn since birth. Carrie lives in a one-bedroom apartment with her mother, father, and brother Ryan.

Episode 1

While her mother works, Carrie is in the care of her grandmother, Evelyn. She is kept warm and dry, and is well fed and cuddled in a calm environment. She listens as her grandmother talks to her. When she is old enough, Carrie will go to Kangaroo Junction Preschool with her brother. At her mother's house, the care is less consistent. Often, there are strange, loud noises and angry voices. Carrie cries when she gets hungry or just wants to be held.

Episode 2

The social worker makes a visit to see Jessica, Carrie, and Ryan. The social worker sees that the living conditions are messy, but the children appear healthy and show no evidence of neglect or abuse. Jessica takes Carrie in for her 2-month well-baby exam and immunizations. **[P]**

Episode 3

Carrie begins going to Kangaroo Junction Preschool with her brother Ryan on the days that Jessica works.

Episode 4

No news this week.

Episode 5

Carrie is frightened by the loud voices and shouting that occur at her mother's home. She cries, expecting for her mother to pick her up and hold her. Casey picks her up, puts her in her crib, and slams the door shut. She cries herself to sleep. **[P]**

Episode 6

The social worker comes by to see Carrie this week. Carrie has no markings on her body that suggest physical abuse and appears to be well fed. While interacting with Jessica, the social worker watches Carrie (who is lying on a blanket on the floor) and notes that she coos, raises her head and chest from a prone position, and expresses interest in objects that come into her visual field.

Episode 7

No news this week.

Episode 8

Carrie is 17-weeks old. She has not been feeling well most of the day. She has been fussy and has not eaten well. Her right ear hurts, although she can't communicate this, except by crying. When her mother picks her up from day care, Jessica is advised that Carrie has a fever and perhaps should be seen by a doctor.

It is late in the afternoon, and Jessica knows she can't go to the pediatrician's office at this point. She takes Carrie to the emergency department at Neighborhood Hospital, where she sees Dr. Gordon. Carrie is diagnosed with otitis media and sent home with a prescription for amoxicillin (Amoxil) and directions for Jessica to treat her fever with acetaminophen (Tylenol) and plenty of fluids. The emergency department nurse notes that Carrie has not yet had her 4-month immunizations and reminds Jessica to schedule an appointment to get those done.

Episode 9

During the middle of the night, Carrie's mother takes her from her crib, wraps her in a blanket, and takes her to a strange house. Carrie does not recognize anybody there. She is placed in a strange crib and goes to sleep.

Episode 10

No news this week.

Episode 11

Carrie and her brother Ryan return to their home. Carrie is delighted to see her grandmother. **[P]**

Episode 12

No news this week.

Episode 13

No news this week.

Episode 14

Carrie is now 6-months old. Evelyn takes her in for a well-baby visit and learns that Jessica never took her in at 4 months for a visit and immunizations. At this visit, Carrie's weight is 15 1/2 pounds, and her head circumference is measured at 42 cm. The nurse observes that Carrie is able to roll over. She tells Evelyn that she can start giving the baby rice cereal. The nurse reviews Carrie's immunization records to determine what she needs to get on this visit. **[P]**

Episode 15

Carrie and her brother move into their grandmother's home.

ROSS AND JARAMILLIO HOUSEHOLD

ROSS AND JARAMILLO FAMILY STORY OVERVIEW

Character	Season 1	Season 2	Season 3
GREG ROSS	Greg lives with his long-time partner Ben. He has inflammatory bowel disease (ulcerative colitis) that is managed with diet and medications. During this season, he has an exacerbation of colitis that is managed on an outpatient basis. Greg wants a child. He is frustrated when he tries to discuss this topic with Ben, because he avoids the discussion. Greg goes to the health fair and learns his blood pressure is elevated.	Greg talks Ben into starting the process of adoption, but they experience discrimination because they are gay. He sees a nurse practitioner about his elevated blood pressure and begins taking antihypertensive medications. Shortly thereafter he notices changes in sexual function. This situation creates personal distress and stress in his relationship with Ben.	Greg figures out that the medication is contributing to his sexual dysfunction. He has an exacerbation of colitis requiring hospitalization. Greg and Ben continue to pursue adoption options and finally find a pregnant teen who agrees to give her baby up after birth.
BENITO JARAMILLO	Ben is a successful financial advisor and an exercise fanatic. He maintains a very active and healthy lifestyle. He lives with his long-time partner Greg. He and Greg frequently take vacations and have a very comfortable lifestyle.	Ben agrees to begin the process of adoption because he knows how important it is to Greg. He notices Greg is less responsive sexually, which leads to many concerns. Ben suffers minor injuries related to his aggressive workout regimen.	Ben becomes angry and frustrated about the ongoing discrimination they experience with the adoption process. Ben has ongoing muscle strains and pains associated with his workouts.

CONCEPTS   *Elimination, Family Dynamics, Immunity, Inflammation, Perfusion, Self Image, Sexuality*

GREG ROSS
Season 1

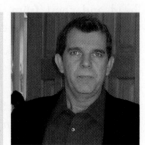

Biographical Information

Greg Ross is a 44-year-old Caucasian male who is in good health. He has inflammatory bowel disease, specifically ulcerative colitis, which was first diagnosed at age 28. His disease is considered mild in severity; it has not progressed, in his opinion, because of his strict adherence to diet therapies, including a low-roughage diet and avoidance of milk products. He takes no specific medication for the colitis when it is in clinical remission, but when he has a "flare-up," he takes antibiotics, corticosteroids, and sulfasalazine. It has been about 2 1/2 years since he last experienced active disease. Greg sees a gastroenterologist once a year or as needed for management of the colitis.

Greg is a sales representative for a large, national manufacturing company. His work requires that he travel 2-3 days a week. Because Greg is very intelligent and has excellent interpersonal skills, he is one of the most successful sales

Continued

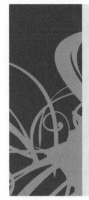

representatives in the company; he has been in the top 5% of sales reps nation-wide for the past 7 years in a row. His income is based on sales percentages, so he is earning a very high income.

Greg is gay and has been in a monogamous relationship for 10 years with his partner Ben. They own a beautiful home that they share with their two pet dogs, Mitt and Bitt. Greg has been estranged from his family for most of his adult life. His parents and siblings have never accepted the fact that he is gay, so contact with his parents is usually limited to talking with his mother a few times a year. Greg has accepted this situation and gone on to lead his own life. He considers Ben and the dogs to be his family, although he dreams of having children.

Episode 1
Greg comes home after being out of town for 3 days this week. He is happy to share with Ben that he won a 10-day trip for two to Italy because of his sales performance during the past year. He marks the trip dates on the calendar, noting it is only a few months away. He gets online and orders several travel books to Italy.

Episode 2
No news this week.

Episode 3
No news this week.

Episode 4
Greg is out of town for a week-long sales meeting this week.

Episode 5
Greg and Ben have a trip to Hawaii planned at the end of the week for Ben's triathlon competition. Greg spends time during the week visiting a variety of Internet sites to learn as much as he can about the area before their trip. **[P]**

Episode 6
Greg and Ben are in Hawaii this week on vacation following Ben's triathlon. They spend most of their time visiting local attractions and resting on the beach. Greg is glad that Ben is taking most of the week off from training. While on the beach, they watch a father playing in the surf with his young children. Greg comments to Ben that he thinks it would be great to have children together someday. Ben simply responds, "Yeah, kids are cool." **[P]**

Episode 7
Greg wanders into the health fair this week as he is passing by. He stops at the blood pressure screening table and is shocked to learn that his blood pressure is elevated at 138/94 mm Hg. The nurse at the screening writes his blood pressure measurement down and suggests that he have it checked again in the next week or so and to follow up with his primary care physician if it remains elevated. **[P]**

Episode 8
During dinner one night this week, Greg talks with Ben about the possibility of adopting a child or even perhaps fathering a child with a surrogate mother. Ben does not show much interest in the topic and questions Greg about how they will have enough time to raise children; he also points out that they already have everything they need. Greg is frustrated with Ben's lack of interest. **[VC]**

Episode 9
No news this week.

Episode 10
After work, Greg drops by the pharmacy to pick up vitamins and dietary supplements for Ben. He sits down at the automated blood pressure machine and takes his blood pressure. The digital display reads 134/90 mm HG, and he decides that his blood pressure is probably not that bad after all. He also notices a pamphlet about HIV testing. He feels relieved that he is in a monogamous relationship, believing he doesn't have to worry about those issues. **[P]**

Episode 11
No news this week.

Episode 12
Ben and Greg are in Italy this week. Greg enjoys being able to spend so much time with Ben. During the trip, he again tries to talk with Ben about having children. Ben points out that, if they had kids, they would never be able to take lovely vacations like this. Greg is disappointed that Ben is closed-minded about the idea and worries that the relationship may never evolve to the point of raising a family together.

Episode 13

Ben and Greg are finishing their vacation in Italy this week. Greg experiences abdominal pain and diarrhea on the way back home and blames it on the stress of travel and the lack of a controlled diet. He hopes that the symptoms will subside once he gets home. **[P]**

Episode 14

Greg continues to have pain and diarrhea, and recognizes that he is having an acute exacerbation of colitis. He makes an appointment with the gastroenterologist, who gives Greg a prescription for oral prednisone and sulfasalazine, and advises him to drink plenty of fluids. The physician also comments that Greg's blood pressure is 146/96 mm Hg. The gastroenterologist explains that his blood pressure is higher than it should be, but his abdominal pain might have something to do with it. Greg is told to have his blood pressure rechecked when he is feeling better. **[P]**

Episode 15

Ben is out of town competing in another triathlon. Greg elects to stay home because of ongoing symptoms with his colitis. Because of the frequent episodes of diarrhea, he stays close to home, trying to rest his colon. **[P]**

GREG ROSS
Season 2

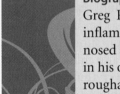

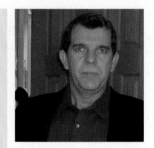

Biographical Information

Greg Ross is a 45-year-old Caucasian male who is in good health. He has inflammatory bowel disease, specifically ulcerative colitis, which was first diagnosed at age 28. His disease is considered mild in severity; it has not progressed, in his opinion, because of his strict adherence to diet therapies, including a low-roughage diet and avoidance of milk products. He takes no specific medication for the colitis when it is in clinical remission, but when he has a "flare-up," he takes antibiotics, corticosteroids, and sulfasalazine. His last "flare-up" was a few months ago. Greg sees a gastroenterologist once a year or as needed for management of the colitis.

Greg is a sales representative for a large, national manufacturing company. His work requires that he travel 2-3 days a week. Because Greg is very intelligent and has excellent interpersonal skills, he is one of the most successful sales representatives in the company; he has been in the top 5% of sales reps nationwide for the past 7 years in a row.

Greg is gay and has been in a monogamous relationship for 10 years with his partner Ben. They own a beautiful home that they share with their two pet dogs, Mitt and Bitt. Greg has been estranged from his family for most of his adult life. His parents and siblings have never accepted the fact that he is gay, so contact with his parents is usually limited to talking with his mother a few times a year. Greg has accepted this situation and gone on to lead his own life. He considers Ben and the dogs to be his family, although he dreams of having children.

Episode 1

No news this week.

Episode 2

The recent exacerbation of Greg's colitis seems to have passed. He is feeling much better again and able to resume his regular business travel. **[P]**

Episode 3

Greg talks to Ben again about considering having a child together—either through adoption or finding a surrogate parent. Greg explains how important it is to him and that he wishes Ben would at least give it some serious thought. He points out that, with their income, they can afford whatever they need to make things work; there's no reason to think they would be unable to continue doing the things they enjoy. Greg offers many suggestions, including hiring a nanny to stay in their home with their child while they work or travel out of town. For the first time, Greg feels as if Ben actually is listening to his point of view. **[VC]**

Episode 4

Greg and Ben discuss the possibility of finding a surrogate mother. Ben suggests asking his sister-in-law if she would consider being a surrogate parent for them. Greg likes the idea of having a child who is biologically related to Ben.

Greg follows up on the advice of the physician and checks his blood pressure at the drug store. He is surprised when 142/94 mm Hg is displayed on the monitor and nearly assumes the blood pressure machine isn't accurate. Just the same, he makes an appointment with the family practice clinic. **[P]**

Episode 5

Greg makes a visit to the family practice clinic and sees the nurse practitioner. His blood pressure is measured at 144/94 mm Hg. Given his recent history of elevated blood pressure and the blood pressure measurement during this office visit, the nurse practitioner gives him a prescription for Lopressor/HCT 100/25 to take one every day. He is asked to make an appointment for a follow-up visit. **[P]**

Episode 6

No news this week.

Episode 7

Greg has been gone most of the past two weeks traveling for work and is very tired when he gets home. He has been taking the blood pressure medication for a several weeks. At a follow-up visit, his blood pressure is down to 136/88 mm Hg. When asked if he has experienced any problems with the medications, he says he does not think so. In reality, Greg is uncomfortable mentioning that his erections have recently not felt the same. He decides the symptom is probably related to being overly tired.

Episode 8

After talking with a few of their gay and lesbian friends who have children, Ben and Greg decide to look into adoption. Greg spends hours on the Internet learning as much as he can about the process. He learns of the many challenges that gay and lesbian couples wanting to adopt face, and this causes him to feel stressed. He learns that the first step is to find an agency to work with. Greg locates several agencies in the area and makes plans to contact a few of them to determine whether they will be able to help. **[P]**

Episode 9

This week Greg and Ben are in Spain for 5 days attending a festival as guests of one of Greg's influential clients. Greg has a noticeable problem with sexual performance this week—in fact, Ben asks him what the problem is. Greg is very distraught about this and worries about Ben's reaction. He tells Ben that he is just feeling tired from traveling, and it has nothing to do with him. Ben is a bit "standoffish" for the rest of the week. **[P]**

Episode 10

Greg continues to experience problems with sexual functioning. He is now quite sure it is not due to fatigue. He reads about erectile dysfunction on the Internet and finds that some of the common causes include blood pressure medications and stress. He wonders if the blood pressure medication he is taking is the problem, but can't specifically remember if the onset of the symptoms coincided with the time he began taking the medication. He makes a point to try to reduce his stress level and relax. He signs up for a massage once a week and decides to try to get more exercise to reduce his stress level. He is very embarrassed about the situation and avoids talking to Ben about it. **[P]**

Episode 11

No news the week.

Episode 12

Greg and Ben meet with a private adoption agency this week. Greg learns that, although the agency works with gay and lesbian parents, they would not be considered a "priority" for infant adoption placements. The agency representative makes it clear that they would be more likely have a child placed with them if Ben and Greg were willing to consider a child with special needs or a "hard to place" child. Greg is frustrated by what he learns; this frustration is further impacted by his ongoing sexual response issues.

Episode 13

Greg and Ben are at the beach for a 3-day weekend. It is a stressful weekend for both of them because of the adoption issues and Greg's ongoing problems with sexual response. Greg goes out of his way to avoid physical contact, and Ben is visibly angry with him. Greg finally shares with Ben that, although he is not sure, he thinks the blood pressure medication he has been taking might be causing his decreased sexual response. Greg tells Ben that he quit taking the medication last week to see if his "problem" would go away.

Episode 14

Greg and Ben meet with another adoption agency this week. When they acknowledge that they are a gay couple, the agency tells claims it will not be able to help.

Greg is disappointed in their closed-minded attitude toward them. He is beginning to wonder if he might have better luck trying to adopt a child as a single man and not mention that he is gay.

Episode 15

Greg and Ben go to an art show over the weekend. While at the show, Greg buys a quilt from Pam Allen whom he learns is a cancer survivor. He spends several minutes talking with the woman and her son Gary, who has Down syndrome. [P]

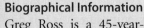

GREG ROSS
Season 3

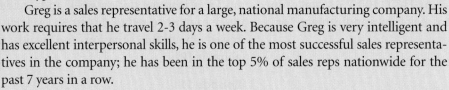

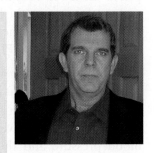

Biographical Information

Greg Ross is a 45-year-old Caucasian male who is in good health. He has inflammatory bowel disease, specifically ulcerative colitis, which was first diagnosed at age 28. His disease is considered mild in severity; it has not progressed, in his opinion, because of his strict adherence to diet therapies, including a low-roughage diet and avoidance of milk products. He takes no specific medication for the colitis when it is in clinical remission, but when he has a "flare-up," he takes antibiotics, corticosteroids, and sulfasalazine. He also has recently been diagnosed with hypertension.

Greg is a sales representative for a large, national manufacturing company. His work requires that he travel 2-3 days a week. Because Greg is very intelligent and has excellent interpersonal skills, he is one of the most successful sales representatives in the company; he has been in the top 5% of sales reps nationwide for the past 7 years in a row.

Greg is gay and has been in a monogamous relationship for 10 years with his partner Ben. They own a beautiful home that they share with their two pet dogs, Mitt and Bitt. Greg considers Ben and the dogs to be his family, although he dreams of having children. In recent months, they have been exploring their options to adopt a baby.

Episode 1

Greg has validated what he suspected might be wrong—the blood pressure medication was causing his sexual dysfunction! He quit taking the blood pressure medication several weeks ago and now has no problems with his sexual response. He is relieved that it was such a simple solution and decides that taking the medication is just not worth it. He makes another appointment with the family practice clinic to discuss alternative blood pressure management. [P]

Episode 2

Greg's blood pressure is 148/96 mm Hg when he is seen at the family practice clinic. The nurse practitioner clearly explains that having blood pressure this high is not acceptable, and other options must be explored. Greg suggests that perhaps he can just avoid salt and increase his exercise. The nurse practitioner tells him that these changes alone are unlikely to reduce the blood pressure enough, but that those measures, in addition to taking medication, will be helpful. The nurse practitioner gives him a prescription for lisinopril (5 mg daily) and hydrochlorothiazide (25 mg daily).

Greg and Ben visit with another adoption agency and are again discouraged when told they should not get their hopes up about adopting an infant. Greg insists on knowing the reason for this. The agency representative tells them that Greg and Ben would not be considered as stable as a traditional married couple. They decide to continue exploring other agency options. **[P]**

Episode 3
No news this week.

Episode 4
Greg has a sudden and somewhat severe acute exacerbation of colitis this week. On one day, he passes several small, loose, bloody stools with cramping. On the following day, he has severe abdominal pain and nine episodes of bloody diarrhea stools with mucus by noon. He takes his temperature and notes that he has a fever.

Ben takes him to the emergency department, where he is treated by Dr. Gordon. While there, Dr. Gordon learns that Greg has not been screened for HIV in several years and suggests running this test. Greg does not think it is necessary, given his monogamous relationship, but agrees to the test when Dr. Gordon pushes the point. He feels somewhat angry, knowing it is unlikely that Dr. Gordon routinely does this. Greg is treated with IV fluids, oral prednisone, and sulfasalazine, and then sent home. He cancels his out-of-town travel for the next 2 weeks to allow time to rest. **[MR] [P]**

Episode 5
Greg follows up with his gastroenterologist, because he is still experiencing bloody diarrhea with mucus. The physician recommends admission to the hospital for IV prednisone, IV fluids, and bowel rest by maintaining an NPO status. Additionally, he recommends that Greg be evaluated for possible surgical evaluation. The physician shares with Greg that his HIV screening done in the ED the previous week was negative.

Episode 6
Greg is back home and feeling much better. He goes with Ben to visit another adoption agency and is again told that gay adoptive parents are not given priority for infant placement. Ben suggests that they hire an attorney in order to be adequately represented through the adoption process. Greg is beginning to think that adoption may not be worth it, but agrees with Ben that hiring an attorney might help.

Episode 7
No news this week.

Episode 8
Greg is back to his regular work and travel schedule, although he is still not feeling 100%. He is still passing several semi-formed stools with small amounts of blood every day. This makes holding meetings with clients and traveling rather difficult. Greg and Ben meet with an attorney, who suggests that they work with a private adoption agency or directly with birth parents. Greg and Ben decide to do this. **[P]**

Episode 9
No news this week.

Episode 10
Greg is thrilled to meet Terry Clark, a pregnant teen who has agreed to give her baby to them for adoption.

Episode 11
Greg has a follow-up visit to see the nurse practitioner this week and is glad to learn that his blood pressure is down to 134/86 mm Hg. The change in medications to lisinopril and hydrochlorothiazide seems to have done the trick, and Greg has no side effects.

Episode 12
Greg accompanies Ben to a physician's office to have his leg evaluated. He feels badly when he realizes that Ben will have to cancel another event.

Episode 13
No news this week.

Episode 14
Greg and Ben are off to Alaska for a cruise. They have a wonderful time together and talk about the many plans they have for the baby. Greg is so happy that things seem to be coming together. He is excited about all of the changes that are about to occur in their life and dreams about being a father.

Episode 15
Terry Clark, the pregnant teenager, changes her mind about putting her baby up for adoption. Greg learns that she was "forbidden" by her parents to give her baby to a gay couple. He is further saddened to learn that the woman whom he bought a quilt from several months ago has died. He remembers her son Gary and the love the two of them shared. Because he feels Gary should have the quilt, Greg tracks down Gary's address and mails the quilt to him. The act of kindness lifts his spirits. **[P]**

BENITO JARAMILLO
Season 1

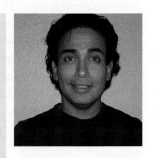

Biographical Information

Benito (Ben) Jaramillo is a 41-year-old Hispanic male in excellent health. He has a very successful career as a financial manager and consultant. He works long hours, but has a great degree of flexibility in his schedule, allowing him to take time off whenever he needs to. His motto has always been "work hard, play hard." He has no medical problems and takes no prescribed medications.

Ben's primary outside hobby and interest is athletic training—in fact, many consider Ben to be an exercise and health fanatic. He participates in many athletic-related events, such as running, cycling, skiing, and triathlon events. To maintain his competitiveness, Ben trains five hours a day on most days. His training schedule includes a two-hour workout early in the morning, an hour over lunch, and two hours after work. In addition to the aggressive training schedule, Ben eats a healthy diet and consults with a nutritionist regularly. He takes herbal preparations and vitamins to optimize his health. He has never been a smoker and has one alcoholic beverage almost nightly.

Ben lives with his long-time partner Greg and their two canine "children," Mitt and Bitt. Although Ben and Greg have very different personalities and interests, they get along very well, providing each other with companionship and balance; they particularly enjoy taking vacations together. Their relationship is monogamous. Ben gets along well with his parents and siblings. Although Ben's parents know he is gay, they refer to Greg as Ben's "special friend." Ben's siblings consider Greg part of the family. He very much enjoys all of the things in his life that his comfortable income offers.

Episode 1
Ben has been training more aggressively this week for an upcoming triathlon in Hawaii. Ben and Greg had previously decided to spend one week there for vacation after the event. Greg announces that they are also going to go to Italy in a few months; Ben enjoys traveling, but is secretly wondering if going to Italy for 10 days will interfere with training for another triathlon that he plans to compete in the month after they go to Italy. **[P]**

Episode 2
No news this week.

Episode 3
No news this week.

Episode 4
Ben takes advantage of the fact that Greg is gone all week and uses the time alone to train for the upcoming triathlon. He spends 7 hours a day each day this week training in addition to maintaining a regular work schedule. **[P]**

Episode 5
Ben continues to train very hard this week until the day before they leave. He knows he won't win, but hopes that he can improve on his personal best time. **[P]**

Episode 6
Ben competes in the triathlon this week. Although his time is a personal best, he is disappointed that it is only an improvement of about 25 seconds. With the exception of early-morning runs on the beach, Ben decides to take a week off from training. He is annoyed when Greg talks about children and deliberately does not respond to Greg's comments; although he likes children, he has never had a strong desire to have one of his own. He wonders why Greg keeps bringing up the subject.

Episode 7
Over the weekend, Ben goes on a day-long bike ride with a group from the cycling club.

Episode 8
Ben is annoyed when Greg again talks with him about the possibility of adopting a child or fathering a child with a

surrogate mother. Ben does not think Greg has any idea of the commitment involved with raising children. Ben asks Greg, "Who would stay home to raise a baby?" Ben does not understand why Greg would want to add such a complication to their lives.

Episode 9
No news this week.

Episode 10
Ben pulls a muscle in his groin this week while training. He is angry that this injury will keep him from running for at least a week. He compensates by spending more time in the swimming pool.

Episode 11
No news this week.

Episode 12
Ben is in Italy this week with Greg. He has never been to Italy and finds the place fascinating. Greg brings up the "children" discussion again, so Ben points out that, if they have kids, they won't be able to take vacations like this. Ben wishes he would just drop the subject and not ruin the vacation.

Episode 13
Greg experiences abdominal pain and diarrhea on the way home from Italy. Ben knows these symptoms tend to occur when he experiences stress, and he blames himself for not being more sensitive to Greg's feelings. This week, he begins an aggressive training schedule for an upcoming triathlon. **[P]**

Episode 14
Ben spends 7 hours a day each day this week training for another triathlon. **[P]**

Episode 15
Ben participates in the triathlon this weekend; he is very pleased with his performance and is very happy to come in second place in his age group. He is disappointed that Greg is unable to come with him to watch. **[P]**

BENITO JARAMILLO
Season 2

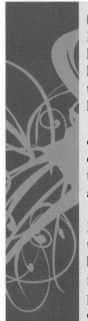

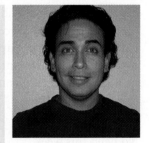

Biographical Information
Benito (Ben) Jaramillo is a 41-year-old Hispanic male in excellent health. He has a very successful career as a financial manager and consultant. He works long hours, but has a great degree of flexibility in his schedule, allowing him to take time off whenever he needs to. His motto has always been "work hard, play hard." He has no medical problems and takes no prescribed medications.

Ben's primary outside hobby and interest is athletic training—in fact, many consider Ben to be an exercise and health fanatic. Ben eats a healthy diet and consults with a nutritionist regularly. He takes herbal preparations and vitamins to optimize his health. He has never been a smoker and has one alcoholic beverage almost nightly.

Ben lives with his long-time partner Greg and their two canine "children," Mitt and Bitt. Although Ben and Greg have very different personalities and interests, they get along very well, providing each other with companionship and balance; they particularly enjoy taking vacations together. Their relationship is monogamous. Ben gets along well with his parents and siblings. Although Ben's parents know he is gay, they refer to Greg as Ben's "special friend." Ben's siblings consider Greg part of the family.

Episode 1
No news this week.

Episode 2
Ben has been very happy about his progress in physical conditioning and performance at the various events in which he participates in. He wishes he could pursue these activities on a full-time basis, but recognizes the reality of lost potential in his highly competitive career and decides it would be a poor decision on his part.

Episode 3

Ben is increasingly aware of how important it is to Greg to have children. Although he has never really thought it through, he comes to realize that it is logistically possible to raise a child together, and he agrees to give it serious consideration.

Episode 4

While visiting his brother's home, Ben asks his sister-in-law Shelly for her opinion about Greg's idea of having a baby. She says she doesn't think it is a bad idea, but wonders just where they thought they would get a baby. Ben asks her if she would consider being a surrogate parent for them. She says she might consider it, but is sure her husband would never go along with the idea and points out to Ben that it could be pretty complicated. She adds that, although Ben's parents are supportive of his sexuality, they might not be thrilled with this idea. Shelly says she will talk about it with her husband, but also suggests they either look for a surrogate who is not a relative or consider adoption. **[VC]**

Episode 5

Shelly calls Ben this week to tell him that her husband is definitely against the idea of her being a surrogate parent. Ben is not surprised and wonders if it is because his brother is against the idea in general or against the idea for a gay couple. This comment bothers Ben, but he decides against taking it up with his brother. He has learned over time that many individuals superficially accept that he is gay, but when it comes down to it, they really are not fully accepting. **[P]**

Episode 6

No news this week.

Episode 7

Ben has been training hard during the past few weeks for another upcoming triathlon event. He hopes to win this time and is trying a new high-protein nutritional supplement that he read about in a sports magazine to enhance his performance in distance events. The supplement purports to help the body convert its extra stored proteins into energy sources during distance races. **[P]**

Episode 8

Ben competes in another triathlon this week. During the cycling portion of the event, he develops severe muscle cramps and is very disappointed when he is unable to finish the race. He tries to work through the cramps, but it is obvious that he is not going to be able to continue. Ben wonders if he failed to train adequately. **[P]**

Episode 9

Ben is on vacation with Greg this week in Spain. He is glad to have a week off from training. Ben is aware of Greg's recent problems performing sexually and is not sure what to make of it. He asks Greg what the problem is, but Greg obviously doesn't want to talk about it. Ben wonders if there is a problem between them that he does not know about. **[P]**

Episode 10

Ben notices that Greg has been increasingly unresponsive to affection and almost seems to avoid sexual contact. This is a very dramatic change in their relationship, and Ben is frustrated with Greg's unwillingness to discuss it. Ben is pretty sure that Greg is not seeing somebody else, because he keeps talking about adopting a child; still, their ability to be close is somehow different.

Episode 11

No news this week.

Episode 12

Ben accompanies Greg to an adoption agency. They discuss the various alternatives, such as adopting an older child as opposed to a very young child or infant. The adoption agency suggests that they consider adopting a young child or a child with special needs, because it can be a difficult transition for older children who have preconceived notions about homosexuality. They are told that younger children tend to adjust more easily to a home with gay parents. After listening to the discussion, Ben wonders if adoption is something they should just forget about. **[P]**

Episode 13

Ben spends the weekend surfing and relaxing on the beach with Greg. He is relieved to know that Greg is finally talking with him about his lack of sexual responsiveness. Ben was really beginning to wonder if their relationship was coming to an end and if the adoption idea was a last-ditch effort in Greg's mind to save their relationship. **[VC]**

Episode 14

Greg and Ben meet with another adoption agency this week. When they acknowledge being a gay couple, the agency tells them that it will not able to help them. Ben feels very angry. He knows they are capable of being good parents—in fact, better parents than many couples, especially considering the economic resources they have available. Ben sprains his knee while training this week. **[P]**

Episode 15

No news this week.

BENITO JARAMILLO
Season 3

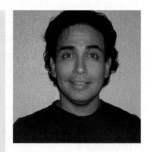

Biographical Information

Benito (Ben) Jaramillo is a 42-year-old Hispanic male in excellent health. He has a very successful career as a financial manager and consultant. He works long hours, but has a great degree of flexibility in his schedule, allowing him to take time off whenever he needs to. His motto has always been "work hard, play hard." He has no medical problems and takes no prescribed medications.

Ben's primary outside hobby and interest is athletic training—in fact, many consider Ben to be an exercise and health fanatic. He participates in many athletic-related events, such as running, cycling, skiing, and triathlon events. To maintain his competitiveness, Ben trains five hours a day on most days. He has never been a smoker and has one alcoholic beverage almost nightly.

Ben lives with his long-time partner Greg and their two canine "children," Mitt and Bitt. Although Ben and Greg have very different personalities and interests, they get along very well, providing each other with companionship and balance; they particularly enjoy taking vacations together. Recently, they have decided to try to adopt a child and are still in the process of finding an agency that will work with them.

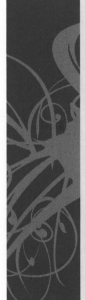

Episode 1

Ben is glad that Greg's sexual response has returned to its previous level. This has tremendously helped reduce the stress they were experiencing within their relationship. Ben has his eye on another triathlon next month and begins extensive training. **[P]**

Episode 2

Ben learns from Greg that his blood pressure is pretty high, and he needs to try other medications. Ben suggests that Greg try herbal supplements from the nutrition store. He goes with Greg to visit another adoption agency. Although encouraged by the fact that the agency agrees to work with them, Ben and Greg are discouraged when told they should not get their hopes up to adopt an infant. Greg and Ben decide to continue exploring other agency options, but Ben feels underlying anger with the whole process.

Episode 3

No news this week.

Episode 4

Ben takes Greg to the emergency department. They are there for 9 hours between waiting to be seen, waiting for tests and treatments, and waiting to be discharged. Ben cannot understand how it could take so long to be seen and wonders what the wait would be for someone critically ill.

Episode 5

Greg is admitted to the hospital this week. Ben cancels his plans to participate in the triathlon. Although disappointed, his priority is to be with Greg. While at the hospital, Ben picks up a magazine with an article in it about gay and lesbian adoptions. The article reads:

> *"The adoption hierarchy places healthy infants and young children with white, married, middle- or upper-middle class couples first; the less preferred children then go to unmarried couples of all kinds, single individuals, and gay people. The children are less preferred, and the recipients are less preferred."*

This makes him feel angry, but he finds that reading the article validates their experiences with various agencies. Ben feels he is not being discriminated against because he is gay, but because he is a Hispanic gay man. **[P]**

Episode 6

Ben feels increasing anger and frustration about the lack of progress with the adoption agencies. He suggests to Greg that they hire a private lawyer who specializes in adoptions to help them through the process.

Episode 7

No news this week.

Episode 8

Ben is back to training for another distance event, this time a mountain terrain extreme race. This week, Ben and Greg meet with an attorney who agrees to help them find a child for adoption and suggests they do a private, open adoption. **[VC] [P]**

Episode 9

No news this week.

Episode 10

The attorney introduces Ben and Greg to a 16-year-old teenager who agrees to put her baby up for adoption. They agree to provide financial support to her until the baby is born and help pay for medical expenses associated with the delivery. **[VC] [P]**

Episode 11

Ben steps up the intensity of his workouts in preparation for the high-adventure event. He goes to the neighborhood high school football stadium and spends 2 hours running up and down the stadium stairs and running laps on the track.

Episode 12

Ben develops what he thinks is muscle pain that gets worse over several days. By the end of the week, his leg hurts when he walks on it. He sees a physician, is diagnosed with tendonitis, and is told to rest the leg. Ben must cancel his plans to participate in the mountain terrain event. **[P]**

Episode 13

Ben feels frustrated by what seem to be constant injuries. He does not understand why these injuries keep occurring and considers hiring a personal trainer to help him.

Ben becomes increasingly excited about the baby that he and Greg will soon adopt. He purchases some baby clothes from the store and shows them to Greg when he gets home. **[P]**

Episode 14

Ben and Greg are on a 2-week Alaskan cruise vacation. During the cruise, they spend a great deal of time talking about their plans for the baby. Although Ben at first was reluctant to commit to raising a child, he now is looking forward to his new role as a parent and feels relieved that all of their problems have resolved.

Episode 15

Ben is furious when their attorney calls to tell them that Terry has decided to keep her baby. He feels as if all of their plans and dreams have vanished and even wonders if Terry was just trying to take advantage of them. He also feels very angry at Terry's parents for forcing their views of homosexuality on her. **[P]**

YOUNG HOUSEHOLD

YOUNG FAMILY STORY OVERVIEW

Character	Season 1	Season 2	Season 3
STEVE YOUNG	Steve is a well-educated, devoted father and husband. He is a supportive father who is aware that his wife is a perfectionist. He is healthy and has a good job as an accountant. He is smoker and makes an unsuccessful attempt to stop smoking. His wife becomes pregnant with their third child.	Steve becomes a father for the third time during this season. He attempts to quit smoking again, but is unsuccessful. When Kelsey has an asthmatic episode, Angie accuses Steve of contributing to the problem and bans his smoking, even outdoors. Angie makes an effort to control for other environmental triggers by getting rid of the family cats, which makes Steve angry.	Steve makes another attempt to give up smoking (as a result of Angie's constant nagging). He is devastated when Marcus is injured in a bicycle accident. He and Angie work together to take care of the family.
ANGIE YOUNG	Angie is a stay-at-home mother who devotes all of her time and energy to making a perfect home for her husband and children. She adores her husband, but does not like the fact that he smokes. She is involved with Kelsey and Marcus' school and frequently arranges outings for the family. She has the children involved in childhood art and music lessons. Angie gets pregnant with her third child.	Angie has very routine and uncomplicated prenatal care and an uncomplicated delivery of her son, Eric. In addition to caring for a new infant, Angie attempts to do whatever she can to minimize the environmental factors affecting Kelsey's asthma, including getting rid of the family cats and banning Steve's smoking.	When Marcus is hit by a car and injured, Angie is a protective and highly critical parent in the hospital. Later, Angie becomes politically active regarding street safety in their neighborhood and attempts to get speed bumps installed on their street.
KELSEY YOUNG	Kelsey is a happy, healthy second grader who has intermittent problems with asthma. She has inhalers, which she uses periodically. She takes piano lessons and, although she does not enjoy the piano very much, she is very good about practicing. She is also involved with gymnastics.	Kelsey has a fairly significant exacerbation of her asthma that is not resolved by her inhaler, requiring a trip to the pediatrician's office. Because of her asthma, Kelsey's mother gets rid of the family cats. This upsets Kelsey, and she feels it is all her fault. Kelsey is thrilled when her baby brother Eric is born.	Kelsey's asthma remains fairly well managed with her inhaler; Angie constantly stresses over exposure to things in the environment and begin to unnecessarily limit things Kelsey can do. Kelsey is very sad when her brother is injured in an accident.
MARCUS YOUNG	Marcus is a healthy 6-year-old boy in the first grade. During this season he is sent home from school with "pink eye." He takes piano lessons, but is really not interested in playing the piano—this is his mother's idea. Practicing the piano causes conflict between Marcus and his mother.	Marcus learns to ride a bike and rides his bike most days after school. He continues to have battles with his mother over practicing the piano. He loves to go to Saturday art classes. Marcus is excited about the birth of his brother Eric.	Marcus is hit by a car while riding his bike. He is admitted to the Pediatric Intensive Care Unit with skeletal trauma. Pain management and dealing with a frantic, perfectionist mother are the issues facing nurses at the hospital.

ERIC YOUNG	Not born yet	Eric is born in an uncomplicated birth. Most of the story describes infant care and age-appropriate behaviors in the context of the family and daily routine.	During this season, Eric has a bout of diarrhea that requires a trip to the pediatrician's office. Later he has a viral upper respiratory infection. Most of the story describes age-appropriate behaviors in the context of the family and daily routine.

CONCEPTS   *Addiction, Coping, Elimination, Fluid and Electrolytes, Immunity, Infection, Inflammation, Interpersonal Relationships, Mobility, Oxygenation, Pain, Reproduction, Stress, Sexuality*

STEVE YOUNG
Season 1

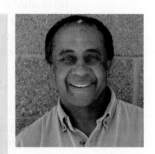

Biographical Information

Steve Young is a 41-year-old African-American male who is in excellent health. He has been married to his wife Angie for 8 years. He has two children with her, Kelsey and Marcus. Angie and Steve met in college and were married shortly after Steve graduated with a degree in accounting. Following graduation, he took the CPA exam and has worked for a large corporate accounting firm ever since. He has been extremely successful and has an income that easily supports his family. He is pleased that his wife is able to be a stay-at-home mother, but his success requires that he work very long hours at the office. Steve has few outside activities and rarely exercises—his world pretty much revolves around work and home. He recognizes that his inactivity has led to weight gain over the past few years, but is not concerned about it.

Steve began smoking at age 17 and, at this time, he has a 10 pack-year smoking history. He knows he should quit smoking, but he likes it—and he figures he can probably get away with it for a little while longer. Because he knows it is a source of irritation for his wife, he plans to quit smoking eventually.

Steve loves spending time with his wife and children in the evenings and on weekends. He is more than happy to help Angie with evening family activities, but he sometimes feels that her perfectionism is overbearing and secretly worries about the effect it may have on the children. He has attempted to discuss this concern with her, but she gets defensive, and he does not want her to perceive that he doesn't appreciate her efforts.

Episode 1
Steve goes with his family to the museum and out to lunch. He enjoys spending time with his children. He does not agree with Angie's demand that the children practice the piano and read as soon as they arrive home, because he believes they should be given an opportunity to play. He does not voice his opinion and lets it go.

Episode 2
Angie discusses Marcus' lack of progress playing the piano with Steve. He suggests to her that she "back off

and let the kids be kids." She reminds him that the kids need discipline and structure. He notices she is a bit "standoffish" the rest of the evening. **[VC]**

Episode 3
Steve and Angie discuss having another baby. Although he is perfectly happy with two children, Steve is not opposed to the idea and believes their income can accommodate a third child. He tells Angie that he's in support of it and is pleased with how happy it makes her.

Episode 4
Steve decides this week that he is going to quit smoking—not so much because he wants to, but because he is tired of Angie nagging him about it. On Monday morning, he throws his cigarettes away and decides to quit smoking "cold turkey." **[P]**

Episode 5
Steve has not smoked for a couple of weeks now, and he feels miserable. He literally thinks about cigarettes from the time he wakes up until the time he goes to sleep at night. He even dreams about smoking. He feels very edgy and is in a bad mood all of the time. To satisfy his craving, he snacks constantly at work and at home—and then finds himself worrying about weight gain. He tries nicotine gum, but ends up chewing the gum constantly. **[P]**

Episode 6
This week, one of the guys in the office announces his engagement. After work, Steve goes with a group from the office to briefly celebrate at a bar before going home. While having a beer with his friends, Steve has a cigarette, and it is one of the most pleasurable things he can imagine. The next morning he buys a pack of cigarettes on the way to work. **[P]**

Episode 7
Steve takes Angie and the kids to the local Health Fair. He had hoped to watch a sporting event on television, knowing that Angie would likely nag at him for failing to quit smoking. He walks right past the American Cancer Society and American Heart Association booths, because he does not want to be bothered with the smoking cessation information he'd find there. But when he gets home, Steve finds smoking cessation literature in his bag. **[P]**

Episode 8
Steve learns that Angie is pregnant this week and is very happy to know they will have another child together.

Episode 9
Steve receives a phone call from Angie at 2 p.m. today, informing him that she is taking Marcus to the doctor. He will need to pick up Kelsey from school at 3 p.m. and get her to her art class by 3:45. Steve is able to cancel a couple of appointments so he can take care of Kelsey. **[P]**

Episode 10
No news this week.

Episode 11
Steve goes with Angie and the kids to the open house at the elementary school.

Episode 12
No news this week.

Episode 13
Steve is out of town all week on a consulting job with a potential new client. He talks with Angie two to three times each day, concerned that she might need his help. **[P]**

Episode 14
No news this week.

Episode 15
Steve takes Angie and the kids on a weekend trip to his mother's house for a visit. Steve's mother is very pleased about the pregnancy and very excited for them.

STEVE YOUNG
Season 2

Biographical Information

Steve Young is a 42-year-old African-American male who is in excellent health. He has been married to his wife Angie for 9 years. They have two children, Kelsey and Marcus, and are expecting a baby in the upcoming months.

Angie and Steve met in college and were married shortly after Steve graduated with a degree in accounting. Following graduation, he took the CPA exam and has worked for a large corporate accounting firm ever since. He has been extremely successful and has an income that easily supports his family. He is pleased that his wife is able to be a stay-at-home mother, but his success requires that he work very long hours at the office. Steve has few outside activities and rarely exercises—his world pretty much revolves around work and home. He recognizes that his inactivity has led to weight gain over the past few years, but is not concerned about it.

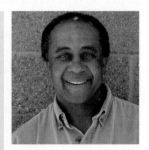

Continued

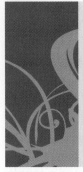

Steve began smoking at age 17 and, at this time, he has an 11 pack-year smoking history. Although he still likes to smoke, he knows he needs to quit smoking. He has vowed to stop smoking before the baby is born.

Steve loves spending time with his wife and children in the evenings and on weekends. He is more than happy to help Angie with evening family activities, but he sometimes feels that her perfectionism is overbearing and secretly worries about the effect it may have on the children. He has attempted to discuss this concern with her, but she gets defensive, and he does not want her to perceive that he doesn't appreciate her efforts.

Episode 1

Steve accompanies Angie to childbirth classes. He wonders why they have to go through all this, considering that they already have had two children. Steve thinks that he and Angie pretty much have it figured out; frankly, he would rather stay home after working all day. **[VC]**

Episode 2

Steve continues to go with Angie to childbirth classes this week. Going to the classes has motivated Steve to stop smoking. He throws his cigarettes away and tells Angie he is going to quit. **[P]**

Episode 3

Marcus tells his Dad that he would like to have a bike to ride like all his friends. Steve talks with Angie about it, and at first she is resistant to the idea, voicing her concern that Marcus might get hurt. When Steve points out that Kelsey got her first bike at the same age, Angie reminds him that Kelsey is more attentive than Marcus. In the end, Steve gets Angie's approval and takes his son shopping. **[P]**

Episode 4

Steve retrieves the crib and other baby accessories from the attic for Angie so she can start putting a nursery together. Steve is very irritable because he wants a cigarette. He goes outside to have just one. One cigarette turns into two the next day and four the following day. Soon, he is back to smoking. He knows this disappoints Angie, but she just doesn't understand how hard it is to quit. **[P]**

Episode 5

Steve is concerned about Kelsey and glad she is improving with the medications.

Episode 6

Steve has a rare fight with Angie this week. She yells at him for being a smoker and causing Kelsey's breathing problems. She tells him that his cigarettes are banned from the house—he may not even bring them inside. She also argues with him about getting rid of the cats, because

Steve does not share her belief that the cats are to blame. He is angry with her because she doesn't seem to recognize how devastating this decision is to the kids. Steve feels angry for several days following the argument. **[VC]**

Episode 7

Steve remains angry with Angie when she takes the cats to the animal shelter. He does his best to comfort his children.

Episode 8

No news this week.

Episode 9

Steve is awakened at 3 a.m. by Angie, who says she is going into labor. He asks her how often her contractions are, and she tells him every 20 minutes. Steve falls back asleep. He gets up at his usual 6 a.m. time and finds Angie in the shower. Her contractions have progressed. He gets the children up, makes them breakfast, and helps them get ready for school. He makes arrangements with their close friends to pick up the kids after school, if needed, drops them off at school, and returns home to be with Angie.

In the late morning, Steve takes Angie to the hospital when she tells him it is time. He coaches her through her labor and accompanies her to the delivery room, where he is thrilled to watch the birth of his son.

Later that day, Steve brings his children to the hospital to see the baby. Kelsey and Marcus ask many questions about the baby and how it was born. Steve's mother and Angie's parents come by the hospital to see the new baby as well. Steve feels grateful for his wonderful family. **[P]**

Episode 10

Steve is back at work this week after taking several days off to be at home with Angie and the new baby. Steve's mother-in-law has been staying at the house, so he is relieved to get away and go to work. **[P]**

Episode 11

No news this week.

Episode 12

Steve helps Marcus learn to ride his bike in the late afternoon before dark. He is excited when Marcus finally catches on and starts riding.

Steve makes another attempt to stop smoking. This time, he decides to follow a plan he read about in a magazine. He plans to cut his smoking down by 1/2 every week until he has quit completely. **[P]**

Episode 13

No news this week.

Episode 14

Steve takes Kelsey and Marcus to the Bicycle Safety Awareness activity. He enjoys watching his children on the bikes. After they are finished, he takes them to McDonalds for a Happy Meal.

Steve continues his smoking reduction plan and is now down to four cigarettes a day.

Episode 15

No news this week.

STEVE YOUNG
Season 3

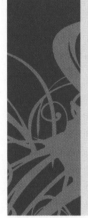

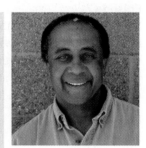

Biographical Information

Steve Young is a 42-year-old African-American male who is in excellent health. He has been married to his wife Angie for 9 years. He has three children with her, Kelsey, Marcus, and Eric. Angie and Steve met in college and were married shortly after Steve graduated with a degree in accounting. He has been extremely successful and has an income that easily supports his family. He is pleased that his wife is able to be a stay-at-home mother, but his success requires that he work very long hours at the office.

Steve began smoking at age 17 and, at this time, he has an 11 pack-year smoking history. He has tried to quit smoking several times, but has just not been able to quit. He knows it is a serious irritation to his wife and is currently attempting to quit by gradually cutting back on the number of cigarettes per day.

Episode 1

Steve has an incredibly stressful week at work, because several fiscal reports are due for several of his clients. He is at work from 6:30 a.m. until 9 p.m. several days this week, and feels badly about not being able to help Angie with the kids. He is down to just a few cigarettes a day, but has not been able to stop yet; he is just glad he has cut back as much as he has.

Episode 2

Angie tells Steve about the immunization issue. He is glad she agrees to the immunizations. Although he doesn't say it, he sometimes wonders what his wife is thinking and why she is so overly protective all the time.

Episode 3

Steven runs to the store at Angie's request to get Pedialyte solution for the baby. Angie looks exhausted. He takes the kids to piano and swimming lessons, allowing her to stay at home with Eric and get some rest. He decides to stop and pick up a pizza on the way home so they will not have to hassle with dinner. The kids are thrilled with the idea of having pizza. **[P]**

Episode 4

No news this week.

Episode 5

Steve receives a phone call from Angie in a panic, telling him that Marcus was hit by a car. Steve tries to get some basic information out of her, but Angie is too upset to communicate clearly. Angie tells him to meet them at the Neighborhood Hospital emergency department (ED).

When Steve arrives at the ED, he asks the receptionist about his son. He is told to have a seat in the waiting room and that somebody will be with him. After 10 minutes, he gets up and again asks about his son. A nurse overhears him asking, clarifies that he is Mr. Young, and escorts him into the trauma room. Angie is relieved to see him; he holds her while they stand back and let the trauma team care for Marcus. On the way home that evening, Steve is so stressed out that he smokes 3 cigarettes, one after another. **[P]**

Episode 6

Steve tries to convince Angie to come home at night, offering to stay with Marcus himself. Angie insists that she needs to stay with her son. He is embarrassed by the way she treats the nurses and wishes she would just go home and get some rest.

Steve is thankful to have Angie's mother at the house to help with the kids. He realizes how difficult it would be to work full-time and manage all of their activities by himself. He wonders how families with two working parents do everything. Steve feels so tempted to start smoking regularly again, but resists the urge. He limits himself to 2–4 cigarettes a day this entire week. **[VC]**

Episode 7

Steve is glad that Marcus is back at home. He sets a bed up for Marcus in the living room so that he can interact with the family during the day and evening. He is able to put him in his own bed at night so that he has a little variety in his surroundings. **[P]**

Episode 8

No news this week.

Episode 9

Steve has not had a cigarette now in a week. He decided that he had been at his 2–4 cigarettes a day long enough that it was time to take the final step and quit. He craves smoking constantly, but this time he wants to be successful. He does not believe Angie has noticed yet—at least she has not said anything.

In the evenings, Steve helps Marcus get up and around. He is amazed at the ability of a child to adapt to obstacles.

Episode 10

Steve continues to work very long hours at work. He has been able to stay away from cigarettes now for 3 weeks. Angie has not yet commented on the fact that he quit, and he wonders if she has noticed yet. Steve finds that he has more energy after quitting and vows never to start smoking again. **[P]**

Episode 11

Steve accompanies Angie and the kids to the petition drive organized by Angie. He can tell many people are not interested in signing, but his wife has a way of getting their signatures just the same. Steve lets Angie do all the talking while he carries Eric or pushes him in a stroller and does his best to keep Marcus and Kelsey entertained on the outing. **[P]**

Episode 12

No news this week.

Episode 13

Steve believes his wife made a fabulous presentation to The Neighborhood Council; he knew, however, that there was no way they were going to place speed bumps on the street. He was not surprised at the opposition from other members of the community.

Episode 14

Steve recognizes that Angie is trying to prevent Kelsey from taking a field trip and is back to insisting that Marcus play the piano. He advocates for his children and talks her into letting Kelsey go on the field trip and not forcing Marcus to play piano. He is pleased that Angie actually agrees to something like this without getting defensive. **[VC]**

Episode 15

Marcus asks Steve about getting a new bike and getting a dog. Steve knows he will have to work on Angie for a while to make that happen. It has now been a couple months since Steve smoked a cigarette. He is so happy that he quit and now realizes that many of his clothes smelled like cigarettes. Angie has not said anything about it, but he is quite sure she has noticed.

ANGIE YOUNG
Season 1

Biographical Information

Angie Young is a 29-year-old African-American female who is in excellent health. She has been happily married to her husband Steve for 8 years, and they have two children, Kelsey and Marcus. Angie and Steve met in college and got married shortly before she graduated with a degree in nutrition. Following graduation, she worked for a nursing home facility as a dietician, but left this position shortly before her oldest child was born. Since that time, she has been a stay-at-home mother. Angie adores her husband Steve, although she is annoyed

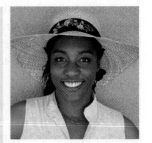

Continued

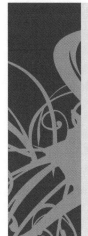

by the fact that he is a smoker. She does not understand why he continues to smoke when it is so obvious that it is physically harmful.

Angie is a perfectionist. She strives to have a perfect home for her family and is committed to offering her children many opportunities to ensure that they excel in life. She has a highly structured routine that includes getting up in the morning and making a nutritious breakfast for the family and nutritious lunches for the children to take to school; getting the children to school; going to the gym to work out for two hours a day; taking care of errands and house cleaning; picking up the children up from school; and taking them to after-school activities. In the evening, she makes dinner, helps the children with homework and piano lessons, makes sure they take baths, and gets them in bed by 9:00 p.m. Angie also volunteers at the school on a regular basis by helping in the classrooms and being available for field trips. She loves being involved with her children's lives.

Episode 1

Angie arranges a family outing to the Natural History Museum on Saturday as an educational activity for her children. They spend a couple of hours at the museum and go to a restaurant for lunch. After lunch, Angie directs her children to read and practice the piano before being allowed to play. Shortly after Marcus begins to practice, she hears him talking and then finds him on the living room floor playing with the cats. She disciplines him by sending him to his room for 1 hour.

Episode 2

Angie notices that Kelsey is experiencing seasonal allergy symptoms. Three times this week, she hears Kelsey coughing a little bit during the night, and she says her throat is a little bit "twitchy." Angie has experience managing Kelsey's symptoms; she gives her an albuterol inhaler (with spacer) and over-the-counter Claritin syrup. Over the course of a week, Kelsey's symptoms subside.

Angie gets frustrated with Marcus this week for failing to practice his piano lessons for at least 30 minutes a day. She also notices he does not seem to be progressing as well as his sister Kelsey. When she discusses this with Steve, he suggests that she lighten up a bit and tells her to "let the kids be kids." She responds, "Children need discipline, and Marcus will never improve if he does not practice." **[P]**

Episode 3

Angie finds herself longing for another baby. She talks with Steve about it, and they both decide to have another child. Angie decides that at the end of her next menstrual cycle she will stop taking birth control pills.

Episode 4

Angie talks with Ramona (the piano teacher) about the differences in progress she has noted in her children and asks if she thinks Marcus is progressing adequately. Ramona tells Angie that every child's ability is where it lies, and that every child is different—talent cannot be predicted or measured. She also tells Angie that boys do not focus as well as girls at this age. Angie asks Ramona if she should make Marcus practice more so that he will improve, but Ramona suggests just the opposite, saying that 10 to 15 minutes a day of practice time is appropriate for his age. Ramona adds that, if Angie puts too much pressure on him, Marcus might resist even more and not want to play at all.

Episode 5

Angie has decided to reduce the practice time she requires of the children to 20 minutes. She sets the kitchen timer so they will know when practice time is up.

She is pleased that Steve has decided to quit smoking and encourages him, although she points out that his constant snacking will cause him to gain weight. She wishes he was not so crabby and tells him that his crabbiness is just another sign of how bad cigarettes are for him. Angie has her period this month and is disappointed that she is not pregnant. **[P]**

Episode 6

No news this week.

Episode 7

Angie arranges for the family to go to the Health Fair. They stop at a nutrition evaluation booth that offers a calculation of body mass index (BMI), bioelectric impedance analysis (to estimate lean body mass and body fat composition), and waist-to-hip ratio measurement. She is pleased to learn her

BMI is 22 kg/m², her total body fat is estimated at 28%, and her waist to hip ratio is 0.62. At another booth, she picks up smoking cessation literature and places it in Steve's bag.

Episode 8
Angie has missed her period and notices fullness in her breasts. She buys a home pregnancy test kit, checks her urine, and finds the test is positive. Angie is ecstatic. She calls Steve at work and then calls her mother to share the news. She shares the news with her children when they come home later that day. **[P]**

Episode 9
Angie notices discharge around Marcus' eye while helping him get ready for school. She determines he must have had something in his eye during the night and thinks nothing more of it. In the afternoon, she receives a phone call from Violet Brinkworth, the school nurse, informing her that Marcus might have an eye infection. Violet advises Angie to pick up Marcus from school and take him to the family doctor. Angie calls Steve and asks him to pick up Kelsey from school and take her to her art class.

Angie takes Marcus to the pediatrician's office and is told he has conjunctivitis. The nurse practitioner tells Angie it is very contagious and that he should stay home from school for the next day. She writes a prescription for eye drops and tells Angie to administer two drops every 2 hours for the first 12 hours, and then twice a day for 4 days. They leave the office, go to the drugstore to get the prescription filled, and then come home, where Angie makes dinner. All evening and into the night (up until 5 a.m.), Angie administers the eye drops. She is very tired the following day and wonders if she'll be able to handle infant feedings during the night once the baby comes.

Episode 10
Angie makes an appointment with her gynecologist, Dr. Mary Howe, for her initial prenatal work-up. **[MR] [P]**

Episode 11
Angie attends the open house at school; she is very proud to know all of the teachers and office staff. **[P]**

Episode 12
Angie goes to the Neighborhood Women's Health Specialists for prenatal care. **[MR] [P]**

Episode 13
Kelsey has another episode with allergy symptoms; Angie can hear her coughing during the night three times this week. She manages Kelsey's symptoms with the albuterol inhaler and Claritin syrup. Angie also is a chaperone for Marcus' field trip to the roller rink this week. She is amazed at how quickly he learns to skate and wishes he would display the same natural talent on the piano. **[P]**

Episode 14
No news this week.

Episode 15
Angie goes to the Neighborhood Women's Health Specialists for prenatal care. She goes with Steve and the children on a weekend trip to visit her mother-in-law. Angie enjoys an excellent relationship with her and is always glad to go. **[MR]**

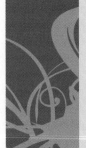

ANGIE YOUNG
Season 2

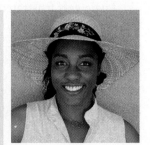

Biographical Information

Angie Young is a 30-year-old African-American female in excellent health. She has been happily married to her husband Steve for 9 years, and they have two children, Kelsey and Marcus; she is pregnant with their third child.

Angie and Steve met in college and got married shortly before she graduated with a degree in nutrition. Following graduation, she worked for a nursing home facility as a dietician, but left this position shortly before her oldest child was born. Since that time, she has been a stay-at-home mother. Angie adores her husband Steve, although she is annoyed by the fact that he is a smoker. She does not understand why he continues to smoke when it is so obvious that it is physically harmful.

Continued

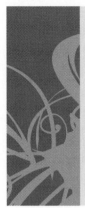

Angie is a perfectionist. She strives to have a perfect home for her family and is committed to offering her children many opportunities to ensure that they excel in life. She has a highly structured routine that includes getting up in the morning and making a nutritious breakfast for the family and nutritious lunches for the children to take to school; getting the children to school; going to the gym to work out for two hours a day; taking care of errands and house cleaning; picking up the children up from school; and taking them to after-school activities. In the evening, she makes dinner, helps the children with homework and piano lessons, makes sure they take baths, and gets them in bed by 9:30 p.m. Angie also volunteers at the school on a regular basis by helping in the classrooms and being available for field trips. She loves being involved with her children's lives.

Episode 1

Angie has a prenatal visit this week. She has felt good, but has been annoyed with constipation and bloating. She also hates the fact that she is developing unsightly varicose veins. Through it all, she continues to keep the children in their regular school activities and is taking childbirth classes with Steve. **[MR] [P]**

Episode 2

No news this week.

Episode 3

Steve talks with Angie about getting Marcus a bike. Angie is concerned that he might get hurt riding it, but Steve points out that Kelsey got her first bike at about the same age. Angie agrees to the idea. **[VC]**

Episode 4

Angie has her 32-week prenatal visit this week. She cleans out the guest bedroom (which has ended up being a "junk room") to make way for a nursery. She gets Steve to retrieve the crib and all of the baby accessories from the attic, and decides the room needs a fresh coat of yellow paint. Angie paints the room this week. **[MR] [P]**

Episode 5

Angie hears Kelsey coughing during the day and at night, and notes that the cough is worse than before. When she is awake, Angie can hear a faint wheezing sound with breathing. Angie treats her 4 mornings in a row with Claritin syrup and the albuterol inhaler before sending her to school. On the fourth day of her symptoms, Angie receives a call from the school nurse, reporting that Kelsey has coughed continually all day in class; the nurse recommends that she be seen by her pediatrician.

Angie takes Kelsey to the pediatrician's office. She is told the pediatrician is booked, but Kelsey can see the nurse practitioner (NP). Angie wishes she could just see a doctor instead. Angie tells the Carolyn Marquette, the nurse practitioner, that Kelsey's symptoms only happen at this time of year; this time, it is just a little worse. Angie says, "With the air pollution this week, it is amazing anybody can breathe."

The NP tells Angie to give her daughter nebulizer treatments every 4 hours at home until tomorrow and check the peak flow. She also gives Kelsey a prescription for prednisone. Angie tells the nurse she is not in favor of her daughter being on steroids. The NP spends a great deal of time explaining current treatment guidelines to Angie. She assures her that the short dose of steroids will not have long-lasting effects, and they will make her daughter feel much better. Angie asks the NP if this is what the doctor would prescribe. On the way home, Angie picks up the prescription and nebulizer and treats her daughter as directed. **[VC]**

Episode 6

On Monday morning, Angie takes Kelsey back to see Carolyn Marquette, the NP. Angie learns that Kelsey has asthma, rather than reactive airway disease. This upsets Angie; she wants to know what caused the condition and wants to do everything in her power to keep Kelsey well. She is not happy about the medication treatment, but after assurances from the NP and the pediatrician in the office, and after looking up information on the Internet herself, Angie realizes that the treatment prescribed follows the American Pediatric Academy's guidelines.

Angie becomes highly regimented in the treatment of Kelsey's asthma. She checks her peak flow religiously every day and gives her the control medications. Angie also looks for things at home that might trigger airway problems. She talks with Steve about needing to protect Kelsey from environmental triggers and tells him he MUST quit smoking—even outside. She also decides that the cats must go.

Episode 7

Angie has her 36–week prenatal visit. An ultrasound is done during the visit, and she learns that she will be having another boy. Angie is thrilled to see the baby and eagerly anticipates the birth, not only out of excitement for the baby, but also because she is tired of being pregnant. She has had increasingly more trouble sleeping because she can't seem to get comfortable. She also feels short of breath because the baby is pushing up against her lungs.

Angie takes the cats to the Animal Humane Center while the kids are at school. She knows they will be very upset, so she decides to take the cats away when the children aren't home to see it. Angie feels very badly for them and for herself. She hates being the "bad guy," but in her opinion, this is something she must do for Kelsey's health. **[MR] [P]**

Episode 8

No news this week.

Episode 9

In the early morning hours on Wednesday, Angie wakes up when she has a moderate contraction. She experiences another contraction about 20 minutes later, which lasts about 30 seconds. She wakes Steve up and tells him she has started her contractions and is annoyed when he falls back asleep.

Several hours later, Angie's contractions are occurring regularly every 6–7 minutes. They are also becoming progressively stronger and lasting about 45 seconds. Steve takes Angie to the hospital, where she is admitted to the labor and delivery unit. Upon admission, her contractions are moderate to strong, occurring every 4–5 minutes and lasting just under 1 minute. Her cervix is 7 cm dilated, and

her membranes are ruptured. About 45 minutes later, she delivers a son in an uncomplicated birth. Angie stays at the hospital overnight and is discharged with her infant Eric the following day. **[P]**

Episode 10

Angie is adjusting to caring for a new infant, along with keeping up with all of her other obligations. Her mother has stayed for the better part of the week to help her with the baby and kids while Steve is at work. Angie doesn't remember feeling so tired after the birth of her other children. **[P]**

Episode 11

Angie has a postpartum follow-up visit with her physician this week. She reports that she is feeling good and that breastfeeding is going well.

Episode 12

Angie takes Eric for his 1-month well-baby check-up. He has gained an appropriate amount of weight, and his immunizations are given to him. Angie encourages Kelsey and Marcus to help her take care of Eric with age-appropriate tasks. Kelsey is always willing to help, but Marcus is less interested.

Episode 13

Kelsey has a mild cough this week. Angie monitors her peak flow several times a day to keep an eye on her status. She is pleased when Kelsey's symptoms do not progress. In her mind, this provides the justification she needs regarding the decision she made about the cats, as unpopular as it was. **[P]**

Episode 14

Steve takes Kelsey and Marcus to a bicycle safety awareness activity at the local school. Angie is glad to have the house to herself with Eric. She is hopeful that she can take a nap while everyone is gone, but Eric is awake the entire time, requiring her attention.

Episode 15

No news this week.

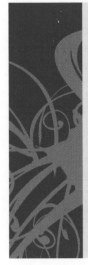

ANGIE YOUNG
Season 3

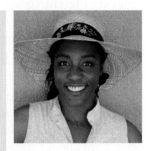

Biographical Information

Angie Young is a 30-year-old African American female who is in excellent health. She has been happily married to her husband Steve for 9 years, and they have three children, Kelsey, Marcus, and Eric. Angie is a stay-at-home mother. She adores her husband Steve, although she is annoyed by the fact that he is a smoker. She does not understand why he continues to smoke when it is so obvious that it is physically harmful.

Angie is a perfectionist. She strives to have a perfect home for her family and is committed to offering her children many opportunities to ensure that they excel in life. Although she likes to maintain a highly structured routine, she has found it to be much more difficult with a new baby. Angie is enjoying her infant son, but finds that it is more work than she remembered with her other two children. Angie has stopped volunteering at the school for the time being, but plans to do it again when Eric is a little older.

Episode 1

Angie has signed Kelsey and Marcus up for swimming lessons at the Neighborhood Pool. She likes the facility because it can accommodate indoor and outdoor swimmers—thus allowing for year-round swimming. Neither Angie nor Steve ever learned to swim, but she wants her children to have this skill. It is her belief that all children should be taught to swim.

Episode 2

Angie takes Eric in for his 2-month well-baby exam. The nurse practitioner (NP) tells Angie that he is due for his immunizations. Angie tells the NP that she is not so sure about immunizations after reading about some of the problems they cause. She tells the NP that she has heard about babies who develop autism as a result of immunizations. The NP reinforces the benefits of immunizations and explains that thiamazole is no longer used in vaccinations; she emphasizes that there really is no evidence to support the connection to autism anyway. Angie agrees to the immunizations. She is not sure if she likes the NP or not. **[VC]**

Episode 3

Eric becomes very fussy and quits eating. Angie notices that he has very frequent, watery stools. She tries to give him water over the course of the day, but the diarrhea continues. She asks Steve to run to the store for Pedialyte in the evening.

Eric continues to have diarrhea throughout the night, so in the morning Angie takes him back to the pediatrician's office. The NP sees Eric and reassures Angie that she is doing everything right. Eric is a little dehydrated, but it is nothing that can't be treated at home with the Pedialyte solution. The NP reminds Angie to monitor his diapers for evidence of adequate urinary output. Angie tells the nurse that she thinks this whole situation probably resulted from the immunizations he received the previous week. The NP attempts to explain that viral diarrhea is not something that is caused or prevented by immunizations. Angie is relieved when Eric's diarrhea stops later that evening. **[VC]**

Episode 4

No news this week.

Episode 5

Angie is breastfeeding Eric when she hears screeching tires outside. She doesn't give it another thought until, a short while later, she hears sirens. A neighbor knocks on the door to tell Angie that Marcus had been hit by a car. Angie runs outside, leaving Eric in the house with Kelsey. She sees Marcus's body lying in the median of the street and begins to scream, believing he is dead. Paramedics have just arrived and are assessing Marcus when she reaches him. A large man holds Angie back while the paramedics attend to her son until she calms down. Angie then spots two teenage boys standing to the side. One of them is crying, and she knows that these are the boys who hit Marcus. She begins walking toward them, screaming, and asking them how they could hurt an innocent little boy. The large man again holds her back, saying, "Not here, not now." After Angie is able to see that Marcus is stable, she runs back to the house to call Steve. She asks one of the neighbors to attend to Kelsey and Eric. Angie gets into the ambulance to go to the hospital with Marcus.

Angie and Steve are permitted to be in the trauma room in the emergency department while the trauma team stabilizes Marcus. Angie is so thankful to be allowed to be with her son during this time and grateful that Steve is so strong throughout the ordeal. **[P]**

Episode 6

Angie's mother comes to stay with them to care for Kelsey and Eric so that Angie can spend as much time as possible with Marcus at the hospital. She is persistent with the orthopedic team about letting her take Marcus home as soon as possible. Angie spends most nights at the hospital with Marcus, but leaves periodically during the day to spend time with Kelsey and Eric. Angie watches everything the nurses do and questions them constantly, checking to make sure they know what they are doing. She insists that everyone washes their hands the minute they enter the hospital room, because she doesn't want Marcus to get an infection. Late in the week, Charles, the young man who almost killed her son, comes to visit Marcus with his friend. Angie is furious at first—how dare he come to see Marcus? However, as the two young men talk, she can see that Charles is deeply sorry about what happened. As it turns out, Angie appreciates their efforts.

Episode 7

Angie is able to convince the physicians to send Marcus home this week. He requires a great deal of care, but Angie is sure she can better take care of him and her other children if Marcus is home. Angie's mother has agreed to stay as long as she is needed.

Kelsey comes home from gymnastics lessons with a cough that is easily treated with the rescue inhaler. Angie tells Kelsey that she might have to stop taking gymnastics because it seems to be bad for her breathing.

Episode 8

No news this week.

Episode 9

Angie is angered by news that the boy driving the car that hit Marcus got off so easily—a charge of recklessness and the loss of his driver's license until age 20. She believes she needs to do something to prevent other people from getting hurt. She writes to her Congresswoman to complain about speed limits in the Neighborhood and determine what she can do to slow down speeding cars.

Episode 10

Angie is surprised by the quick response from the Congresswoman. She encourages Angie to follow up with local officials regarding speeders, but claims that there is nothing that she can do officially on the state level. The Congresswoman wishes Marcus a speedy recovery. Angie begins making phone calls to city officials.

During the week, Eric develops a runny nose, cough, and fever. He is very fussy and not interested in eating. Angie takes him to Neighborhood Pediatrics and again sees the NP. She cannot believe the NP won't give Eric a prescription for antibiotics and questions the NP about the reason. Angie has read about the overuse of antibiotics, but is concerned that, in Eric's case, he might really need them.

Episode 11

Angie learns that there is nothing she can do to get the speed limit changed on their street. She is told that one option for her is to get signatures on a petition asking for speed bumps to be placed on the streets. Angie organizes a Neighborhood petition campaign and takes her entire family on an outing with her to help her collect signatures. **[P]**

Episode 12

No news this week.

Episode 13

Angie takes the signed petition to the Neighborhood Council Meeting this week. She is disappointed when several people come to the meeting to speak out against her proposal, citing that speed bumps will damage their cars' suspensions. She does not understand why people are more concerned with their cars' suspensions than the safety of their children.

Kelsey brings a permission slip home from school for a hayride on a farm 20 miles south of *The Neighborhood*. The hayride is part of a pioneer learning experience with her class and will be held later in the month. Angie tells her Kelsey that she should not go because of her asthma. **[P]**

Episode 14

Angie asks Marcus if he is ready to start taking piano lessons again. She is not surprised when he tells her that he doesn't want to do it. Steve intervenes on his behalf and tells her that they really need to stop pushing the children, and Marcus should be allowed to drop that activity. He also talks to her about letting Kelsey go on the hayride. After much discussion, Angie agrees to call the nurse and ask her opinion. The NP suggests that Angie premedicate Kelsey with albuterol and Claritin before the hayride.

Episode 15

Angie takes Eric to Neighborhood Pediatrics this week for his 6-month visit. She sees the NP again, whom she has come to trust. On this visit, she does not argue about the immunizations and is just happy to talk to the nurse about her son. Angie appreciates the fact that the nurse asks Angie how Marcus has been doing.

KELSEY YOUNG
Season 1

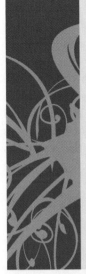

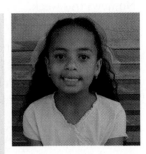

Biographical Information

Kelsey Young is the 7-year-old daughter of Angie and Steve Young. She is a pretty typical girl who is in enrolled in second grade at Neighborhood Elementary School. She likes her teacher and has many friends—especially Keisha. She has a very stable home life and is close to her parents and brother Marcus. Kelsey loves animals, especially the family cats, Chico and Kiekie. Her favorite places to visit are the pet store and the zoo. She loves to read stories and see movies that involve animals. She has never been particularly active physically, but after watching gymnastics on TV, she has taken an interest in this activity. She takes piano lessons, but has little interest in it.

Overall, Kelsey is healthy, but she has ongoing problems with reactive airway disease. This condition does not make her feel badly, except when she has periodic episodes, which seem to be seasonal. Her mother typically manages her symptoms with an albuterol inhaler with a spacer and over-the-counter Claritin syrup. She is up to date on her immunizations and sees a dentist every six months.

Episode 1

Kelsey goes with her family to the Natural History Museum and then out to lunch on Saturday. Kelsey likes the mammal display the best. In the afternoon, her mother insists that she practice the piano for 30 minutes and then read for 30 minutes before going outside to play with Keisha. She complies with her mother's demands and is glad she didn't make her mother mad, like Marcus did. **[P]**

Episode 2

Kelsey experiences allergy symptoms this week and coughs periodically during the night three times this week—although the coughing is not severe enough to wake her. Her mother administers her inhaler and gives her other medication to treat her symptoms. She feels well enough to go to school.

Episode 3

No news this week.

Episode 4

Kelsey is invited to a birthday party for her friend, Samantha, at Big Red's Pizza Parlor this week. The party, however, conflicts with her music lesson. Kelsey wants to go to the party, but her mother insists that she go to the lesson instead. Angie compromises by taking Kelsey to the birthday party late—after the piano lesson. By the time she arrives, the children have already eaten pizza and opened presents, and are playing the arcade games. Kelsey feels very disappointed and is angry that she missed most of the party.

Episode 5

No news this week.

Episode 6

Kelsey goes to the zoo on a field trip with her second-grade class. She is very excited to see all of the animals. Because her mother is one of the chaperones, she makes sure her best friend Keisha gets to ride to and from the zoo with her. Before they leave the zoo, Kelsey's mother buys her *Animals of the Jungle*, a coloring poster kit with markers. As soon as she completes her homework that evening, she spends time with her father coloring a lion poster. **[P]**

Episode 7

Kelsey goes to a health fair with her family this week. Her favorite activity is an apple puzzle game at a booth that teaches children about healthy snacks. She notices her brother is not interested in the game and instead eats the apple slices. **[P]**

Episode 8

Kelsey is told by her mother that she has a tiny baby growing in her stomach, and Kelsey will soon have a new brother or sister. Kelsey tells her mother that she hopes she gets a baby sister.

Episode 9

Kelsey is surprised and delighted to see her Daddy at school to pick her up—she is used to only seeing her mother at school. He tells her that he is taking her to art class, and on the way he stops at an ice cream store for an after-school treat. Kelsey thinks she has the very best Daddy in the world. **[P]**

Episode 10
No news this week.

Episode 11
Steve and Angie attend the open house at the grade school this week. Angie, of course, knows Kelsey's second-grade teacher very well, but Kelsey is especially excited for her Daddy to meet her teacher.

Episode 12
No news this week.

Episode 13
Kelsey has another week with allergy symptoms and has episodic coughing three nights this week, although the coughing does not wake her up. Her mother gives her the inhaler and the Claritin syrup. **[P]**

Episode 14
No news this week.

Episode 15
Kelsey goes with her family on an out-of-town trip to see her grandmother. Every time they go there, she gets to make cookies with her grandmother—this is their special activity. Her grandmother also has a dog that Kelsey loves to play with, and a man who lives down the street has horses. Her father takes her on a walk each day to give carrots to the horses. **[P]**

KELSEY YOUNG
Season 2

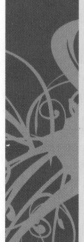

Biographical Information

Kelsey Young is the 7-year-old daughter of Angie and Steve Young. She is a pretty typical girl who is in enrolled in second grade at Neighborhood Elementary School. She likes her teacher and has many friends—especially Keisha. She has a very stable home life and is close to her parents and brother Marcus. She knows there will be a baby in the house soon and looks forward to taking care of it. Kelsey loves animals, especially the family cats, Chico and Kiekie. Her favorite places to visit are the pet store and the zoo. She loves to read stories and see movies that involve animals. She has never been particularly active physically, but after watching gymnastics on TV, she has taken an interest in this activity. She takes piano lessons, but has little interest in it.

Overall, Kelsey is healthy, but she has ongoing problems with reactive airway disease. This condition does not make her feel badly, except when she has periodic episodes, which seem to be seasonal. Her mother typically manages her symptoms with an albuterol inhaler with a spacer and over-the-counter Claritin syrup. She is up to date on her immunizations and sees a dentist every six months.

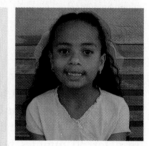

Episode 1
The weather turns cold this week, and Kelsey has a "flare-up" of her reactive airway disease. Her mother gives her the albuterol inhaler and the cough syrup, but she does not feel well for several days. She coughs frequently day and night for 3 days. Although she feels well enough to go to school, she does not feel like running around on the playground. She and Keisha sit on the swings and talk about horses until some boys start to throw sand at them. Rather than chasing the boys, Kelsey just gets off the swings and walks away with Keisha, informing the boys that she is going to tell the teacher.

Episode 2
No news this week.

Episode 3
Kelsey talks with her mother about the baby. She is fascinated by the fact that the baby is inside her mother's stomach and tries to imagine what the baby looks like and what it is doing in there. Kelsey likes to touch her mother's stomach, especially when she can feel the baby move. She asks her mother how the baby breathes inside, but does not understand her mother's explanation. She hopes the baby will be a girl. **[P]**

Episode 4
No news this week.

Episode 5
Kelsey has another round of allergy symptoms, but this time it is worse. Her coughing keeps her (and the rest of the family) awake at night. When she is awake, she has a subtle wheeze with breathing. Her mother gives her Claritin and the inhaler before school each morning. By Friday (the fourth day of her symptoms), her classroom teacher sends her to Violet Brinkworth, the school nurse, who then calls her mother. She hears the nurse tell her mother, "Kelsey should be seen by her primary care provider."

Kelsey is seen by a nurse practitioner. Her peak flow is assessed and found to be in the yellow zone, prompting an immediate nebulizer treatment. Kelsey thinks the treatment is strange—it makes a weird sound, and white smoke comes out the end. She thinks it looks like smoking a funny pipe.

Following treatment, Kelsey is better, but her peak flow shows that she is still in the yellow zone. She gets a second nebulizer treatment, and this improves her breathing significantly. Kelsey feels much better. On the way home, she and her mother stop at the drugstore to pick up medications and a little machine. **[MR] [P]**

Episode 6
On Monday, Kelsey returns to see Carolyn Marquette, the nurse practitioner. It has been a few days since her breathing episode. She has been feeling well all weekend and has slept well. Her mother gives her another breathing treatment a little while before going to the office. Her peak flow is checked by the NP and found to be 200, which is in the green zone. **[MR] [P]**

Kelsey is devastated when she hears her mother announce that the family cats must go to prevent Kelsey from getting sick again. She believes this situation is all her fault. She loves the cats and cannot bear the thought of giving them away. She is also upset by the fact that her mother and father are fighting. She is not used to this. Kelsey is very sad and cries for hours.

Episode 7
The family cats are gone when Kelsey gets home from school. She goes into her room and cries. She tells her mother that she doesn't mind having problems breathing—she just wants her kitties to come home. Kelsey is angry with her mother and angry that she has a problem with breathing. **[P]**

Episode 8
No news this week.

Episode 9
Kelsey is excited when she learns that her new baby brother was born. She talks to the baby and tells him she is his big sister and she will take care of him. Kelsey asks her mother if she has changed the baby's diaper yet. She is intrigued by the appearance of the umbilical cord. **[P]**

Episode 10
Kelsey looks forward to coming home each day to see the baby. She likes it when her mother lets her sit in a chair to hold Eric, and stands on a chair next to the changing table to watch her mother or grandmother change the diapers. She also enjoys watching the baby get a bath in the tiny bathtub. She thinks about her cats often and wonders how they are. **[P]**

Episode 11
No news this week.

Episode 12
Kelsey plays with Eric as he lies on a blanket on the floor while her mother takes a shower. Kelsey loves playing with the baby.

Episode 13
Kelsey has a mild cough this week, but it does not progress any further. Angie tells Kelsey that it is a good thing that the cats no longer live with them, or she might have ended up in the hospital.

Episode 14
Kelsey goes to the Bike Safety Awareness class with her brother and father. She has fun, but thinks she is a little bit "old" for the activity. She perceives it as an activity for little kids. The best part of the outing is that her Daddy took them to McDonalds for a Happy Meal. **[P]**

Episode 15
No news this week.

KELSEY YOUNG
Season 3

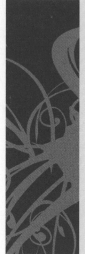

Biographical Information

Kelsey is the 8-year-old daughter of Angie and Steve Young. She is a pretty typical girl who is enrolled in third grade at the elementary school. She likes her teacher at school and has many friends—especially Keisha. She has a very stable home life and is close to her parents and her brothers, Marcus and Eric. Kelsey loves her new baby brother and enjoys helping her mother take care of him. She also loves animals and is still angry with her mother about getting rid of the cats. She loves to read stories and see movies that involve animals. She takes gymnastics, swimming lessons, and piano lessons.

Overall, Kelsey is healthy. She has asthma and takes Advair Diskus 100/50 in the morning and evening. If she has an acute breathing problem, she takes a rescue medication, albuterol metered dose inhaler (MDI) with a spacer—2 puffs, wait 15-20 minutes, and then repeat. She has not needed to use her albuterol in months. She is up to date on her immunizations and sees a dentist every 6 months.

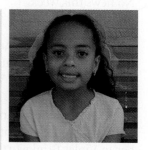

Episode 1

Kelsey and her brother Marcus are taking swimming lessons at Neighborhood Pool starting this week. Kelsey enjoys swimming, but does not like getting in the cold water. **[P]**

Episode 2

Kelsey plans to spend the night with Keisha. This is her first time spending the night away from her home. Kelsey does fine all evening, until it is time to go to bed, when she starts to feel very sad and wants to go home. After a call from Keisha's mother, her father drives to Keisha's house to pick up Kelsey and bring her home. **[P]**

Episode 3

Kelsey is aware that the baby is sick, and she is worried. Kelsey's father takes her to her piano and swimming lessons so her mother can take care of the sick baby. Kelsey experiences some coughing after being in the pool. When she gets home, her mother checks her peak flow, and it is found to be 200. Her mother does not give Kelsey albuterol, and the coughing subsides shortly thereafter. **[P]**

Episode 4

No news this week.

Episode 5

Kelsey hears her mother screaming outside and runs to the door to look. She is unable to see anything but an ambulance down the street. She becomes frightened, thinking that Marcus is hurt. When Eric begins to cry, Kelsey does not know what to do and tries to comfort him. Finally, a neighbor comes to the house and tells Kelsey

that her brother was injured and is on the way to the hospital. The neighbor makes Kelsey supper and helps her with her with homework. Kelsey is so happy when her Daddy comes home several hours later. **[P]**

Episode 6

Kelsey has been to the hospital to see Marcus, but only once in the lobby. She is told she is not allowed to go into his hospital room because she is too young. She feels sorry for her brother when she sees his casts and the pins in his hips. She asks Marcus if it hurts, and he tells her yes. Kelsey is happy that her grandmother is at the house this week. Because she has watched her mother over the past few months, she knows the routine and helps her grandmother take care of Eric.

Episode 7

Kelsey goes to her gymnastics lessons with her Dad. After the lesson, Kelsey starts to cough. When she gets home, her mother checks her peak flow and finds it is 190. She administers the rescue medication (albuterol with spacer); a few minutes later, her peak flow is 220, and Kelsey stops coughing. Kelsey's mother tells her that she might have to quit gymnastics because of the asthma. Kelsey tells her mother she likes gymnastics. **[P]**

Episode 8

No news this week.

Episode 9

Kelsey is disappointed when her mother decides to take her out of swimming lessons. She hears her mother talk about her asthma to other people on a regular basis and decides that she must have a bad disease, yet she does not feel too badly. Kelsey is still in gymnastics class and hopes she does not have to quit gymnastics, too. She wishes the asthma would prevent her from playing the piano.

Episode 10
Kelsey is happy that Marcus is back at school with her. She helps him get to his class and tries to take care of him. She often sits with him at recess. At home, Kelsey reminds her mother that Marcus has his cast off now and wants to know when he is going to have to practice the piano.

Episode 11
Kelsey accompanies Marcus, Eric, and her mother and father on a petition-signing event to get speed bumps placed on the streets. She is not happy about going because she wants to go play at Keisha's house.

Episode 12
No news this week.

Episode 13
Kelsey's teacher at school announces to the children that they will be going on a hayride for a learning activity as part of the Pioneer Unit later in the month. Permission slips are distributed, and the children are instructed to return the signed slips by next week. Kelsey is angry when her mother tells her she should not go on the hayride because of her asthma. Kelsey feels like asthma ruins everything for her.

Episode 14
Kelsey is delighted when her mother gives her the signed permission slip for the hayride. She can't wait to tell Keisha that she is going to be going after all. **[P]**

Episode 15
Kelsey goes on the hayride with her class at school. They learn about shoeing a horse, milking cows, and building log homes. Kelsey liked the hayride the best because she was able to watch the horses as they pulled the wagon.

MARCUS YOUNG
Season 1

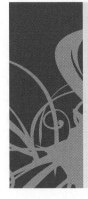

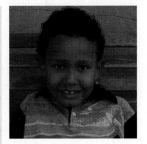

Biographical Information

Marcus Young is the 6-year-old son of Angie and Steve Young. He is a pretty typical boy who is in enrolled in the first grade at the elementary school. He likes his teacher at school and has many friends. He has a stable home life and is close to his parents and sister Kelsey. Marcus loves his pet cats, Chico and Kiekie. He also enjoys going to the park and playing on the playground equipment. He is very interested in sports and wants to play football and baseball someday. He takes piano lessons, but is not interested in this activity at all. Marcus has no health-related problems; he is up to date on his immunizations and sees a dentist every 6 months.

Episode 1
Marcus goes with his family to the Natural History Museum and then out to lunch on Saturday. He likes the dinosaur and volcano displays the best. In the afternoon, his mother insists that he practice the piano for 30 minutes and then read for 30 minutes before he can go outside to play. He sits in front of the piano and plays for about 10 minutes before getting distracted by his cat, Chico. His mother finds him playing with the cat and sends him to his room for 1 hour for failing to practice. **[P]**

Episode 2
As soon as Marcus comes home from school this week, his mother makes him sit down to practice the piano before he gets an afternoon snack, believing this might motivate him more. Marcus protests, but sits down to practice. He practices for about 10 minutes before he gets distracted his sister. He is sent to his room without a snack until dinner for failing to practice. **[P]**

Episode 3
No news this week.

Episode 4
After his piano lesson, Marcus overhears his mother talking to Ramona (his piano teacher) about his practice habits. Marcus and his sister see a lady walking her dog on the sidewalk and run out of the house to pet the dog and talk to the lady. **[P]**

Episode 5

Ever since Marcus started first grade, he has been jealous of the things other kids get to eat for lunch. He tells his mother that he would like to have cookies, chips, or Twinkies in his lunchbox, like the other kids get. His mother tells him that those foods are not nutritious, and he should be happy to have the lunch he gets.

Episode 6

No news this week.

Episode 7

Marcus goes to a health fair with his family this week. Overall, he finds the fair pretty fun, especially the children's section. They visit a booth that teaches children about healthy snacks (but his mother does this at home), a place where they are weighed, and a place where they learn to take care of their teeth. Marcus is happy to get a new red toothbrush. His favorite booth involves jump roping and then counting his heartbeat in his wrists. He used to think jump roping was for girls, but decides after trying it at the health fair that it is pretty fun.

Episode 8

When he arrives home from school, Marcus is told by his mother that she has a tiny baby growing in her stomach, and he will soon have a new brother or sister. He looks under Angie's blouse at her stomach and is unimpressed. He tells his mother that he would like a snack.

Episode 9

Marcus wakes up in the morning with a sticky sensation and crust around his left eye. His mother cleans his eye before he goes to school. While at school, his eye is itchy, and he rubs it frequently. As the day progresses, his eye begins to hurt. He is sent to the nurse's office by his teacher, who then calls his mother to come pick him up.

His mother takes him to the pediatrician's office, where he is seen by a nurse practitioner. Marcus is told that he has pink eye, but he doesn't think his eye is pink.

A prescription for Ciloxan ophthalmic drops is written. On the way home from the office, they stop at the drugstore to fill the prescription. When they get home, Kelsey tells Marcus, "Daddy got me ice cream today on the way to art class." Marcus feels sad and wishes Daddy would have taken him to the doctor so he could have had ice cream on the way home.

Episode 10

No news this week.

Episode 11

Marcus continues to take piano lessons with Ramona at his mother's insistence. He has come to really hate playing the piano and admits this when Ramona (the piano teacher) asks him if he enjoys it. Marcus tells Ramona that she'd better not tell his mother, because she might get angry with him. He tells Ramona that he wants to play on a baseball team instead.

Marcus goes to the school open house with his parents. While there, he goes outside to play with a basketball with his Dad and sister. They have fun until Angie puts a stop to it. **[P]**

Episode 12

No news this week.

Episode 13

Marcus goes to a roller skating party with his first-grade class this week. He is not so sure he wants to go because he thinks roller skating is for girls. After he puts on the skates and figures out how to keep his balance, he decides he likes it. He spends most of his time with his friend, Darren, acting like monsters and chasing the girls around the roller rink. **[P]**

Episode 14

No news this week.

Episode 15

Marcus goes with his family on an out-of-town trip to see his grandmother. He loves his grandmother and wishes she lived closer. There is a fort in the backyard that he loves to play in—and there is no piano.

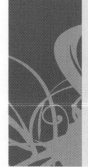

MARCUS YOUNG
Season 2

Biographical Information

Marcus Young is the 6-year-old son of Angie and Steve Young. He is a pretty typical boy who is in enrolled in first grade at the elementary school. He likes his teacher at school and has many friends. He has a stable home life and is close to his parents and sister Kelsey. He loves to read and go to the park to play on the playground equipment. He is very interested in sports and wants to play football and baseball someday. He takes piano lessons, but is not interested in this activity at all. Marcus has no health-related problems; he is up to date on his immunizations and sees a dentist every 6 months.

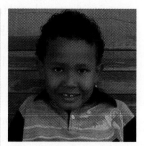

Episode 1

Marcus goes to a birthday party at his friend's house. They play on a trampoline. Marcus thinks it is the best thing ever. When he comes home from the party, he asks his mother if they can have a trampoline. His mother says they are dangerous and reminds Marcus to practice the piano before dinner. **[P]**

Episode 2

No news this week.

Episode 3

Many of Marcus's friends are getting bikes, so he asks his father if he can get a bike as well. His father takes him to the store and gets a bike with training wheels. He tells his father that he doesn't want the training wheels, but is told that he must first learn to ride safely with the training wheels, and then they can take them off. **[P]**

Episode 4

No news this week.

Episode 5

Marcus knows his sister had to go to the doctor because she had a bad cough and watches with interest when his sister breathes in the white smoke while having a treatment. He tells his mother that he would like to do that, too, and is disappointed when he learns the machine is just for Kelsey. Angie suggests that he practice the piano instead. **[P]**

Episode 6

Marcus is upset when he hears his mother say that they need to get rid of the family cats to prevent Kelsey from getting sick. He hears his mother and father arguing about it, which makes him feel very sad. He goes to his room to pet Kiekie. **[P]**

Episode 7

Marcus is very sad when he comes home from school and learns that the cats are gone. He is told that they went to another home to live and that they will be well cared for. This does not comfort Marcus one bit. He wants his cats. Although he was told to practice his piano lesson, he goes to his room instead and spends the rest of the afternoon lying on his bed feeling very sad. His father later comes into his bedroom and attempts to comfort him. **[P]**

Episode 8

No news this week.

Episode 9

Marcus is excited when his father picks him up from their friend's home after school and announces that he has a new baby brother. Marcus is intrigued when he meets his new brother at the hospital. He knows the baby was in his mother's stomach, but has a hard time understanding just how it got out. Marcus touches the baby's head and hands; he is surprised at how small the baby is.

Episode 10

Marcus has adjusted to having a new baby in the house. He likes having his grandmother at the house and likes looking at the baby. He is a little disappointed that the baby is too small to play with. Marcus is glad that his mother has been too busy with the baby to notice that he has not been practicing the piano. Marcus misses the cats and asks his father about getting a dog.

Episode 11

No news this week.

Episode 12

Marcus learns to ride a bike without training wheels this week. He had been working very hard to learn to ride and suddenly figured out how to keep his balance. He spends every day after school riding his bike up and down the sidewalk in the front of their home. Marcus stays on the sidewalk because his mother told him that, if she caught him in the street, she would take his bike away.

Episode 13

Ramona (the piano teacher) senses complete disinterest in and a lack of concentration in Marcus during the past several lessons. She talks with him about what kinds of things are going on with him. He tells her about learning to ride a bike without training wheels, about the cats, and about the new baby. Having this information is helpful to Ramona, who now has a better understanding of his lack of focus. **[P]**

Episode 14

Marcus, Kelsey, and Steve go to the Bike Safety Awareness class. Marcus loves the activity because he gets to demonstrate his skill riding through orange cones and around other obstacles. Marcus is proud of the fact that he is able to do this more efficiently than his sister—even though his training wheels just recently came off.

Episode 15

No news this week.

MARCUS YOUNG
Season 3

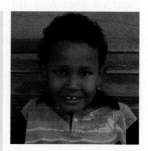

Biographical Information

Marcus Young is the 7-year-old son of Angie and Steve Young. He is a pretty typical boy who is in enrolled in the second grade at the elementary school. He likes his teacher at school and has many friends. He has a stable home life and is close to his parents, his sister Kelsey, and his new baby brother Eric. He loves to read and go to the park to play on the playground equipment. He is very interested in sports and wants to play football and baseball someday. He takes piano lessons, but is not interested in this activity at all. Marcus has no health-related problems; he is up to date on his immunizations and sees a dentist every 6 months.

Episode 1

Marcus and his sister Kelsey are now taking swimming lessons at the pool. Marcus likes swimming and wishes he could just take swimming lessons instead of piano lessons. Marcus sees a dog that belongs to some people up the street occasionally. He asks his parents about getting a dog.

Episode 2

Marcus rides his bike after school nearly every day. He has learned how to navigate over the curbs along the sidewalk. Because his mother requires that he practice the piano before he can ride, Marcus is highly motivated to get this done as soon as possible after school. His friend, Darren, also now has a bike. **[P]**

Episode 3

Marcus is happy that his father is taking him to after-school swimming and piano lessons this week while his mother stays home with the sick baby.

Episode 4

No news this week.

Episode 5

One day after school this week, Marcus and Darren are riding their bikes up and down the sidewalk. A big black dog runs out of its owner's yard and begins to chase them. The boys get scared and ride faster. Marcus darts off the sidewalk and around a parked car to get away from the dog. He never sees the speeding red car driven by Charles (Randall Johnson's best friend). Charles sees Marcus at the last minute and attempts to miss him.

Marcus is struck from behind. The impact throws him through the air more than 30 feet. He is fortunate to land in a grassy spot in the median of the roadway, but sustains a pelvic fracture, a right leg fracture, a left leg laceration, and a left arm laceration. He briefly loses consciousness, but does not sustain a head or spinal cord injury.

Marcus does not remember much about the incident. He wakes up in the intensive care unit at Neighborhood Hospital with his mother and father at his side. He has tremendous pain in his hips, legs, and arm. He is very frightened.

Episode 6

Marcus remains at Neighborhood Hospital. He wants to go home soon and misses going to school. He is still restricted to bed rest and is bored. He has lost interest watching cartoons on TV. The nurses and other hospital staff attempt to keep him occupied by providing a variety of activities for him, such as coloring and other crafts. He gets cards and balloons from his classmates at school. He watches as his mother decorates the hospital room with the colorful cards.

Two teenage boys visit Marcus at the hospital. One of the teens tells Marcus his name is Charles, the driver of the car that hit him. He tells Marcus that he feels very badly about hurting him, but is glad to see that he is going to get better. Charles gives Marcus a handheld video game to play with. Marcus likes Charles and his friend, Randall. **[P]**

Episode 7

Marcus is now home from the hospital. His leg remains in a cast, and his pelvis is still pinned; thus, he remains confined to bed. A home health nurse comes to see him every couple of days. Marcus is miserable being stuck in bed, but he is much happier at home than he was in the hospital. He is very happy to eat his mother's cooking and see his sister and brother Eric. His father moves a bed into the family area so that Marcus can be involved in all the family activities.

A lady from the school comes to see Marcus every day so he does not fall behind in school. Fortunately, he is right-handed, so he is able to complete writing assignments with assistance. Several of his classmates make a surprise visit to see Marcus, and he is very happy to see them. When they leave, he feels sad for missing out on going to school.

Episode 8

No news this week.

Episode 9

Marcus still has pins in his pelvis and a splint on his leg. He is able to get up and move a little bit now and is so happy to be out of bed and up and around. The lady from school continues to come to his house to help him with school work. Although he likes her, he misses being at school and is looking forward to going back soon. He goes to a clinic a couple of times a week to do exercises with hospital people. He likes to go because they make the exercises fun. Marcus has some pain in his leg and pelvis with the exercises, but not as much as he used to. **[P]**

Episode 10

The pins are now out of his pelvis, and Marcus is finally able to go back to school. He is unable to run on the playground at this point, but is happy to go outside at recess and watch the kids play. He shows the kids at school the scars from where the pins were and tells them the pins went all the way into the bones. The kids at school think it is gross. He is very tired when he comes home from school and needs to take a nap. He is glad that his mother does not make him practice the piano. **[P]**

Episode 11

Marcus is quickly regaining his agility with his movement. To watch him, you would not know he had been so severely injured a few months ago. Although he fell a little bit behind in his school work, the teacher has developed a plan that will help him catch up within a few weeks. Marcus goes around the neighborhood with his mother to collect signatures for speed bumps. He wishes he could stay home.

Marcus loves to play with Eric. He likes to put his face near Eric's and make noises, because this makes Eric laugh.

Episode 12

No news this week.

Episode 13

Marcus is embarrassed when his teacher asks him in front of the class about his mother being in the newspaper regarding the speed bump issue at city hall. He did not know she was in the paper and wonders why they put her picture there.

Episode 14

Marcus dreads it when his mother asks him if he is ready to take piano lessons again. He has not played in several months and has not missed it one bit. He had hoped his mother forgot about it. Marcus is so glad when his father talks his mother out of making him start the lessons again. **[P]**

Episode 15

Marcus asks his Dad about getting another bike and getting a dog. His dad promises to talk with his mother about it. **[VC]**

ERIC YOUNG
Season 2

Biographical Information
Eric Young is the newborn infant of Angie and Steve Young. He was born at 38 weeks' gestation in an uncomplicated birth.

Episode 9

Eric Young is born this week in an uncomplicated labor and delivery. He is placed on his mother's abdomen immediately after birth and covered with a warm blanket to maintain his body temperature. His Apgar scores are 8 and 10 at 1 and 5 minutes, respectively. He weighs 3.3 kg (50th percentile), is 51 cm long (50th percentile), and has a head circumference of 35.2 cm (50th percentile). Shortly after birth, Eric is cleaned and examined, and erythromycin ophthalmic ointment and tetracycline ophthalmic ointment are placed into his eyes. A dose of phytonadione and hepatitis B vaccine are administered intramuscularly.

Eric has no problems or complications following birth and is discharged home with his mother and father the next day. Prior to discharge, a heel stick is performed to obtain a blood specimen for routine newborn screening. By the time he is discharged, he is breastfeeding about eight times a day and has had seven wet diapers and a large meconium stool. His umbilical cord is dry, and the clamp has been removed.

Episode 10

Eric continues to adapt to his new surroundings. He is comforted by his mother's smell and voice. He breastfeeds well, and then he sleeps.

Episode 11

Eric is seen at Neighborhood Pediatrics for a 2-week well-baby visit. His weight is 3.6 kg. **[MR]**

ERIC YOUNG
Season 3

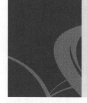

Biographical Information

Eric Young is the newborn infant of Angie and Steve Young. He was born at 38 weeks' gestation in an uncomplicated birth. He is 6 weeks old and is in perfect health. He is a breastfed infant who lives in his home with his parents and two siblings, Kelsey and Marcus.

Episode 1

No news this week.

Episode 2

Eric is now 2 months old, and his mother takes him back to Neighborhood Pediatrics to see the nurse practitioner (NP) for a well-baby check. He weighs 5.0 kg (45th percentile), his head circumference is 38.6 cm (48th percentile), and his length is 55.6 cm (50th percentile). The NP notes that he smiles responsively and holds his head well when in an upright position. He gets immunizations during this visit (HBV, DTaP, Hib, IPV, PCV). He experiences pain and cries when given an injection in the leg. **[P]**

Episode 3

Eric spends time this week at the nursery at the local fitness club while his mother works out. A few days later, he has an emesis and then very watery diarrhea. He becomes cranky and cries a lot—more than usual for this typically happy baby. He is given water throughout the day by his mother and continues to have diarrhea. In the evening, his mother gives him Pedialyte. During the night, he continues to have diarrhea; by morning, Angie recognizes that he just does not look right.

The following morning, Angie takes Eric to the pediatrician's office, and he once again sees the nurse practitioner

(NP). His weight is down only a little bit, but he has an elevated temperature, and his skin has decreased turgor. His diaper is dry. The NP suggests that Angie continue to give the baby Pedialyte and monitor his fluid output. She explains to Angie that he should have at least four wet diapers a day.

Over the course of the next 12 hours, the diarrhea slows down and eventually returns to his normally loose stools. Eric eagerly breastfeeds for the next few days.

Episode 4

No news this week.

Episode 5

Eric has become quite the chatterbox. He is very happy and babbles and coos to the delight of his parents and grandmother. He is completely unaware of the events that have occurred within his family.

Episode 6

No news this week.

Episode 7

No news this week.

Episode 8

Eric's mother takes him to Neighborhood Pediatrics for his 4-month well-baby check. On this visit, he weighs 6.4 kg (40th percentile), his head circumference is 42 cm

Episode 12

Eric lies on a blanket and listens to his sister talk to him. He is unable to focus on her face, but he can see generally the shape and knows intuitively this person is not his mother.

Episode 13

No news this week.

Episode 14

Eric is spending noticeably greater amounts of time awake than before. He is a happy baby who is rarely fussy. He enjoys being held by his mother and father.

Episode 15

No news this week.

(50th percentile), and his length is 63 cm (40th percentile). He gets immunizations during this visit (DTaP, Hib, IPV, PCV). He experiences pain when given an injection in the leg and cries.

The NP notes that Eric actively grasps objects when offered to him and inspects his hands. She also notes that he lifts his head easily when in the prone position and looks around the room; she does not observe head lag when she pulls Eric to a sitting position.

Episode 9
No news this week.

Episode 10
Eric develops a runny nose, cough, and fever this week. He is very fussy and does not eat well. His mother takes him to Neighborhood Pediatrics and, once again, he sees Carolyn Marquette, the nurse practitioner (NP). The NP examines Eric and tells Angie that he has a viral upper respiratory infection and that she just needs to give him Infant Tylenol and keep him well hydrated.

Episode 11
Eric's father puts him in a stroller and takes him out with the family to gather signatures for Angie's speed-bump campaign. Eric watches with interest the changes in his surroundings, but eventually gets bored. Steve tries to please him with a pacifier and various toys, without luck; Eric is only happy once he is carried by his father. He eventually falls asleep during the outing.

Episode 12
Eric is now able to distinguish various members of his family. He loves it when his siblings play with him. He smiles regularly and makes many sounds now (to everyone's delight).

Episode 13
No news this week.

Episode 14
To the delight of his family, Eric has begun to "talk" when he is interacting with Steve and says "Ma" or "Da." When Steve or Angie appears, he recognizes them and often holds his arms up to be picked up. He has now also begun to search for items that he drops.

Episode 15
Eric's mother takes him to Neighborhood Pediatrics to see the Nurse Practitioner for his 6-month well-baby check. On this visit, he weighs 7.4 kg (37th percentile), his head circumference is 44 cm (50th percentile), and his length is 67 cm (40th percentile). He gets immunizations during this visit (DTaP, Hib). He cries when the injection is given in his leg.

NURSE CHARACTERS

NEIGHBORHOOD HOSPITAL

NEIGHBORHOOD HOSPITAL NURSES OVERVIEW

Character	Season 1	Season 2	Season 3
KATE SWANSON	Kate is a newly graduated nurse working on the medical-surgical unit. Due to increased patient loads, Kate ends up staying late after her shifts to finish patient charting. She also agrees to pick up extra shifts to help out with the staffing situation. Kate becomes extremely fatigued and overwhelmed at times.	Kate receives good feedback from her nurse manager, Pat. Her confidence continues to build as a nurse, yet she is still exhausted at the end of the day from working so much. Kate has problems with another nurse and suspects substance abuse.[en]Kate also has problems within her relationship with her fiancé.	An accused rapist and murderer is one of Kate's patients, and Kate finds it very difficult to care for him. The nurse's union goes on strike, leaving Kate to work many extra shifts. She continues to have problems in her relationship and decide to call off the wedding.
PATRICK RICHMAN	Pat is the nurse manger on the medical-surgical unit at Neighborhood Hospital. Morale is low, and Pat's staff is unhappy and overworked. Positions are available, yet nurses are not applying. He constantly worries about work and his staff's ability to provide safe, effective care to their patients. Pat receives a complaint from a patient about one of his nurses.	The staffing situation has gotten worse. Due to the Neighborhood forest fire, more hospital beds are needed, and mandatory overtime has been implemented in the hospital. One of his nurses has been found to be working under the influence of drugs.	Pat is under a lot of stress with the staffing shortage and is working 70 hours a week. The strike ends, and Pat hires two new nurses.
BOBBY SCHOFIELD	Bobby is frustrated with the staffing problems on the unit. He also becomes fed up with his coworkers and gets into an argument with one nurse when comments are made about the way he cares for his patients. To relieve his stress and unwind, Bobby drinks beer, gets stoned, and parties with friends. One day, he shows up to work drunk and stoned; no one seems to notice, and Bobby takes great pleasure in knowing that he was not caught.	Bobby begins to regularly take narcotics from work. Bobby's co workers begin to notice his constant mood swings and report his questionable behavior to Pat. Finally, Bobby is asked to provide a urine sample for drug screening, tests positive, and is reported to the Board of Nursing. He must go through the Diversion Program to keep his nursing license.	Bobby does not believe he has a substance abuse problem, but pretends to go along with the Diversion Program in order to keep his job. Eventually Bobby's license is suspended. He finally realizes the need for help and makes a serious effort. He knows he has a long recovery ahead of him, but feels truly committed this time.

CONCEPTS   *Advocacy, Ethics, Leadership, Organizations, Professionalism, Professional Organizations Self-management, Substance Abuse.*

KATE SWANSON
Season 1

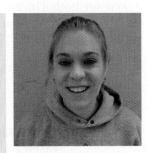

Biographical Information

Kate Swanson is a 23-year-old nurse from a small, rural community. Kate graduated from nursing school a few months ago and took a job working on a general medical-surgical inpatient unit at Neighborhood Hospital. At some point, her goal is to work in an adult Intensive Care Unit. She recently received a sign-on bonus and looks forward to buying her first new car. Kate lives alone in an apartment. To keep healthy, Kate has always watched what she eats and has maintained a regular workout routine. She has been dating Cruz Romero for 2 months.

Episode 1

Kate has a busy week. Because of increased patient admissions, she has seven to eight patients of her own. She has trouble managing her charting with all of the patient care she must do and ends up staying up to 2 hours after each shift to get it done. Kate's manager Pat talks with her about this problem and reviews the importance of point-of-care charting. The feedback he gives her is generally positive. He also asks Kate if she is available to cover extra shifts. Kate agrees to take a night shift next week and also volunteers at the immunization clinic. **[P]**

Episode 2

No news this week.

Episode 3

Kate covers an extra shift again this week. She and her boyfriend Cruz participate in the "Run for Fish" event in the community. She has not been exercising as regularly as she used to, because she can't seem to find the time to go to the gym. She has started to gain a little weight and is feeling self-conscious. The run is a fun opportunity to be active again. **[P]**

Episode 4

No news this week.

Episode 5

No news this week.

Episode 6

Kate stays to cover part of a second shift and is at the hospital for 17 hours. She is exhausted and must return the following morning at 7 a.m. She feels fatigued and a little overwhelmed, and gets very irritated with her coworker, Bobby, who always seems to have time to take long breaks. **[P]**

Episode 7

No news this week.

Episode 8

Kate is feeling more comfortable and assertive at work. She decides to say something to Bobby when she notices that his call lights are frequently on when he is in the break room. **[VC]**

Episode 9

Kate reads about increased drug use in the paper and finds herself feeling angry with alcohol- and drug-abusing patients. She thinks that they have brought many of their problems on themselves.

Episode 10

One of Kate's patients this week is Mrs. Ocampo, an elderly woman who was admitted to the unit following surgery for a hip fracture. She has Alzheimer disease and is extremely confused. She pulls out her IV, yells frequently, and speaks in a language that Kate can't understand. Mrs. Ocampo needs to be restrained, which only upsets her more. She only seems to be calm when her husband is present. Kate takes a special interest in Mrs. Ocampo and works hard to provide exceptional care to her.

Episode 11

Mrs. Ocampo is still on the unit this week. She has calmed down, but is still combative at times. Kate has formed a rapport with her husband, Dr. Ocampo. She feels proud of the care she's been able to give Mrs. Ocampo and finds other nurses' comments and complaints inappropriate. Bobby, another nurse on the unit, is particularly rude. Kate feels indignant and resolves to take even better care of Mrs. Ocampo. She volunteers at the Senior Center to give flu shots and also buys her first new car this week.

Episode 12

No news this week.

Episode 13

Kate is glad to see that Mrs. Ocampo has finally gotten well enough to be transferred to the rehabilitation hospital. Kate can see the toll this hospitalization has taken on both Dr. and Mrs. Ocampo and hopes that Mrs. Ocampo can go home soon.

Episode 14
No news this week.

Episode 15
Kate and her boyfriend Cruz go out for a romantic dinner. Cruz proposes to her, and Kate is thrilled. She can't help wondering, though, how she is going to find the time to plan a wedding with all of the extra hours she has been working. **[P]**

KATE SWANSON
Season 2

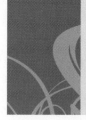

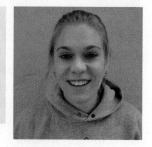

Biographical Information
Kate Swanson is a 24-year-old nurse from a small, rural community. Kate graduated from nursing school last year and has been working on a general medical-surgical inpatient unit at Neighborhood Hospital since that time. At some point, her goal is to work in an adult Intensive Care Unit. Kate lives alone in an apartment. She and her boyfriend Cruz recently got engaged.

Episode 1
Kate continues to receive positive feedback from her unit manager, Pat Richman, and continues to gain confidence as a nurse. She still plans to eventually become an intensive care nurse and wants to start getting experience with more complex patients. She and Pat agree that she will start cross-training for the sub-acute unit. **[P]**

Episode 2
No news this week.

Episode 3
It is another long week at the hospital. Kate takes a night shift and has to work with Bobby. She hasn't gotten along with him since he was rude to Mrs. Ocampo, and she doesn't like working with him. He's competent, but patients often complain about him. She wishes her manager Pat would do something about Bobby, but because of the nursing shortages, even Bobby is better than having no nursing coverage.

Kate is a volunteer organizer for the "Walk for Life" fundraiser. She spends all of her free time this week on final preparations and then the whole weekend at the event. She is so fatigued by Sunday evening that she cancels plans with her fiancé Cruz and spends the evening at home watching TV. **[P]**

Episode 4
This is the second time Kate has picked up a night shift when she takes care of patients that Bobby had during the day shift. On both occasions, her patients complain that they have had a bad day due to poor pain control. Kate looks at the Medication Administration Record and Narcotic Records and sees that Bobby has been giving appropriate pain medications to the patients. Kate can't quite understand this situation, because when she gives pain medications to her patients, they report adequate pain control. **[VC]**

Episode 5
The unit is full of patients with emphysema and asthma because of the Neighborhood forest fire. The emergency department keeps calling for beds, but none are available, so there is pressure to get patients discharged. Kate is kept very busy admitting new patients as soon as others are discharged or transferred to other units. The entire staff is stressed, and morale is low on the unit.

Episode 6
At the monthly staff meeting, a new mandatory overtime policy is announced. This angers most of the nurses, and even Kate feels demoralized. She doesn't know how she can possibly work more than she already does, but she feels uncomfortable with all the complaining. She's nervous about the antagonism on the unit and trusts that administration will find a good solution. She resolves not to get involved in the issue and is determined to just focus on taking care of her patients.

Kate and Cruz haven't been able to spend enough time together lately. It seems like they never go out anymore, but just end up watching movies and falling asleep on the couch. **[P]**

Episode 7
No news this week.

Episode 8
No news this week.

Episode 9
No news this week.

Episode 10
Kate cries when she reads about Dr. Ocampo's death in the Neighborhood Newspaper. She found him to be such a caring man and wonders what will become of his wife Lydia.

Kate and Cruz decide they need to make more time for each other. They go out for dinner and dancing and have a wonderful evening together. Kate decides to focus on wedding plans instead of problems at work.

Episode 11
Kate just can't shake the feeling that something is going on with Bobby. He moves slowly, is tired all of the time, and seems to be spending a lot of time in the medication room. She worries that Bobby may be using drugs or alcohol and schedules an appointment with her unit manager, Pat Richman, to discuss her concerns. **[P]**

Episode 12
Kate takes an extra night shift this week. When she leaves the hospital in the morning, she discovers that someone hit her brand-new car. She breaks down crying at the sight of it. Everything has been so overwhelming and tense lately. She just can't handle one more thing and knows the repairs to her car will be expensive. To make matters worse, Kate and Cruz get into an argument about wedding plans. She wants a big wedding and wants it to be perfect; he doesn't want to go into debt. Kate feels like everything is falling apart. She wants the wedding to be romantic and special. Life has been so stressful lately that she feels like she deserves one perfect day. **[P]**

Episode 13
No news this week.

Episode 14
Kate is shocked when she observes Bobby in report at the beginning of the shift. She decides he is really wasted and calls Pat Richmond, her nurse manager, to share her concerns. She later learns that Bobby tested positive for drug use. She is disappointed, but not really surprised. Because she is the one who made the phone call to Pat about his condition, Kate wonders how the other nurses on the unit perceive her.

Episode 15
Kate's good friends, Nicole and Ramon, get married. The wedding is beautiful, but Kate and Cruz get into an argument at the reception. Things are tense and distant between them. Recently they have had many arguments over little things.

KATE SWANSON
Season 3

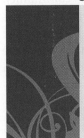

Biographical Information
Kate Swanson continues to work on a general medical-surgical unit at Neighborhood Hospital, but occasionally works on the sub-acute unit as well. Tension is high among the nursing staff due to nursing shortages and mandatory overtime. Kate does not mind an occasional extra shift, but not only does this occur often, but it is expected. Kate is trying to remain positive at work, however, she finds work and the stress associated with planning a wedding very stressful.

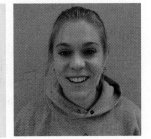

Episode 1
No news this week.

Episode 2
No news this week.

Episode 3
Kate learns that Alvin Cromwell, the man who raped and murdered a local 6-year-old girl, is in the hospital and on her unit. She overhears her colleagues talking about withholding his pain medication and joking about his code status. Kate initially feels strongly about caring for each patient with equal care and feels her coworkers are behaving inappropriately. However, later in the week, Kate overhears Mr. Cromwell make vicious comments about the murdered child while she administers his medications. Kate is so furious that she almost

loses control. She is disgusted with this man. He does not deserve the care he has been receiving! She never considered herself to be the kind of person who would allow her emotional reactions to influence the quality of her care

Episode 4

Kate is assigned to take care of the accused rapist and murderer, Alvin Cromwell, again and does her best to remain impassive. However, she does not take his reports of pain seriously and ignores his call light. Kate has always prided herself on caring for people equally, but finds it is difficult to do so this week. She works an extra shift and, by the end of the week, is completely drained. **[VC]**

Episode 5

The nurse's union is threatening to strike, and Kate doesn't know what to think. Many of her friends have encouraged her to join the union to be protected, but Kate has never believed that professional nurses should join a union.

Episode 6

No news this week.

Episode 7

No news this week.

Episode 8

Kate and Cruz are supposed to go out of town together this week, but they cancel their plans after a blow-up over the guest list for the wedding. Kate agrees to work extra shifts because of the strike and also to keep her mind off of her problems with Cruz.

Episode 9

Kate continues to work several extra shifts this week because of the nursing strike. She is so busy that she would even be happy to see Bobby. She disagrees with the union and cannot imagine abandoning patients. At the same time, it is difficult to walk past many of her striking coworkers when she goes to work. She never imagined that her job would be like this.

Episode 10

Kate is relieved when the strike ends this week. Pat Richman, the unit manager, asks Kate to consider applying for a charge nurse position on the unit. Kate tells Pat that she'll think about it. **[VC]**

Episode 11

While shopping for a wedding dress this week, Kate realizes that she isn't ready to get married and needs to reevaluate her life. She and Cruz have dinner that night, and both agree that they rushed into their engagement. They mutually decide to call off the wedding plans, and Kate is hugely relieved by this decision. They agree to keep in touch, but to take a break from the relationship.

Episode 12

No news this week.

Episode 13

Kate joins a gym this week and takes an aerobics class. She feels renewed and rejuvenated, and realizes how poorly she's taken care of herself lately. She resolves to join a book club and take a vacation. She searches the Internet for cruise specials. **[P]**

Episode 14

No news this week.

Episode 15

Kate learns of an opening in an adult intensive care unit (ICU) at another hospital in a nearby community. Although she eventually wants to work in an ICU, she is committed to Neighborhood Hospital and her peers. She accepts the charge nurse position on her unit. Despite the ups and downs of this past year, she realizes how much she has grown professionally and looks forward to beginning this challenging new position.

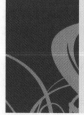

PATRICK RICHMAN
Season 1

Biographical Information

Patrick Richman is a 47-year-old nurse manager who works on the general medical-surgical unit at Neighborhood Hospital. He has been a nurse for over 20 years and has been the unit manager for the past 8 years. Pat considers himself to be a laid-back person and feels he has a good rapport with his staff. He is married and has two sons. He serves as an Assistant Scoutmaster for his son's Boy Scout troop.

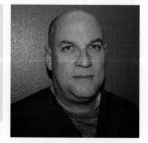

Episode 1

Although Pat has been a successful nurse manager for years, lately he has been feeling like he isn't doing a good job. The staff is overworked and unhappy, and overall morale is low. He has tried to solve the problems with the staff, but the bottom line is that the unit needs more employees, but no one is applying for the empty positions.

Episode 2

Pat talks with Bobby, the acting charge nurse on the unit. Bobby informs him that they are short a nursing tech, and that the nursing supervisor won't find them any help. Bobby seems very upset with Pat when he explains that he will do his best to get help from an agency, but he can't promise him anything. **[VC]**

Episode 3

No news this week.

Episode 4

Pat has another stressful week at work. Mandatory in-services for new intravenous pumps must be scheduled, and all nursing staff must be educated by the end of the week. Because the unit-based educator recently quit, Pat ends up doing much of the training himself.

A new boy by the name of Jason Riley joins the Boy Scout troop this week. Pat can immediately see that Jason is a boy who is picked on by his peers. He puts a stop to the teasing during the meeting, and lets the senior Scoutmaster know of the situation.

Episode 5

No news this week.

Episode 6

Pat always takes his two children to the annual Neighborhood Rodeo, but he can't make it this year because he has been working so much overtime. This week, he even had to pick up a shift on the floor because of staff calling in sick. It was the first shift he had worked in 8 months, and it was exhausting. His staff members have also been working far more than they should, with some nurses working five 12-hour shifts a week and others working extra-long shifts. **[P]**

Episode 7

Pat reads about the problems with the Neighborhood Hospital Emergency Department in the paper. The last thing he needs is the hospital getting bad press while he is trying to attract new nurses to his unit.

Pat enjoys a weekend hiking trip with his son's scout troop. He continues to observe Jason Riley's interactions with the other boys in the troop and wonder what kinds of problems he might be experiencing at school. **[P]**

Episode 8

Pat finds himself worried about work constantly. Difficult working conditions and low wages are causing nurses to leave the hospital. He worries about the ability of his nursing staff to provide safe and effective care to the patients.

At the scout meeting this week, Pat observes Jason Riley go into a rage after being scolded by the senior Scoutmaster for his behavior. Pat attempts to talk with the Scoutmaster about his perceptions regarding Jason and ways to redirect the boy's behavior positively, but the frustrated Scoutmaster simply says, "We are not babysitters, and I don't need troublemakers in this troop."

Episode 9

No news this week.

Episode 10

Pat has received a complaint about Bobby, filed by Dr. Ocampo, the husband of a patient. Dr. Ocampo states that Bobby was rude and was not taking care of his wife properly. Pat knows he needs to address the issue, but will not have time this week. **[P]**

Episode 11

No news this week.

Episode 12

No news this week.

Episode 13

Pat attends a meeting for nurse managers. The managers are informed that the hospital administration is implementing mandatory overtime for nurses in the near future. Pat is told not to say anything to his staff.

Pat missed the Boy Scout meeting last week, but was disappointed to learn that Jason Riley had been kicked out of the troop by the Scoutmaster. He realizes Jason has problems, but wishes he could have had a positive experience in the troop.

Episode 14

No news this week.

Episode 15

Pat reads about the plans for a new cancer treatment facility that will be built at the hospital. He wonders where the administrators plan to get nursing staff for the facility and worries that it will attract nurses away from his unit. He agrees that the new facility is a good idea, but does not think administration is reality-based in their decision. **[P]**

PATRICK RICHMAN
Season 2

Biographical Information

Patrick Richman has been a nurse manager on the general medical-surgical floor at Neighborhood Hospital for about 8 years. Pat considers himself to be a pretty laid-back person and feels that he has a good rapport with his staff. Lately, he has been very concerned about nursing shortages on his unit. Pat has a wife and two sons, and serves as an Assistant Scoutmaster for his son's Boy Scout troop.

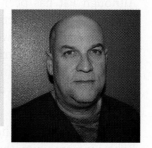

Episode 1

Pat meets with Kate Swanson, whom he considers an ideal employee. She has been doing a great job, and Pat reluctantly agrees to her request to start cross-training for the sub-acute care unit. Although Pat wants to allow Kate other opportunities, he does not want her to leave his unit. He decides to start the cross-training slowly so that he doesn't lose her anytime soon.

Episode 2

The unit is going to be short on staff again. Pat is relieved when Bobby agrees to pick up extra night shifts.

Episode 3

No news this week.

Episode 4

No news this week.

Episode 5

The Neighborhood forest fire has made the entire hospital crazy. There are far more patients needing hospital beds than are available, and the nurses in the emergency department keep calling to the unit, demanding that they make beds available.

Pat becomes really angry when he attends an administrative meeting in which the managers are informed that mandatory overtime will be instituted at the hospital beginning the next pay period. He can't believe how bad their timing is.

Episode 6

Pat holds a staff meeting that he has been dreading the whole week. He announces mandatory overtime to the staff and can feel the tension in the room. He has brought muffins and coffee to try to improve the staff's mood, but can see that this clearly has not helped. The person he thought would be most negative about the news was Bobby, but Pat is surprised that Bobby says little during the meeting. **[P]**

Episode 7

No news this week.

Episode 8

No news this week.

Episode 9

No news this week.

Episode 10

No news this week.

Episode 11

Pat is surprised when Kate makes an appointment with him to talk about Bobby. Kate tells Pat that she suspects Bobby may be working under the influence of drugs. Although Pat has never seen Bobby as a model employee, he certainly never suspected anything like this. **[P]**

Episode 12

Pat has decided to keep a close eye on Bobby without letting anyone know. He spends more time on the unit when Bobby is working. Additionally, Pat interviews some of Bobby's patients to learn about their perceptions of his care. **[P]**

Episode 13

Pat continues watching Bobby. He has not actually caught Bobby doing anything wrong, yet he strongly suspects he is taking narcotics. Pat knows what he must do, but is feeling overwhelmed with all that has been going on lately. Pat contacts his supervisor, the area director, to make sure he handles this situation appropriately. **[VC]**

Episode 14

Pat receives a phone call from Kate Swanson at 7 a.m., informing him that she thinks Bobby is "messed up." After observing Bobby for a few minutes, Pat relieves him of his duties and orders Bobby to submit a urine sample for a drug screening. Pat is extremely disappointed, but not surprised, when he is notified that Bobby tests positive for several types of drugs. In addition to having to deal with this, Pat is now down yet another nurse. **[P]**

Episode 15

Pat learns that Bobby has decided to enter the Diversion Program. He is hopeful that Bobby will be successful and will be able to return to his unit.

PATRICK RICHMAN
Season 3

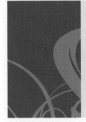

Biographical Information
Patrick Richman has been a nurse manager on the general medical-surgical floor at Neighborhood Hospital for about 9 years. Pat considers himself to be a pretty laid-back person, but the past several months have been very stressful. He has seen a lot of changes at the hospital in the past 5 years, but has a feeling that bigger changes are still to come.

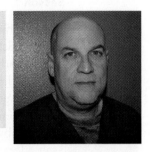

Episode 1
No news this week.

Episode 2
Pat has a meeting with Bobby about his treatment plan. Bobby tells him that the meetings are going well, and he thinks he will be back to work soon.

Episode 3
Pat feels like he just can't get a break. In addition to the nursing shortage and the situation with Bobby, now a disgusting pervert who raped and killed a 6-year-old child has been admitted to his unit. He starts to wonder if life really needs to be this stressful and resolves to think about looking for a new position with less responsibility. He laughs to himself when he thinks about what a position at the new cancer treatment facility would be like.

Episode 4
Although he knows he will have to deal with it, Pat can't believe that the accused rapist would have the nerve to complain about the care he has received from nurses on his unit. Does he expect to be treated like royalty? As far as Pat is concerned, any pain and suffering that he has experienced serves him right. It is only a fraction of the pain that the little girl's family must be feeling.

Episode 5
Just when Pat thought things couldn't get any worse, they have. Bobby's drug test was positive again, and he will probably lose his nursing license. In addition, the nurse's union is threatening to strike. Although he can't say that he blames them, he has no idea what this is going to mean for him and his unit.

Episode 6
No news this week.

Episode 7
Pat has not heard anything further about the strike. He figures no news is good news. Unfortunately, he has heard news about Bobby. His license has been suspended, and there is nothing Pat can do about it. He has been so nervous lately that he has been getting headaches. **[P]**

Episode 8
This week, the nurses at Neighborhood Hospital stage a walk-out. Pat had to work on the unit again and call in anyone off duty who was willing to come in. He cannot believe that the nurses would neglect the patients and is disappointed by their lack of commitment. **[P]**

Episode 9
The nursing strike continues, and Pat finds himself working 70-hour weeks. He finds it stressful crossing the picket lines with some nurses, whom he considered friends, taunting him.

Episode 10
Pat is relieved that the nursing strike is over and that he has more staff available to cover shifts. Pat has four interviews lined up for nursing positions on his unit. The hospital has offered a sign-on bonus, which has attracted nurses from nearby communities. **[P]**

Episode 11
No news this week.

Episode 12
No news this week.

Episode 13
Pat is pleased with the applicants he has interviewed during the past few weeks. He decides to hire a new graduate nurse and a nurse with many years of experience.

Episode 14
No news this week.

Episode 15
Pat is happy when Kate Swanson accepts the charge nurse position on his unit. Because of her high standards and enthusiasm for nursing, he knows she is just the right person for the position.

Pat is pleasantly surprised when he hears that Bobby has been attending AA meetings regularly and seems to be turning his life around. Pat is also relieved that things finally seem to be turning around at work.

BOBBY SCHOFIELD
Season 1

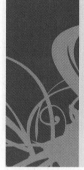

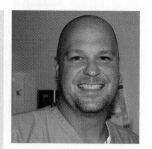

Biographical Information

Bobby Schofield is a 32-year-old staff nurse on the medical-surgical unit at Neighborhood Hospital. Bobby has been a nurse for 5 years. He got into nursing because he thought it would be an easy, flexible, and exciting career with job security and good money. Overall, he likes his job, but lately he has gotten bored. He applied for a position with the flight nurse team, but was not offered the position.

    Bobby is single and, although he has a few close friends, he considers himself a loner. He has never had a close relationship with his family. Although he dates, he is not in a serious relationship. He loves to party and have a good time.

Episode 1

No news this week.

Episode 2

Bobby is the acting charge nurse on the unit this week. On one of the days, he becomes frustrated when a nursing tech calls in sick. Because the unit is full, he contacts the nursing supervisor on call and asks if she can send a tech to the floor to cover the shift. The supervisor tells Bobby he will have to "do without," at least until noon. Bobby also talks with his nurse manager, Pat, who isn't any more helpful than the supervisor.

    After a long, 4-day stretch at the hospital, Bobby is glad to have some time off. He spends his days off partying with friends. **[P]**

Episode 3

This week, Bobby gets into an argument with another nurse on the unit who made a sarcastic comment about his "caring way with patients." Bobby is fed up with all of the pathetic nurses on his unit. Who are they to tell him how to do his job? After work, he really feels a need to unwind. He picks up a six-pack on the way home from work, kicks back in front of the TV, drinks beer, and gets stoned. **[P]**

Episode 4

No news this week.

Episode 5

No news this week.

Episode 6

Bobby partied most nights this week. On one night, he got really wasted. He was out until 4 a.m. and had just enough time to go home, take a nap, and get a shower before getting to work at 7 a.m. He has never gone to work stoned or drunk before and was nervous that someone would notice. Fortunately, the unit was short staffed, and the charge nurse did not seem to notice. Bobby felt a certain pleasure in getting away with it. **[P]**

Episode 7

No news this week.

Episode 8

Bobby has worked several shifts this week. He feels irritable and unfocused at work. All of the whiny patients get on his nerves. He can't stand all of the stupid requests they make constantly, as if he is their personal servant. He is also very annoyed with a new nurse, Kate, who bothers him when he's on his breaks to tell him that his patients need him and a nurse aid who wants help lifting a patient. He wishes they would all just get off his case. **[VC]**

Episode 9

Bobby reads in the paper about the possibility of companies banning smoking breaks. He feels like smoking is the only thing that keeps him sane at work. If Neighborhood Hospital administrators take breaks away, that would be the last straw!

Episode 10

Mrs. Ocampo is one of Bobby's patients this week. She is confused and disruptive, and he finds her behavior to be incredibly frustrating. Bobby initiates the paperwork to get her restrained because she attempts to pull out her tubes. He also obtains an order for lorazepam (Ativan) to settle her down. Her husband is demanding and rude, and keeps interfering. Bobby is completely fed up with both of them. They just don't get it.

Episode 11

Mrs. Ocampo is still on the unit, and she really annoys Bobby. He gives her lorazepam (Ativan) to quiet her down whenever she gets too agitated.

Episode 12

Bobby attends a meeting with the hospital discharge coordinator and Dr. Ocampo. Dr. Ocampo has this idea that he should take his wife home. Bobby can't understand how Dr. Ocampo is unable to see what a bad decision this is. Frankly, he hopes she will be transferred soon.

Episode 13
Bobby has grown very tired of dealing with Dr. Ocampo. He is always asking Bobby questions, which annoys him. Bobby wishes Dr. Ocampo would just stay home once in a while. He is glad when he hears that Mrs. Ocampo is being transferred to the rehabilitation unit.

Episode 14
One of Bobby's post-operative patients, Pamela Allen, was just diagnosed with colon cancer. When her family is not around, she cries all the time. Bobby can hardly stand to go into her room. He is completely fed up with all of his needy patients. **[P]**

Episode 15
No news this week.

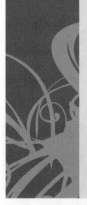

BOBBY SCHOFIELD
Season 2

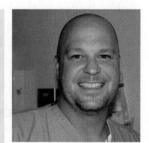

Biographical Information
Bobby Schofield is a 32-year-old staff nurse on the medical-surgical unit at Neighborhood Hospital. Bobby has been a nurse for 5 years. He got into nursing because he thought it would be an easy, flexible, and exciting career with job security and good money. Overall, he likes his job, but lately he has gotten bored.

Although he has a few close friends, Bobby considers himself a loner. He has never had a close relationship with his family. He has always been smart and fiercely independent. Although he dates, he is not in a serious relationship. He loves to party and have a good time. Bobby's recreational drug use has progressively increased, but he thinks he can handle it. He often feels restless and dissatisfied.

Episode 1
No news this week.

Episode 2
Bobby agrees to work a night shift this week. During the shift, he keeps the morphine from a discontinued PCA vial instead of wasting it. When he gets home, he injects the morphine into his vein and finds that it is a great high. It relieves all of his tension and anxiety—and it was remarkably easy to get. **[P]**

Episode 3
No news this week.

Episode 4
Bobby begins to regularly take narcotics from work. He usually takes a portion of the dose of a patient's pain medication. He looks forward to going home, using the drugs, and relaxing. Bobby experiments with a wide variety of drugs, but discovers that he enjoys morphine the most.

Episode 5
No news this week.

Episode 6
Bobby attends a staff meeting where Pat Richman, the unit manager, announces the new mandatory overtime policy. All of the nurses are angry and discouraged. In some ways, Bobby is annoyed with the administration's demands, but he also sees it as an opportunity. After all, he only has access to morphine when he is at work. He volunteers for a couple of extra night shifts, because it's easier to take narcotics on night shifts with fewer people working and less supervision. **[P]**

Episode 7
No news this week.

Episode 8
Bobby becomes increasingly creative in finding ways to steal morphine without getting caught. He removes morphine from pre-filled syringes and replaces it with saline, draws narcotics directly out of IV lines, volunteers to go to the pharmacy, and always makes himself available for narcotic count. Bobby no longer waits to go home before injecting—he sometimes does it on his breaks. He feels smarter than everyone else; the people he works with are so busy and dumb that they don't even notice. **[P]**

Episode 9
No news this week.

Episode 10
No news this week.

Episode 11

Bobby has been feeling particularly edgy and unfocused at work lately, and avoids conversations with coworkers. He is unaware that some of his coworkers are beginning to notice his evasiveness and mood swings.

Episode 12

Bobby's narcotic use continues to escalate; he rarely works a shift now without using a narcotic at least once. He finds he physically feels better when he uses the drugs and is sure nobody notices.

Episode 13

Bobby begins to think about stopping narcotic use—at least at work. Although he thinks of quitting, he feels very anxious and depressed. He decides he is okay for now, but vows to quit soon. **[P]**

Episode 14

Bobby reports to work one day this week stoned. He is looking forward to beginning his shift so he can get a narcotic fix. Bobby is surprised when, out of nowhere, Pat Richman (the unit manager) approaches him, relieves him of his patient care assignment, and tells him he needs to give a urine sample for a drug screening. Bobby knows he will test positive and wonders which of the nurses has been watching him.

Bobby is reported to the Board of Nursing, and he is offered a chance to keep his license if he goes through the Diversion Program. Bobby does not perceive the need to do this, but sees that this is the path of least resistance and agrees to attend the program. **[P]**

Episode 15

Bobby begins the Diversion Program this week.

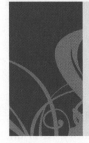

BOBBY SCHOFIELD
Season 3

Biographical Information

Bobby Schofield is a 33-year-old nurse who has recently entered the Diversion Program for substance abuse. He must agree and adhere to a 5-year contract that includes abstinence, treatment, frequent meetings with a supervisor, and drug testing to make sure he has not relapsed. If he follows through with the contract, he will be able to keep his nursing license, his treatment will remain completely confidential, and he will never be reported to the Board of Nursing.

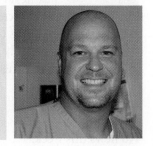

Episode 1

Bobby hates the Diversion Program. He is supposed to admit that he has a substance abuse problem, which he doesn't truly believe. He resents all of the supervision and thinks the Alcoholics Anonymous (AA) and Narcotics Anonymous (NA) meetings are idiotic. **[VC]**

Episode 2

Bobby meets with his nurse manager, Pat Richman, to discuss his treatment plan. Bobby knows he has to pretend to go along with the Diversion Program to keep his job, but he still believes he has everything under control. He thinks abstinence is a joke and that he could probably get away with some very limited use. **[P]**

Episode 3

No news this week.

Episode 4

Bobby tests positive for opiates again. He quits the Diversion Program because he thinks it doesn't do anything for him.

Episode 5

Bobby receives a letter from the Board of Nursing (BON), offering him another opportunity to go through the Diversion Program. If he declines, he must attend a disciplinary hearing. Bobby is sure he will convince the stupid people at the BON that he has stopped using drugs and to let him keep his license. He elects to attend the hearing.

Episode 6

No news this week.

Episode 7

Bobby has his disciplinary hearing this week before the Board of Nursing (BON). His license is suspended. Bobby is in a state of disbelief. He asks the BON members what options he now has. He is told that, if he wants to try the Diversion Program again, and if he shows some real recovery, he may be able to get his license reinstated after 2 years.

Bobby feels shocked by the decision. He wonders how he will be able to make his house and car payments.

He is furious and goes to a bar and drinks there until it closes. He wakes up in a stranger's house, doesn't know where his car is, and has to walk home. Bobby feels depressed and realizes he needs to get his act together. **[P]**

Episode 8
No news this week.

Episode 9
The Board of Nursing hearing was a real wake-up call. Bobby continues to feel depressed and is concerned about making his house and car payments. He goes to an Alcoholics Anonymous (AA) meeting, where he meets an older gentleman named Jim. Bobby immediately likes him and learns that Jim has been in the program for 30 years. Jim takes Bobby out for coffee after the meeting, and they end up talking for three hours.

Episode 10
Bobby goes to the AA meetings three nights this week. His new friend, Jim, tells him that anytime he feels he wants a drink or needs to smoke, he should call him. Bobby calls Jim frequently for support because he finds that Jim understands what he is going through.

Episode 11
No news this week.

Episode 12
No news this week.

Episode 13
Bobby contacts the Board of Nursing and asks to have another chance with the Diversion Program. He agrees to a new contract and feels committed this time. He knows it is his only chance at getting his nursing career back.

Episode 14
No news this week.

Episode 15
Bobby attends meetings regularly and is working closely with his Diversion Program supervisor. He knows he has a long road ahead; every day is a struggle, but he feels a sense of hope. **[VC]**

NEIGHBORHOOD SENIOR CENTER NURSING CLINIC

NEIGHBORHOOD SENIOR CENTER OVERVIEW

Character	Season 1	Season 2	Season 3
KAREN WILLIAMS	Karen works at the Senior Center Nursing Clinic and interacts with a variety of older adults who visit there. She becomes acquainted with Mrs. James during this season. Karen attempts to educate Mrs. James about her medications and how to manager diabetes, but she seems disinterested. Suspecting elder abuse involving Mr. Alden, Karen contacts a social worker from Adult Protective Services to evaluate Mr. Alden's situation at home.	The number of seniors coming to the center is increasing, and Karen feels overwhelmed. Karen learns that Mrs. James has had a stroke and visits her in the hospital, encouraging her to get better. Mary Martin visits with Karen at the center and voices her concerns about having cataract surgery. Karen reassures her that she will have great improvement in her vision.	Karen does a presentation on medication management. Because the Senior Center Nursing Clinic is very busy, Karen writes a letter to the City Council requesting an increase in funding. Mrs. James is now at home recovering from her stroke. She comes to the center to visit with Karen and allows her to check her blood pressure and glucose level.

CONCEPTS   *Advocate, Boundaries, Communication, Cultural Competence, Domestic Violence, Educator, Ethics, Policy, Professional role, Role model, Transitional Care*

KAREN WILLIAMS
Season 1

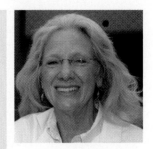

Biographical Information

Karen Williams is 57 years old. She has been a geriatric nurse for 30 years and has worked at the nursing clinic at the Neighborhood Senior Center for five years. Karen's position is supported by funds from the city budget. In addition to providing health screenings and information to seniors, Karen also supervises nursing students who come to the center for their clinical experience. She has noticed an increase in the number of visitors to the center during the past few years, which she attributes to a lack of extracurricular activities available for seniors in the community. Karen knows most of the individuals who regularly come to the center on a first-name basis. They often come to her with their questions and concerns. One thing that Karen enjoys about geriatric nursing is that the seniors are eager to talk, and most of them are very appreciative of her help. Karen is a widow; her husband died suddenly two years ago of heart disease. She finds working at the clinic rewarding, and it provides an opportunity for regular and interesting interactions.

Episode 1

George Murphy shares with Karen that his son and daughter are trying to force him to sell his home and move into an assisted living facility. It makes him angry to think of leaving the house where he and his wife lived for 20 years, but he admits that he can't take care of the house anymore. Karen encourages George to talk with his children about how he feels. When asked if he has visited the assisted living facility, he tells Karen that he refuses to go. She encourages him to consider making a visit just to see what it is like.

Betty, a woman who comes to the Senior Center Nursing Clinic regularly, overhears the conversation George is having with Karen. Trying to be helpful, she suggests that George come to live with her. **[P]**

Episode 2
No news this week.

Episode 3
Karen sees Mrs. James, a newcomer to the Senior Center Nursing Clinic. She has an infected ulcer on her leg that needs treatment. Karen helps her make an appointment with her primary care provider and arranges transportation through the Senior Center.

Episode 4
Mr. and Mrs. Simmons, who have been coming to the Senior Center Nursing Clinic for many months, stop in to ask Karen to check Mr. Simmons' blood pressure. Mrs. Simmons explains to Karen that her husband's blood pressure was elevated at a recent visit to the physician, and he was told that, if it stayed elevated, he would need to take "blood pressure pills." Karen takes his blood pressure as requested and reports to them that it is 128/72 mm Hg. **[P]**

Episode 5
No news this week.

Episode 6
Karen sees Mrs. James again this week at the Senior Center Nursing Clinic. She is proud to show Karen that her leg is healing. Karen attempts to talk with her about her medications and give her information about managing her diabetes, but Mrs. James shows little interest. She encourages Mrs. James to bring a list of the medications she takes on her next visit. Mrs. James is in a hurry to leave so she can get her free lunch.

Episode 7
Karen encourages seniors at the center to attend the upcoming Neighborhood Health Fair. Many of them ask her if they will be giving away any free food or medical supplies at the fair.

Episode 8
No news this week.

Episode 9
Karen helps a group of women from the Neighborhood Senior Center develop a presentation to correspond with Smoking Awareness Week. Their goal is to teach individuals about the hazards of smoking. Karen helps them assemble a plastic "smoking lung" prop from the Lung Cancer Association. Karen helps another woman make a chart of the number of cigarettes her husband smokes per day, per week, and per year, and the cost of all of those cigarettes over a 20-year period. Another group member plans to talk about how she developed asthma from second-hand smoke in her home.

Episode 10
Mrs. James comes into the clinic to see Karen this week. Karen checks her vital signs (blood pressure, 126/92 mm Hg; blood glucose, 124 mg/dL), and asks Mrs. James about her medication list (which she has not brought along with her). When performing an exam on her feet, Karen notices that Mrs. James' shoes are in poor shape. One shoe has been cut down, and the edges are covered with cotton balls and tape. She talks to Mrs. James about the need to wear shoes that fit and suggests that she check at the Senior Center for help obtaining properly fitting shoes. Karen also notes that the wound on her leg has nearly completely healed.

Mrs. James starts to talk about her frustrations with her doctors and all of her appointments, and Karen listens quietly. It seems to her that Mrs. James is quite isolated and does not have many opportunities to talk about her feelings. Karen listens attentively and encourages Mrs. James to call her physicians to inquire about the appointments.

Episode 11
This week, the Neighborhood Senior Center Nursing Clinic is offering flu vaccinations. Karen checks the refrigerator to be sure that adequate vaccines are stocked. As she is preparing for the shot clinic, one of the staff members from the kitchen knocks on the door and asks if her daughter can get a flu shot. Karen encourages her to bring her daughter to the clinic and tells her the cost is $20.

Four nursing students are scheduled to help give flu vaccines at the center. One student admits to Karen that she is nervous about giving vaccinations to some of the ladies because their arms are so thin. Karen reviews the vaccination techniques with the student and reassures her that she will be in the room supervising the entire time. **[P]**

Episode 12
Karen sees Mr. Alden sitting alone with disheveled hair and unclean clothes. She encourages him to have his blood pressure checked. When she asks him to pull up his shirt sleeve, she notices that his arm is purple and appears freshly bruised. He tells her that he thinks he fell down, but when she looks closely at his face, she sees another bruise that is turning yellow. She asks him if he has any other bruises. He reluctantly agrees to show her his abdomen, and it too is very bruised. Karen asks Mr. Alden if he lives with anyone, and he tells her that he lives with his son. When she asks him if he remembers how he got all of the bruises, his reply

is, "I don't know." Based on her observations and his vague answers, Karen contacts a social worker at Neighborhood Adult Protective Services and shares her concerns of elder abuse. The social worker agrees to make a home visit to evaluate Mr. Alden and his home situation. **[P]**

Episode 13
No news this week.

Episode 14
Mary Martin tells Karen that she has been recently diagnosed with osteoporosis and wonders if she will get hurt during the exercise class at the Senior Center. Karen asks if Mary talked about exercising with her doctor; Mary confirms that she saw Dr. Rowe, who said it was fine. Karen explains to Mary that exercising helps to strengthen her bones and can increase her bone density. Karen provides positive encouragement for Mary's participation in the exercise class and tells her that aerobics is an excellent form of weight-bearing exercise.

Episode 15
No news this week.

KAREN WILLIAMS
Season 2

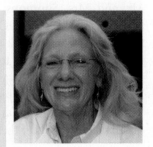

Biographical Information

Karen Williams is 57 years old. She has been a geriatric nurse for 30 years and has worked at the nursing clinic at the Neighborhood Senior Center for five years. Karen's position is supported by funds from the city budget. In addition to providing health screenings and information to seniors, Karen also supervises nursing students who come to the center for their clinical experience. She has noticed an increase in the number of visitors to the center during the past few years, which she attributes to a lack of extracurricular activities available for seniors in the community. Karen knows most of the individuals who regularly come to the center on a first-name basis. They often come to her with their questions and concerns. One thing that Karen enjoys about geriatric nursing is that the seniors are eager to talk, and most of them are very appreciative of her help.

Episode 1
Nursing students are at the Neighborhood Senior Center Nursing Clinic to check blood pressures this week. Karen overhears one of the students agree to give Mrs. Marsh, a 78-year-old woman, a ride home from the center. Karen pulls the student aside and talks with her about the situation, explaining that Mrs. Marsh consistently asks for rides and special favors from the staff. Karen gently points out that the student should not offer to give rides to Mrs. Marsh or any other senior. The student tells Karen that she was overwhelmed and didn't know what to do, so Karen reassures her and tells her that talking and listening to Mrs. Marsh is perfectly fine, but she should not become involved beyond that point. **[P]**

Episode 2
In order to qualify for funding, Karen maintains a log of the number of individuals she sees. By looking through her records, she recognizes that the numbers have defi-

nitely increased, despite the drop in nursing hours. Karen is glad to see that elders in the community use the service, but she is concerned about the time constraints she faces in trying to connect with so many individuals. She also finds that she has limited time for teaching the seniors at the center, which is a part of her job that she enjoys a great deal. **[P]**

Episode 3
The Senior Center Planning Committee organizes a trip to a national park for sightseeing. Karen agrees to go and ensures that the bus has an updated first aid kit. She reminds everyone to bring plenty of water, as well as hats and sunscreen. Most of the seniors attending are fairly healthy, so Karen does not anticipate problems. After arriving at the park, the seniors take a short walk. Mr. Dallion, who has emphysema, returns to the bus short of breath after the walk. Fortunately, he brought his oxygen pack on the bus just in case he needed it. Karen assists Mr. Dallion with the oxygen. On the way

home, she sits with George Raley, who talks to her the entire way home about his stiff knee and shows Karen the scars from his knee replacement surgery.

Episode 4
No news this week.

Episode 5
Karen can see the effects of the forest fire on many of the individuals at the Neighborhood Senior Center Nursing Clinic. Many of the seniors, including Mr. Dallion, have needed to use oxygen more often this week. Mr. Dallion tells Karen that he has had a cough. She advises these individuals to stay indoors to avoid the respiratory irritants. **[P]**

Episode 6
No news this week.

Episode 7
No news this week.

Episode 8
Karen gets a call from Brian James, who tells her that his mother, Norma James, has had a stroke. Karen goes to the hospital to visit her. Mrs. James looks exhausted and complains that the nurses aren't taking good care of her; they make her walk every day and go to "stupid classes." Mrs. James makes it clear that there is no point to any of this. Karen encourages Mrs. James to get better so that she can get home to care for her cats. Mrs. James was unaware that her cats were still alive and being cared for, and now has renewed interest in her own care. **[P]**

Episode 9
No news this week.

Episode 10
Mr. Andrews at Neighborhood Hospital calls to offer Karen a job with excellent pay, which would mean a salary increase of over $20,000 per year. Although Karen is flattered by the offer, she is not surprised, given the well-publicized staffing shortages at the hospital. Karen feels committed to her work with the elders in the Neighborhood community and is really not interested in going back to work in a hospital setting. **[P]**

Episode 11
No news this week.

Episode 12
No news this week.

Episode 13
No news this week.

Episode 14
The Neighborhood Senior Center Nursing Clinic is very busy and crowded this week, and Karen is overwhelmed by the number of individuals who want to see her. She is concerned that a few of the seniors are not being seen by their primary care physicians, because they are reluctant to go. One of the seniors, Betty, complains of ongoing pain throughout her lower abdomen. Karen is concerned when Betty leaves her office without promising that she will see her physician. **[P]**

Episode 15
Mary Martin visits with Karen and talks about needing cataract surgery. She shares with Karen her fears about the surgery—specifically that she heard that she could go blind. Karen tells Mary that cataract surgery is very common, and the risk of blindness is very low. She also tells Mary that many of the seniors have reported great improvements in their vision since having the same surgery. Mary tells Karen that she needs to be able to see well so she can take care of her great-grandson Tyler, going on to say that her daughter-in-law doesn't take good care of him. Karen suggests that Mary talk with some of the other women at the center about their cataract surgery experiences. **[P]**

KAREN WILLIAMS
Season 3

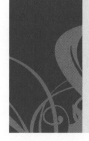

Biographical Information
Karen Williams has been a geriatric nurse for 31 years and has worked at the nursing clinic at the Neighborhood Senior Center for six years. Karen is very committed to her work and believes the center helps to foster healthy community relationships for those individuals who come. As the volume of visitors continues to increase at the center, Karen realizes the need for an additional nurse. She begins to explore funding options to meet this need.

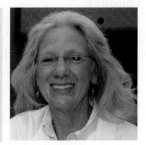

Episode 1

Karen calls Mrs. James at home to see how she is doing and talks with her son, Brian. He shares with Karen that his mother has become very dependent on him, but he will soon need to return home. Karen asks Brian if there are any resources that his mother may need that she could help him to obtain. Brian assures her that he has had plenty of help, and it is now up to his mother to demonstrate her independence. Karen asks Brian to encourage Mrs. James to come back to the Neighborhood Senior Center once she feels up to it. **[P]**

Episode 2

No news this week.

Episode 3

Margaret Herrera, a 64-year-old woman who frequently comes to the Neighborhood Senior Center Nursing Clinic, tells Karen that her doctor prescribed a "water pill" for her a few days ago, but she did not also get a prescription for potassium pills, like her friend Betty Sparks has. Margaret asks Karen if she should go back and demand to receive potassium pills. Karen looks at the prescription bottle and notes that Margaret has been prescribed spironolactone. She reinforces with Margaret the same patient information previously shared by her physician and the pharmacist. **[P]**

Episode 4

No news this week.

Episode 5

Karen does a presentation entitled *Medication Management for the Elderly* this week at the Neighborhood Senior Center. Because it was publicized in the Neighborhood Newspaper, there is a very large turnout. Karen is acutely aware of the challenges that many elderly people face with medication management and adherence. After the presentation, many individuals personally thank Karen for the helpful information, and many of the regulars at the center comment about how pleased they were that "their nurse" was in the newspaper. **[P]**

Episode 6

Karen writes a letter to the City Council requesting an increase in funding for the Senior Center Nursing Clinic, specifically to hire another nurse to assist her during the busiest hours and to extend the hours of service. She also encourages the seniors who regularly visit the center to write letters. **[P]**

Episode 7

Mrs. James pays a visit to the Senior Center clinic and lets Karen check her glucose level and blood pressure. She enjoys talking with Karen about her cats. Mrs. James is visibly annoyed when Mr. Sanchez stands next to them waiting to talk with Karen. Mrs. James gets up and leaves in a bit of a huff. Karen invites Mr. Sanchez to sit down and asks how he is doing. Mr. Sanchez is 80 years old and lives alone. His wife died last year, and he has had a difficult time adjusting to being widowed. He explains that he has been coming to the center less often because transportation has been an issue for him, so Karen talks with him about calling the Senior Ride service. **[P]**

Episode 8

No news this week.

Episode 9

No news this week.

Episode 10

Mrs. James sees Karen at the Senior Center again this week. Although she has become quite a regular participant, she would never admit that she enjoys it. She is visibly annoyed when Karen asks her about her medications and glucose measurements, telling her that everything is fine. Still, she allows Karen to check her blood pressure and glucose. **[P]**

Episode 11

Karen sees Mary Martin this week. Mary explains to Karen how stressful the situation is at her son's home. She describes trying to help care for her grandson Mark, who was recently in an auto accident and left paralyzed. She also describes all of the problems with Anthony and how his mother has driven him away. Karen reminds Mary that she needs to take time for herself to rest, both physically and emotionally. **[P]**

Episode 12

No news this week.

Episode 13

This week, fitness guru Jack Blaine is hosting a free seminar at the Senior Center. In addition to the public seminar, Karen has arranged for Mr. Blaine to meet informally with the seniors during their lunch hour. Karen is pleased with the response Jack receives from the seniors. They are receptive to his suggestions and ask many questions regarding their own fitness routines.

Episode 14

Mrs. James stops in to see Karen early in the week to inform her that she will be leaving to visit her son Brian for a few weeks. Mrs. James explains that she knew Karen would wonder what happened to her, and she didn't want Karen to worry about her absence. Later in the afternoon, Mary Martin stops in for a brief moment to give Karen some flowers to thank her for being so helpful. Although Karen leaves the center feeling tired and sometimes burdened, she feels content. **[P]**

Episode 15

No news this week.

NEIGHBORHOOD WOMEN'S HEALTH SPECIALISTS

NEIGHBORHOOD WOMEN'S HEALTH SPECIALISTS OVERVIEW

Character	Season 1	Season 2	Season 3
CAROL RAMSEY	Carol is a nurse midwife. She loves her career, but because her patient load has recently increased, she is feeling overwhelmed and run down, spending time after hours to finish her work. Carol notices that more teenage girls are coming to the Community Health Clinic seeking birth control. She participates in the community health fair, providing information and promoting sexual health. Carol detects a mass in the abdomen of a patient, which is later diagnosed as cancer. Jessica Riley comes to the clinic for her first prenatal exam.	Carol is sees a variety of patients during this season, including a woman with severe preeclampsia; Terry, a 16-year-old who learns she is pregnant; Kristina Martin, a 15-year-old requesting birth control pills; and Jessica Riley, who is receiving prenatal care. She suspects that Jessica is the victim of domestic abuse. After delivery of her baby, Jessica finally admits to the abusive relationship that she has with Casey, but refuses to press charges. Carol contacts a social worker to follow up on Jessica's case.	Carol's patient load continues to increase, so she is thrilled to hear that another nurse midwife has been hired. Nancy, one of Carol's older pregnant patients, wants her daughter to be present during the birth of her son. Kristina Martin presents to the Community Health Clinic with Chlamydia. Carol gives her a prescription and talks with her about STD prevention. Carol begins to think about opening her own clinic for midwifery and gynecological care.

CONCEPTS   *Advanced Practice, Advocacy, Collaborative Practice, Educator, Ethics, Domestic Violence, Policy, Professionalism, Role model*

CAROL RAMSEY
Season 1

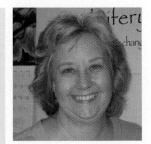

Biographical Information

Carol Ramsey is a 51-year-old certified nurse midwife who works at Neighborhood Women's Health Specialists (NWHS). She has been a midwife for 21 years, after spending the first 8 years of her career as a labor and delivery room nurse. Four physicians and three midwives, including Carol, work at NWHS. In addition to working 4½ days a week at NWHS, Carol works one afternoon each week at the Neighborhood Community Health Department. At NWHS, Carol sees her own patients. The majority of her work involves prenatal, delivery, and postpartum care, although she also provides routine gynecologic care for many of her patients. At the Neighborhood Community Health Department, Carol sees a variety of patients, many of whom are seeking contraception, pregnancy testing, or screening and treatment of sexually transmitted infections.

Episode 1

Carol is not feeling well this week. She has been trying to recover from a mild cold, but it has really zapped her energy. She has a full caseload this week, because one of the midwives in the practice is out on medical leave for the next few months. Carol and the other two midwives at the Neighborhood Women's Health Specialists are working extra patients into their schedule; this is a bit tough, because she feels as if she is already working at full capacity. Carol finds it hard to see extra patients in addition to working at the Community Health Clinic. **[P]**

Episode 2

A new computer upgrade that has been in the works for several months is finally implemented this week. Carol and the other providers feel overwhelmed because of multiple system problems, including the fact that the medical office personnel are unable to transfer the old medical records into the new system. Carol ends up documenting her patient care visits on a yellow legal pad, knowing she will have to spend time after hours getting these data entered into the system later. **[P]**

Episode 3

No news this week.

Episode 4

Carol spends most of her day at Neighborhood Hospital with two of her patients, Donna and Marta, who both happen to be in the labor unit at the same time. Both women presented to the hospital after their membranes spontaneously ruptured, but neither is progressing 12 hours later. Carol attempts to get them to progress through nipple stimulation, walking, and warm baths. Eventually Marta begins to actively progress, and Carol successfully delivers her baby several hours later. The next morning, Carol finds that Donna has still failed to progress, so a Pitocin drip is initiated. After a few more hours without adequate progression, Carol consults with Dr. Tito, the obstetrician. Dr. Tito decides to perform a cesarean section in order to achieve the best outcome for Donna. Donna is devastated, verbalizing that she "failed" to give birth naturally. Carol feels as if she let Donna down. **[P]**

Episode 5

No news this week.

Episode 6

Carol sees an increase in the number of teenage girls who are coming to the Community Health Clinic seeking birth control. She often feels frustrated when she tries to talk with them about safe sex practices and protecting themselves against sexually transmitted infections. Most of the girls are only interested in obtaining birth control pills. **[P]**

Episode 7

Carol participates at the community health fair this week. She is involved with a display promoting sexual health that is sponsored by the Community Health Department. She has information regarding safe sex practices, contraception, and sexual abuse at her table, as well as a container filled with free condoms. Carol notices several middle-aged women pass by the table and give her dirty looks, as if she is promoting evil behavior. By the end of the afternoon, the container is empty. **[P]**

Episode 8

No news this week.

Episode 9

Marcie, a 42-year-old woman, comes into the clinic to be evaluated for pregnancy this week. She is sure that she is pregnant because she has not menstruated for "two or three months," she has gained ten pounds, and she reports fullness in her abdominal area. Marcie has never been seen at the clinic before, and she tells Carol that she moved into the neighborhood about one year ago. A pregnancy test is negative, and a pelvic exam reveals that her ovaries and uterus are normal in size and shape. Carol palpates a mass in her abdomen, just above the ovaries. She also notes that a guaiac test of her stool is positive for occult blood. Carol asks Dr. Tito, one of the gynecologists in the office, to evaluate Marcie, and she agrees with Carol's findings. Marcie is scheduled for a CT scan of the lower abdomen and asked to return to the office the following week. **[P]**

Episode 10

This week, Marcie has a follow-up appointment at the Neighborhood Women's Health Specialists office. Carol is sickened when she reads the radiology report and shares the information with Dr. Tito. The CT scan shows a large mass in the colon that extends into the pelvic area. Although Carol knows a pathology report is necessary to confirm the diagnosis, she feels certain that Marcie has advanced colon cancer. Carol and Dr. Tito talk with Marcie and refer her to a surgeon for follow up. Carol knows she is unlikely to ever see Marcie again, but can't stop thinking about her. **[P]**

Episode 11

No news this week.

Episode 12

17 year-old Jessica Riley comes to the clinic for her first prenatal exam. Carol asks her about previous pregnancies and learns that she already has one son. Carol asks Jessica if she drinks alcohol or smokes; when she finds that Jessica does both, she explains that both are extremely harmful to the developing fetus. She encourages Jessica to try to stop, or at least to cut down drastically on her intake. She conducts an initial prenatal exam. Based on her last menstrual period, size of her uterus, and symptoms, Carol determines that Jessica is about 16 weeks pregnant.

Episode 13
No news this week.

Episode 14
It's been a busy week for Carol. She has delivered eight babies in six days, and has a full schedule all week. She is feeling really worn out. Sometimes a week or two goes by without a delivery, and sometimes all of her patients deliver at the same time. It is never easy to predict what a week will look like. The practice is still down one midwife, and Carol wonders when another person will be hired. She wonders just how long the physicians are going to expect her to carry the additional workload.

Episode 15
No news this week.

CAROL RAMSEY
Season 2

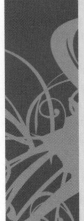

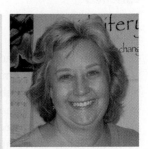

Biographical Information

Carol Ramsey is a 51-year-old certified nurse midwife who works at Neighborhood Women's Health Specialists (NWHS). She has been a midwife for 21 years, after spending the first 8 years of her career as a labor and delivery room nurse. Four physicians and three midwives, including Carol, work at NWHS. In addition to working $4 \frac{1}{2}$ days a week at NWHS, Carol works one afternoon each week at the Neighborhood Community Health Department. At NWHS, Carol sees her own patients. The majority of her work involves prenatal, delivery, and postpartum care, although she also provides routine gynecologic care for many of her patients. At the Neighborhood Community Health Department, Carol sees a variety of patients, many of whom are seeking contraception, pregnancy testing, or screening and treatment of sexually transmitted infections.

Episode 1
Jessica Riley comes to the clinic for her 24-week prenatal visit. Carol asks her how she feels, and Jessica reports that she is less tired than before. Carol asks Jessica if she has given any more thought to quitting smoking and drinking. Jessica says that she has cut back, but her boyfriend Casey gives her a hard time if she doesn't party with him. Carol is beginning to wonder what kind of relationship Jessica has with Casey.

Carol begins teaching another childbirth class this week through Neighborhood Hospital. She donates her time to this effort for community service. **[P]**

Episode 2
No news this week.

Episode 3
Carol sees Sandra, a 28-year-old woman in her 23rd week of pregnancy, this week. Sandra complains of swelling in her hands and face that does not go away, as well as headaches. Carol notes that her blood pressure is 142/96 mm Hg, and her urine protein is 2+. Recognizing the symptoms as preeclampsia, Carol asks Dr. Tito, the obstetrician in the office, to follow Sandra for the remainder of her pregnancy. **[P]**

Episode 4
Carol sees Jessica Riley again this week. When Carol asks her how she is feeling, Jessica reports less fatigue, but she has ongoing constipation. Carol asks her what kinds of fluids she drinks, and Jessica replies that she mainly drinks soda. Carol encourages Jessica to drink at least 8–12 glasses of water a day and eat more fiber, such as raisins, oatmeal, or bran cereals. **[P]**

Episode 5
No news this week.

Episode 6
No news this week.

Episode 7
Jessica Riley comes in for a visit along with her boyfriend Casey. Carol finds Casey to be dominant, insisting on answering questions for Jessica. Carol mentions Casey's visit in her case notes and writes herself a note to remind herself to question Jessica alone the next time she visits.

Later in the week, Carol meets 15-year-old Kristina Martin, who presents to the Community Health Department requesting birth control pills. Kristina admits to Carol that she has been having sex and is scared she could get pregnant. Carol confirms that Kristina is not pregnant with a pregnancy test and menstrual history before writing a prescription. She teaches Kristina how to take her birth control pills and reminds her that the pills will prevent pregnancy, but will not protect her against sexually transmitted infections. **[VC] [P]**

Episode 8
No news this week.

Episode 9
Carol sees Jessica Riley this week. She talks with Jessica about fetal development and reviews the birth process. During the exam, she notices that Jessica has several bruises on her abdomen. Carol has seen these types of injuries before on women who have been abused by their partners.

Carol asks Jessica how she got the bruises. Jessica says that she is very clumsy, and she ran into a table. She denies that anyone has hurt her and repeats that she is just clumsy. Carol makes a note of the injuries in Jessica's medical record. **[P]**

Episode 10
No news this week.

Episode 11
Carol sees Jessica Riley for her 36-week exam. Jessica is accompanied by her boyfriend Casey. Before she examines Jessica, Casey tells Carol that Jessica has bruises on her abdomen because she runs into things. When Casey leaves the room, Carol tells Jessica that, if she needs help, there is information in the restroom about the local domestic abuse shelter for women and children who are being abused by a significant other. **[VC]**

Episode 12
Carol sees Jessica Riley again this week. During the exam she notes that Jessica's cervix is thinning and dilating slightly. She knows Jessica will be having the baby in the next few weeks.

While working at the Community Health Department this week, Carol sees Terry Clark, a 16-year-old female who is concerned that she might be pregnant. Terry tells Carol that she has recently become sexually active with her boyfriend Jeremy, and that she has not had a period "for a while." Terry cries when Carol confirms that she is pregnant, telling Carol that she doesn't know what to do, and that her parents will "kill her."

Carol talks with Terry about her options (having the baby, adoption, or abortion) and suggests that she talk with Jeremy and her parents so she can make the best decision for herself. Terry tells Carol that she doesn't want a baby, but she doesn't want to kill the baby either. Carol refers Terry to Planned Parenthood and offers to provide prenatal care for Terry during her pregnancy. **[P]**

Episode 13
Carol receives a call from the Neighborhood Hospital Labor and Delivery unit, informing her that Jessica Riley delivered her baby. Carol goes to the hospital and learns of the circumstances of the delivery. When Carol talks with her, Jessica breaks down crying and tells Carol about the problems she has with Casey and their abusive relationship. Carol tells Jessica that she can call the police and press charges against Casey, but Jessica insists that Casey loves her and didn't mean to hurt her. Carol sets up a social work consultation for Jessica, explaining that it is standard procedure for social services to follow up any time there is a risk of intimate partner violence.

Episode 14
No news this week.

Episode 15
Jessica Riley comes to the clinic for a postpartum exam. Carol asks her how things are going at home, and Jessica tells her that Casey is being a wonderful father and is treating her and the children very well. Jessica tells Carol that she believes that Casey has changed. Carol encourages Jessica to get more iron in her diet and reminds her to keep taking vitamins. She notices that Jessica's breasts have reduced in size and asks her about breastfeeding. Jessica says she doesn't want to breastfeed, so Carol talks with her about formula feeding. **[P]**

CAROL RAMSEY,
Season 3

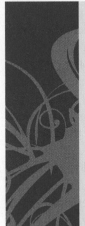

Biographical Information

Carol Ramsey is a 52-year-old certified nurse midwife who works at Neighborhood Women's Health Specialists (NWHS). She has been a midwife for 22 years, after spending the first 8 years of her career as a labor and delivery room nurse. Four physicians and three midwives, including Carol, work at NWHS. In addition to working 4½ days a week at NWHS, Carol works one afternoon each week at the Neighborhood Community Health Department. At NWHS, Carol sees her own patients. The majority of her work involves prenatal, delivery, and postpartum care, although she also provides routine gynecologic care for many of her patients. At the Neighborhood Community Health Department, Carol sees a variety of patients, many of whom are seeking contraception, pregnancy testing, or screening and treatment of sexually transmitted infections.

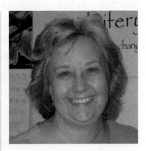

Episode 1

One of the obstetricians at the Neighborhood Women's Health Specialists practice resigned after his malpractice insurance premiums skyrocketed due to a pending lawsuit. Carol and the other midwives now have even more patients to see. Carol is working 10–12 hour per days this week, trying to compensate for the increased patient load. The physician group places a national search for a new obstetrician and a new midwife.

Carol sees Terry Clark, the 16-year-old pregnant teenager, in the office this week. Terry tells Carol that her parents want her to put the baby up for adoption. She is not sure she wants to, but has pretty much decided it is for the best. She also tells Carol that her boyfriend wanted her to have an abortion, and when she refused to do this, he broke up with her. **[P]**

Episode 2

Nancy, a 40-year-old woman, sees Carol for prenatal care. She already has a 9-year-old daughter. The woman tells Carol that she would like her daughter to be present and participate in the birth process. Carol is not against this, but tells Nancy that she will need to clear it with the hospital first. **[P]**

Episode 3

Carol and the nurse manager of the Labor and Delivery unit at Neighborhood Hospital meet with Carol's patient, Nancy, and her 9-year-old daughter Lindsey to discuss Lindsey's presence during the birth of her mother's baby. Carol tells Lindsey what birth is like, and that she might feel frightened if she sees blood and or thinks that her mother is hurt. The girl says that she would like to be

there when her little brother is born, and Nancy insists that Lindsey has been watching birth shows on television. Carol and the nurse manager approve Nancy's request to allow Lindsey to be present during the birth. **[P]**

Episode 4

No news this week.

Episode 5

Kristina Martin comes into the Community Health Department to see Carol this week. Carol remembers writing a prescription for birth control for Kristina several months ago. Kristina tells Carol that her boyfriend told her to get tested for Chlamydia, but she isn't sure what that is. Carol explains that Chlamydia is a common sexually transmitted infection and then examines Kristina. She gives her a prescription for doxycycline and instructs Kristina to take the whole prescription for ten days and abstain from sex during that time. Carol also talks with Kristina about measures she can take to prevent sexually transmitted infections and reinforces the need to take the birth control pills. [**VC**—cross link with Kristina Martin, L3W5]

Episode 6

Carol sees Terry Clark and her mother this week for a prenatal visit. Terry's mother tells Carol that there is no way Terry is old enough to raise a baby, and she is not interested in doing it either. The family has a friend who knows an attorney, and they are going to explore private adoption. Terry's mother hopes that they can get the adoptive family to help pay for Terry's medical bills. Terry verbalizes that she is too embarrassed to go to school, so she is being home-schooled for the rest of the year. **[P]**

Episode 7

A new certified nurse midwife is hired this week. Carol is thrilled to have another colleague in the office and agrees to orient her. **[P]**

Episode 8

No news this week.

Episode 9

Carol sees 16-year-old Terry Clark and her mother this week for a prenatal visit. Carol learns that an adoptive family has been located, and Terry has agreed to give the baby up for adoption. Because Carol knows that this is what Terry's parents have been pushing for, she asks Terry how she if feeling about the decision. Terry tells Carol that, "It is probably fine," and she is going to meet the adoptive family sometime in the next couple of weeks. She has been told they are really nice. **[P]**

Episode 10

While on-call for the practice, Carol gets a phone call from Dr. Gordon, the ED physician, asking her to see a patient. Reyna, a 13-year-old girl, presented to the ED with abdominal pain and heavy, bloody vaginal discharge. A pregnancy test ordered by Dr. Gordon is positive.

After examining Reyna, Carol informs the girl and her mother that she is pregnant and having a miscarriage. The mother is in shock. Reyna denies that she is pregnant and tells Carol that she couldn't be pregnant because she's never had sex. **[P]**

Episode 11

No news this week.

Episode 12

Nancy, the patient who wants her 9-year-old daughter Lindsey present during her delivery, goes into labor. Carol is present during the birth and notices that Lindsey chooses not to watch the actual birth, but she stays in a corner of the room. After the baby is born, Carol wraps him up in a receiving blanket and shows him to Nancy. Lindsey shyly comes to the bedside and peeks at her baby brother. She asks to hold him. Nancy thanks Carols for her flexibility and says she is glad Lindsey was allowed to witness her brother's birth. **[P]**

Episode 13

Carol has a very busy week. She delivers seven babies within 4 days. Carol and the new midwife still have more patients ask for their services than they can accept, but they have added several new patients to their caseloads.

Episode 14

Carol begins to wonder if she could open her own clinic for midwifery and gynecological care. Her state allows certified nurse midwives to work independently of physicians, and she has prescriptive authority. She has a friend who is also a midwife in another state who is thinking of moving to Carol's state because she wants to open her own clinic.

Episode 15

Terry Clark is in the office for her 39-week visit. Carol learns that Terry will not be giving the baby up for adoption after all. Terry tells Carol that her mother and father found out that the adoptive family was really two men, and they could not stand the idea that their grandchild would be adopted and raised by a gay couple. Carol feels badly that Terry's parents control her life in this way and grieves for the two men who were anticipating adopting the baby. **[P]**

NEIGHBORHOOD PUBLIC SCHOOLS

NEIGHBORHOOD PUBLIC SCHOOLS OVERVIEW

Character	Season 1	Season 2	Season 3
VIOLET BRINKWORTH	Violet is the nurse at the elementary, middle, and high schools. She observes the unhealthy foods and snacks that the children are buying at school and talks to the principals about offering more nutritious choices at the snack bars. Jason Riley gets in a fight with -another student. He is also having trouble with schoolwork; Violet wonders if he has a learning disability. Marcus Young comes to school with pink eye.	Two new health aides are hired to help Violet with the three schools. Violet continues to interact with Jason Riley. She has been asked to complete a questionnaire that will help to assess whether Jason has a learning disability. Kelsey Young comes into the nurse's office coughing and having trouble breathing. Violet also interacts with Jenna Riley and becomes concerned about her weight gain. The school board announces a ban on all "junk" food sold at the schools.	Because many parents and students are angry about the "junk" food ban, the principal tells Violet that she is considering bringing back some of the more popular items. Violet calls Jenna Riley's mother when she is concerned about her need to see a physician. Violet has a run-in with the middle school principal about a sexuality unit she is planning to teach. A female student is found on the floor with difficulty breathing. Violet is reprimanded for calling an ambulance to come to the school.

CONCEPTS   *Advocate, Collaborator, Educator, Health Promotion, Policy, Professionalism, Role Model*

VIOLET BRINKWORTH
Season 1

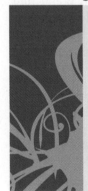

Biographical Information

Violet Brinkworth is a 41-year-old nurse who works for the Neighborhood Public School System. She has been married to her husband Richard Brinkworth for 15 years. Because Richard is often away on business trips, Violet decided to become a school nurse 6 years ago so she could be on the same schedule as her son, who is now 12 years old. For the first few years, Violet worked full time at Neighborhood Elementary School. However, because of budget cuts, Violet now also covers Neighborhood Middle School and Neighborhood High School. Fortunately, the schools are close to one another. Despite this, Violet finds it difficult to be an effective nurse because each school has so many needs.

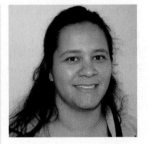

Episode 1
No news this week.

Episode 2
While in the teacher's lounge, Violet overhears two teachers talking about Jason Riley, a fifth grader at Neighborhood Elementary School. One teacher comments that Jason was in another fight this week and that his mother Evelyn must be out of touch with her son's behavior. Violet knows Jason well; he often tries to get out of class and come visit her. Because she knows that Jason has trouble with his peers and schoolwork, Violet is interested to hear the perceptions of the teachers.

Episode 3

No news this week.

Episode 4

Violet screens all of the Neighborhood Elementary School students for vision and hearing problems. When Jason Riley comes in to be screened, Violet notices that he can only read the 20/100 line of the eye chart in both eyes. She then tests Jason's hearing, which is within normal parameters. She calls Jason's mother Evelyn Riley and suggests that Jason be taken to an optometrist for a vision exam. **[P]**

Episode 5

Violet asks to meet with the administrators from Neighborhood Elementary, Middle, and High Schools to discuss the problems associated with trying to "cover" three schools. There is just not enough time to address the needs of all of the students. The administrators agree to look at possible solutions, including hiring a health aide. Violet does not think this is a very good idea, because the district does not require health aides to have any training other than first aid.

Episode 6

Violet spends a lunch hour observing the kids at the middle school to see what they are buying for lunch. She notices that most kids buy foods such as pizza slices, French fries covered with cheese sauce, nachos with cheese sauce, cheeseburgers, and fried burritos from the snack bar. Potato chips and other snack foods are also popular. She notices that dill pickles are the only food offered at the snack bar that represents the vegetable food group. Violet talks with the cafeteria manager and asks him if fresh fruits and vegetables could be offered. Violet is told that those food items are expensive and end up being thrown away because so few of the students buy them. **[P]**

Episode 7

Violet sees Jason Riley in the hallway and notices he is wearing new glasses. She asks him if he is happy with the change. Jason shrugs his shoulders and says that his headaches are better, but he still is too "dumb" to do his schoolwork. Violet wonders if Jason has ever been tested for learning disabilities.

Episode 8

No news this week.

Episode 9

Marcus Young, a first-grade student at the Neighborhood Elementary School, is sent to the office by his teacher. The teacher is concerned because Marcus has been rubbing his left eye all day and now complains that it hurts. Violet examines Marcus' eye and sees that it is red, irritated, and has discharge. She calls Marcus' mother Angie Young and explains that Marcus could have an infection in his eye and that it might be contagious. She asks his mother to pick Marcus up from school as soon as possible and take him to his health-care provider for treatment. Violet sends a note to the classroom teacher to keep an eye out for other children with similar symptoms and to ask all of the students to wash their hands. Violet types up a quick information sheet about pink eye for the students to take home to their parents. **[P]**

Episode 10

Violet sees Sam, a fifth-grade student with scrapes and bruises after an altercation with Jason Riley on the playground. Sam tells Violet that Jason is "such a loser." Violet asks Sam what caused the fight, and he tells her that Jason just started to beat him up for no reason.

Episode 11

Violet makes herself available three evenings this week for the Neighborhood Elementary, Middle, and High Schools open houses on different nights. Only a few people stop to say hello, making Violet feel somewhat invisible. **[P]**

Episode 12

Violet talks to the Neighborhood Middle and High School principals about stocking the student snack bar with more nutritious choices of food and drinks, citing several studies that link childhood obesity with childhood onset type 2 diabetes. The principals agree that the food could be more nutritious and say they will review the foods sold in the snack bar. However, they explain that the school district has a contract with a company that will provide each school with a $2,000 donation plus a percentage of sales if the school sells its products for the school year. The principal of the high school tells Violet that the girl's soccer team desperately needs new uniforms, and the donation has been earmarked to cover that expense. **[P]**

Episode 13

This week Violet reviews the medication plans of students in her schools to ensure that she has up-to-date information. Because she has three schools to cover and no help, this takes several days to complete. **[P]**

Episode 14

No news this week.

Episode 15
Jenna Riley, an eighth-grade student at Neighborhood Middle School, comes to the nurse's office and asks Violet if she can sleep for a while. She says she is very tired and not feeling well. Violet does not know Jenna, but recognizes that she is Jason's sister. Violet assesses Jenna for fever, and finds that she does not have one. She asks Jenna if she feels badly enough to call her mother and go home, but Jenna says she'll be okay if she can just nap for a while. Violet lets her stay in the office for an hour and then sends her back to class.

VIOLET BRINKWORTH
Season 2

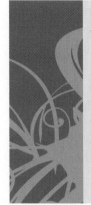

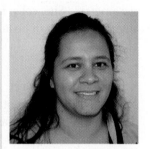

Biographical Information
Violet Brinkworth is a 41-year-old nurse who works for the Neighborhood Public School System. She has been married to her husband Richard Brinkworth for 15 years. Because Richard is often away on business trips, Violet decided to become a school nurse 6 years ago so she could be on the same schedule as her son, who is now 12 years old. For the first few years, Violet worked full time at Neighborhood Elementary School. However, because of budget cuts, Violet now also covers Neighborhood Middle School and Neighborhood High School. Fortunately, the schools are close to one another. Despite this, Violet finds it difficult to be an effective nurse because each school has so many needs.

Episode 1
The principal of the Neighborhood High School meets with Violet to inform her that the school board approved a proposal to hire two health aides to help her cover the elementary, middle, and high schools. Violet tells her she appreciates the fact that her request for help was heard, but feels it would be better to hire another nurse. The principal tells Violet that they cannot afford another nurse, and they could not justify the expense. Violet looks at the salary range for health aides and knows it will be difficult to find good help. **[P]**

Episode 2
Jason Riley comes to the nurse's office for the third time this week claiming to have a stomachache. As Violet talks with Jason, she learns that he has been kicked out of Boy Scouts for biting another scout. She also learns that he has been in another fight this week.

Episode 3
The school counselor consults with Violet about Jason Riley. She asks Violet to complete an assessment questionnaire; two other school staff members have been asked to complete the questionnaire as well. The questionnaires will be used to assess Jason for learning problems. **[P]**

Episode 4
Violet is disappointed, but not surprised, that there are no applicants for the school health aide positions this week.

Episode 5
A teacher sends Kelsey Young, a second-grade student, to the nurse's office because she has been coughing. Violet notices that Kelsey has an increased respiratory rate, is coughing frequently, and has wheezing in her lungs. Kelsey tells Violet that she has problems breathing. Because Kelsey does not have an inhaler at school, Violet calls Mrs. Young to pick Kelsey up from school and suggests that she be seen by her doctor. When Mrs. Young arrives, Violet encourages her to send an inhaler to school that can be kept in the nurse's office, but Mrs. Young seems reluctant to do this. **[P]**

Episode 6
A teacher at Neighborhood Middle School tells Violet that one of her students, Jenna Riley, has gained a lot of weight recently and wants to know if she has any medical conditions. Violet vaguely remembers Jenna, but does not recall anything specifically, so she tells the teacher she will look into the matter. When Violet pulls Jenna's file, she sees there is no history of any medical problems and that she is up to date with her immunizations. **[P]**

Episode 7
No news this week.

Episode 8
Violet gets a phone call from the school board president wanting to know how Violet feels about the food

choices at school. The president explains that she is tired of seeing children eating "crappy" food. Violet explains that she has attempted to get more healthy alternatives into the school snack bar, but has not had any luck. The school board president asks Violet to gather information on the nutritional value of some of the more popular snack bar items and to create a presentation for the next school board meeting in three weeks. Violet agrees to this. **[P]**

Episode 9
No news this week.

Episode 10
Violet goes to the school board meeting to present her findings on the nutritional value of the popular items that are sold at the snack bars at Neighborhood Middle and High Schools. She stresses to the board that there are not enough healthy items, such as fresh fruits and vegetables, available to the students.

Violet is reminded of the contract the schools have with a supplier. Violet suggests that the vending machines in the schools be filled with bottled water or juice, as opposed to soda, since the supplier carries both. The cafeteria worker, who is also at the meeting, disagrees with Violet and claims that the snack bar would lose a large amount of money if she were to sell fruits and vegetables as opposed to popular foods. No decision is made at the meeting, but the board says it will study the issue further.

Episode 11
At long last, two health aides have been hired. Violet spends the week orienting them to their new jobs. She clearly explains to them their scope of practice, teaches them basic first aid measures, and reviews the medication policies. She explains that they can dispense prescription medications to students who have supplies at school, but they may not give any student over-the-counter medications, such as Tylenol or cold medicines. **[P]**

Episode 12
No news this week.

Episode 13
The school board appoints Violet to a task force charged with reviewing food choices at the schools. The task force is directed to submit a recommendation to the school board within 2 weeks.

Episode 14
No news this week.

Episode 15
Based on recommendations from the task force to which Violet belongs, the school board announces a ban on all "junk" food sold at the schools. The supplier agrees to switch drinks from sodas to water, tea, lemonade, and fruit juice. Many of the students and parents at the school are furious about the ban and vow to fight it. One angry mother and her daughter learn that Violet was on the task force and share their displeasure with her. Violet is surprised by the response. **[P]**

VIOLET BRINKWORTH
Season 3

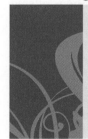

Biographical Information
Violet Brinkworth is a 42-year-old nurse who works for the Neighborhood Public School System. She has been married to her husband Richard Brinkworth for 16 years. Because Richard is often away on business trips, Violet decided to become a school nurse 7 years ago so she could be on the same schedule as her son, who is now 13 years old. She sometimes feels frustrated with her job because of the lack of support from the school principals.

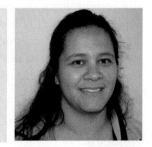

Episode 1
Violet sees Jason Riley in her office at lunchtime so that he can take his Ritalin. He tells Violet that he doesn't want anyone to know he takes medication because he doesn't want to be teased.

Meanwhile, several angry students and parents have signed a petition demanding that the Neighborhood Schools bring back the original menu items in the snack bars and vending machines. The students and parents argue that the kids are old enough to make their own decisions and don't need the school deciding what they should or should not eat. The principal tells the parents that she will consider their demands and determine if a compromise can be reached. She explains to Violet that she wants to support the task force and the decision that was made, but since many parents are upset, they should probably bring back the most popular items that have been removed from the menu. **[P]**

Episode 2

Jenna Riley comes into the nurse's office this week complaining of a twisted ankle. Violet does not see any indication of an ankle injury, so instead talks to Jenna about other things. Jenna tells Violet she is unhappy about her weight, which reminds Violet of Jenna's teacher's remarks about her weight gain. She asks Jenna if she has been really thirsty or hungry lately, and Jenna admits that she's been drinking a lot more soda because she's "always thirsty." Violet tells Jenna that she should see her family doctor and gets Jenna's permission to call her mother.

Episode 3

No news this week.

Episode 4

Violet visits with Mrs. Keller, the principal of the Neighborhood Middle School, about her intention to include information about sexually transmitted infections and pregnancy in a health unit that she is preparing. The principal is resistant to the idea, because she knows that there is a local group of churches that is mounting a campaign against books and materials that they deem to be too inappropriate and immoral to be allowed in the schools. Violet wonders how much of this argument is really coming from the community groups as opposed to Mrs. Keller herself. Violet reminds the principal that the school requires each student to turn in a signed permission slip before he or she is eligible to be present when she teaches on these topics. **[P]**

Episode 5

No news this week.

Episode 6

Mrs. Keller, the middle school principal, informs Violet that the school board is not comfortable with the topics of the presentations she was planning, and that she needs to limit her focus to abstinence only. Furthermore, she asks Violet not to discuss sexually transmitted infections and instead to create a brochure that will be made available to the students. Violet is furious and argues that she is doing the students a disservice by withholding information that they need to keep themselves safe. Grudgingly, she agrees to focus on abstinence. **[P]**

Episode 7

Out of 120 seventh-grade students, only 6 have returned notes from parents asking that their children not participate in the sexuality unit. As an alternative assignment, Violet gives them a packet to work on that focuses on obesity and nutrition. These students are sent to the library to work on the packets during class time.

During this same week, Violet notices a large stack of the sexually transmitted infection brochures that she created and made available for students in the trash can in the teachers' lounge. She knows that only teachers and staff have access to the lounge and is distressed that someone would intentionally throw away important information that the students need. Violet suspects that Mrs. Keller, the principal, is behind this, but says nothing. **[P]**

Episode 8

Two eighth-grade students come to Violet's office this week to ask her how to get condoms or birth control for "their friends." Violet tells them to let their friends know that the Neighborhood Health Department Clinic offers birth control and exams for sexually transmitted infection for free or at a reduced cost. She wishes that she could give this information to all of the students and hopes that the students who came to her are able to pass along the information to the others.

Episode 9

Violet receives a call from Mr. Anderson at the Neighborhood Hospital with a job offer. She is well aware that the nurses are currently on strike, citing increased patient loads and unsafe working conditions. She is offered considerably more money than she earns at the school, but turns down the offer in order to keep her schedule and take care of her son. **[P]**

Episode 10

This week, Violet writes a letter to the parents of all of the eighth graders, asking for official copies of shot records and reminding them that their children will not be allowed to begin high school if their immunization records are not up to date. As she reviews the records, she finds several students who are missing one or more of their scheduled immunizations. She makes a list of these students' names and waits to see if they bring in new or updated records. **[P]**

Episode 11

No news this week.

Episode 12
No news this week.

Episode 13
While working at Neighborhood High School, a student comes running into Violet's office and tells her that one of the students is sick in the hall outside the girls' locker room. Violet hurries out and finds a female student lying on the floor awake. When Violet asks her what happened, the girl does not respond. Violet notices that the pupils of the girl's eyes are dilated, and she is having trouble breathing. She sends a student to the main office to tell someone to notify the principal and then calls 9-1-1 on her cell phone. She asks the girl if she has taken any medicine or drugs recently. She does not respond, but her friend tells Violet that she had taken a "whole bunch" of her pills, and hands her a medicine bottle labeled Ritalin. The paramedics arrive and take the student to Neighborhood Hospital. Violet writes up a detailed incident report and submits it to the office. **[P]**

Episode 14
Violet is called into the principal's office at Neighborhood High School and reprimanded for calling an ambulance to come to the school. The principal tells Violet that in the future she needs to allow her to decide whether or not an ambulance is needed and make the call. Violet tells the principal that there was no time to try to find her, and she used her professional judgment and decided to call an ambulance based on her assessment of the situation. She tells the principal that she is very willing to inform her of the need to call for emergency help if she is easy to find; however, she will use her judgment as to whether or not there is time to find the principal before she calls an ambulance if she is not nearby. The principal tells Violet that she is expected to follow the school policy. It is on days like this that Violet wonders if she would be better off working at Neighborhood Hospital. **[VC]**

Episode 15
The school year has come to an end. Violet spends the last week of school chaperoning students as they engage in various end-of-year activities. She also spends time reorganizing her files and preparing her year-end reports. She is very tired, and is looking forward to several weeks of rest before the next school year starts. **[P]**

NEIGHBORHOOD NEWSPAPER

SEASON 1 NEWS

EPISODE 1

Free Immunizations Peak Interests [P]
by M. Lee

The Neighborhood Health Care Clinic is offering free immunizations today from 8:00 AM to 4:00 PM, provided that citizens bring a copy of their immunization records. "Our primary interest is a healthy community," said Jade Scott, MD, the physician organizing the immunization program. "Providing treatment at a fraction of a price is one thing, but providing it at no price is the best way to encourage people to get immunized," Dr. Scott added. The clinic's offering marks the second occurrence of an annual immunization program enabling individuals in the community to be immunized at no cost.

Immunizations Hit All-Time Low
by A. Lowell

According to local medical professionals, the number of individuals receiving immunizations is dwindling. "State immunizations have hit an all-time low," said Dan Sibray, MD, head of the immunization program at Neighborhood Hospital. The local hospital recently started discounting prices of routine physical examinations and immunizations, hoping to bring people back to the hospital. "Our worry is that if parents do not spend the time and money to bring their children into the hospital for routine procedures, they will end up spending more money on medicine, or worse, the emergency department," added Dr. Sibray. Statewide, medical professionals seem to agree with Sibray. "It's a real problem, and we hope that the discounts we're offering will encourage parents to bring their children in for immunizations. Our job is not to put a price on children's well-being, but with these new solutions, we hope to lessen the burden on citizens."

Medical Phobia Results in Tragedy
by N. Mckinney

Last night, a 3-month old Ruralton boy died after a battle with pertussis. Thomas O'Brien was admitted to Neighborhood Hospital on Wednesday after being ill at home the previous day, and died on Friday while in the pediatric intensive care unit. Joseph Descloitres, MD, the attending physician to the infant, reported that the mother refused to vaccinate her child, citing personal opposition. "Her feelings toward immunization were not positive," said Dr. Descloitres. "She felt that certain immunizations could cause her child to develop autism, and despite the rapid deterioration of her son's health, we had to honor these wishes," he added. The hospital has the authority to overturn a parent's decisions, but according to medical reports and given the rapid progression of the illness, obtaining a court order would have been difficult.

See Tragedy on page 4

Local Immunization Protest Ends in Arrest
by G. Johnson

While talk indicates that immunizations may be at an all-time low, one group thinks that the low rate of immunization is a positive outcome. Members of the local group, People Against Injecting Sickness, or PAIS, believe that medical institutions are injecting patients with latent forms of various diseases and only to meet their high patient quotas. "Immunizations have led to many illnesses, such as autism, and sometimes they cause the very diseases they claim to prevent," said Mark Bowie, leader of PAIS. Local physician, David Jackson, MD, feels differently, "The idea that institutions are immunizing patients to increase their number of patients is preposterous. While every treatment has its side effects, these effects are not intentional. In actuality, the cases in which side effects as severe as PAIS is suggesting are

See PAIS on page 7

EPISODE 2

Can Blood Drive Eliminate Hospital's Shortage? [P]
by P. Roberts

The Neighborhood Library will be holding a blood drive on Saturday from 8:00 AM to 4:00 PM. Last year's blood donation event at the library resulted in a record number of donations, and hospital officials are hoping for the same outcome this year. "It is good to know that the citizens care about other members of their community," Clancy Long, MD, a physician at Community Hospital, said during a meeting announcing the event. "While the supply intake last year was more than we could have hoped, the recent increase in traumatic injuries has caused the supply to dwindle once again," Dr Long stated. He added that although publicly announced donation events always result in good turnout, people do not only have to donate when there is an event. Long added, "People should know that donations can be given at any time—even during a lunch hour." Statistically, donations throughout the year are scarce, leading to shortages when doctors need the blood most. Despite the substantial blood donations received during city-sponsored events, these events only supply one day of donations.

Low Blood Supplies Alarm Medical Professionals
by G. Johnson

The belief among many state and local medical professionals is that blood donations have hit an all-time low. Several members of the medical community have asserted that the cause of the low blood supply is the recent rise in traumatic injuries throughout the state. Erik Goldsmith, MD, a physician at Neighborhood Hospital, suggests that people make an effort to donate blood, regardless of when or the amount they donate. "The recent rise in traumatic injuries in the state is not something known to only the medical professionals," said Dr. Goldsmith. "People know that injuries are increasing because they are the people receiving the injuries," he asserted. The rise in the number of traumatic injuries has left health officials baffled as to why more people are not donating, since the problem affects the community directly and

See Shortage on page 2

Budget Cuts Increase Strike Concerns
by A. Lowell

Given the recent budget cuts in health-related fields, it appears that even companies that garnered awards are not permitted a saving grace. The local company Neighborhood Manufacturing, which won an award last year for the innovation of a workplace health promotion program, has been forced to shut down this promotion program. The closure came as a sudden shock to all, but no shock was greater than that of the employees. The president of the company, Albert Black, expressed his shock. "I came into work like any other day, and I received a conference call from the Financial-Handling Department and my bosses," Black stated. "While I cannot divulge the contents of that call, I can say that I was left with only one option—shutting down our health promotion program." Employees, on the other hand, do not

believe that this was the only option and think that their superiors should have tried harder to keep the promotion program. These feelings have led to rumors and threats that soon the workers will begin to strike and

See Cuts on page 6

"Karate Kids Lack Discipline," Say Elders
by N. Mckinney

The recent encouragement by local schools to have their students participate in more extracurricular and fitness activities has seemed to have a negative effect on the community, according to the elderly population. "I come outside in the morning and I find the boards on my fences either damaged or destroyed by kids who recently learned how to kick and hit in their violent program," said retired U.S. Army veteran Ross Webb. Police reports state that no children have been apprehended in relation to these allegations, but that law enforcement personnel are keeping a close eye on the issue. Master Nguyen of the local karate program High Kicks, Strong Discipline suggests that it is impossible that these labeled children are his students. "My program teaches defense and discipline. Just because there is a karate program in town does not mean that it should be the first to blame," said Nguyen. "The percentage of children who might have seen such an act on television is much higher than the chance that one of my students committed such a crime." Officer Wilson of the local police department

See Karate on page 3

EPISODE 3

Run—Not Swim—for Fish
by N. Mckinney

While there may seem be some underlying irony in holding a running race to benefit aquatic creatures, enthusiasts suggest otherwise. "This event allows citizens of the Neighborhood to better themselves and their community," said head of the event, Kira Fort. The event Fort is referring to is the annual "Run for the Fish" fundraiser. The fundraiser's main objective is to clean up Neighborhood Lake, which has seen great deterioration and pollution increase since the recent manufacturing growth in the town. For an entry fee of $20.00, all participants receive a T-shirt and water bottle and the chance to participate in the run later that afternoon, which will span the lake's 5-mile perimeter. Citizens are allowed to participate in the run even if they are not interested in donating $20.00 to the cause, and donations are welcome from those choosing not to participate. "We just want to gather support, and if we gather donations along the way, then that is twice as good," said Fort. Last year's run raised approximately $5,880 with around 294 participants. Fort added that, "Even if a person does not donate to the fund, we still know that since that person shows interest, we will have an extra pair of hands when it comes to actually cleaning the lake."

See Run on page 3

Officials Confirm Pollution Worries [P]

by M. Lee

At last night's City Council meeting, Mayor Nathan Brice confirmed what many environmental activist groups have been proclaiming for months—Neighborhood Lake's concentration of pollutants has reached critical levels. Local resident Elton Bentley was quoted saying, "[The pollution] is too bad...I remember fishing here as a kid when the waters were pristine." Officials say that concerns that newer generations will be unable to enjoy the waters recreationally as Bentley did are the least of the community's worries. "Right now, our main concern is the town's water supply," said Councilman Richard Bradley. "This a concern because rather than affecting the newer generation's aesthetic view of the community, the severe pollution could affect their health and well-being". The mayor declined to comment directly to the press on the issue, but insisted that he was taking steps to correct

See Pollution on page 2

Police Report: Local Man Dies, Cause Unknown [P—Sheriff Shuster]

by L. Deacon

"I assure you it wasn't the polluted water that killed him," joked Sheriff Mark Shuster. Local mechanic Jon Smith died in his home 2 nights ago of unknown causes, according to the initial police report. Shuster insists that jokes aside, the police department is taking this case very seriously. "While it may seem quick to jump to suspicions, there are too many variables to just toss this one aside to a death from natural cause," Shuster added. "The man was relatively young to die from natural causes, and although he was a smoker, his death came too suddenly to be blamed on either of these without further investigation." Police have questioned several neighbors of the Smith household, but their primary area of focus has been Smith's wife, Karen, who has been questioned several times since her husband's death. Shuster stated that "We do not want to jump to conclusions, and right now we're focusing on getting all the facts."

EPISODE 4

Hotline Puts Families at Ease [P]

by A. Lowell

Recently, the state government passed a bill that opens up all cities to a convenience once enjoyed only by major cities—a poison hotline—and the Neighborhood is one of these towns that is now benefitting from this convenience. People can reach the hotline by dialing 1-800-POISONS on any model of phone. The hotline, which services the state 24 hours a day, 7 days a week, informs callers of how to deal with both foreign and domestic poisons. Local parent Sally Franken was put at ease, since the service provides her with a "comfort that is readily welcomed, especially given the rise of pollution in our community's most revered locations." Local physician Dan Sibray, MD, shared similar sentiments to Ms. Franken. "[The hotline] provides citizens with information that could save them a visit to the hospital and the bills involved with such a visit." Although a majority shares a positive perspective regarding the availability of a hotline, local activist group PAIS (People Against Injecting Sickness) suggests that the service is biased and is only giving information that would

See Hotline on page 2

Terrorism Concerns Reach Community

by G. Johnson

In a recent press release, the U.S. Department of Homeland Security declared that chemical warfare has topped their list as the most serious threat to U.S. citizens following a string of terrorist threats against the nation. Local officials have declared that although the Neighborhood is smaller than neighboring cities, it is not immune to attacks. "The chances of an attack here are slim, but there is no harm in being prepared," said Councilman Richard Bradley. In response to the Department of Homeland Security's press release, local officials have released this precaution and preparation list in the event of an attack, which they define as an inexpensive means to stay safe:

- Ensure a sufficient supply of water and food (canned food is recommended due to its extended shelf-life)
- Maintain a healthy diet and keep immunizations current
- Organize an assortment of simple tools and mechanical supplies (hammer, screwdriver, duct tape, etc.)
- Create an evacuation plan or list of what to do in the event of a terrorist attack; a plan of action can sometimes eliminate indecisiveness due to panic

See Concerns on page 7

Police Report: Woman Arrested, Accused of Husband's Murder [P—Sheriff Shuster] [P—Karen Smith]

by L. Deacon

"It is not the synopsis of a Hollywood film, nor creative, but sick and twisted," said Sheriff Mark Shuster during an interview announcing the arrest of Karen Smith in relation to the murder of her husband, Jon Smith. Shuster announced that his deputies apprehended Mrs. Smith late Thursday evening, after the autopsy of her husband revealed a concentration of arsenic so high that it could kill several people. Mrs. Smith's defense lawyer claims that his client was cleaning the kitchen that day and misplaced the arsenic in with an assortment of cooking spices. Scoffing at this defense, Shuster stated, "Given the concentration of poison found in Mr. Smith's body, there is no way this act was accidental. Such a defense is insulting to the memory of the deceased." Subsequent to the arrest of Mrs. Smith in suspicion of murder, police obtained a search warrant for her home, where they found an assortment of poisons in a shoebox under Mrs. Smith's bed. This assortment included several types of pesticides, but most prominently, arsenic. After this discovery, the Neighborhood Police Department officially charged Mrs. Smith with murder in the first degree (premeditated, with malice, and intent to kill).

See Report on page 2

EPISODE 5

Town Meeting Will Focus on Drunk Driving [P]

by G. Johnson

"Statistically, with an increase in population, we see an increase in crime," said Neighborhood police officer John Capote. Although parents have been expressing a concern with this increase, no crime is more of a concern to both police and parents than drunk driving. The concern expressed will be the focus of this week's town meeting, which is scheduled for Thursday night at 7:00 PM. The discussion at the meeting will determine whether or not the local government pursues legislation against drunk driving—specifically, the imposing of harsher sentences and punishments if a person is convicted of drunk driving.

Accident Ends in Death of Two

by A. Lowell

An accident that occurred this past weekend claimed the lives of two of the Neighborhood's citizens—Myrna Ogdon, 24, and her son, Raymond Ogdon, 10 months. The crash took place Saturday night near Neighborhood Lake. Police report that the accident was apparently the result of drunk driving. The occupants of the other car, Amy Price, 16, and Carrie Rivera, 17, were declared drunk and arrested after Sheriff Mark Shuster administered a sobriety test that both young women reportedly failed. The Ogdons were struck head-on by Price's car, a sport utility vehicle, crumpling Ogdon's small sedan.

See Accident on page 2

Police Report: Wife Denies Baking Poison Pie [P—Jon Smith] [P—Karen Smith]

by L. Deacon

A crime that seems more like the plot of a Hollywood movie is appearing to have its share of plot twists. Karen Smith, who was arrested recently in relation to the murder of her husband, Jon Smith, has reportedly changed her story, placing the blame on the local church. Smith delivered a new account of the crime at a press conference yesterday afternoon. This new account states that the pie was purchased from a bake sale at Neighborhood Church. Smith contended that someone at her church made the poison-laced pie and she bought it, not knowing its fatal contents. Initially, Smith claimed that while cleaning the kitchen, she misplaced a small container of arsenic among other spices, claming that the similarity between the containers caused her to mistake arsenic for one of her many spices. Smith's defense attorney, Nicholas Ocoada, claims that this scenario was forced upon Smith in order for police to obtain a confession. "A woman whose husband has just been declared dead is not in the proper state of mind to make rational choices, and I motion that the police constructed a confession and in her emotional state, she accepted it," Ocoada said.

See Report on Page 5

EPISODE 6

Mosey Down to the Rodeo Grounds [P]

by N. Mckinney

The annual Neighborhood Rodeo is taking place this week, every night from 7:00 PM to 11:00 PM. The Rodeo Daze competition is being held again as well. Entry into the competition is free, and every person who participates is guaranteed a prize—ranging from a free hat to a grand prize of $500. There is, however, an admission fee to the Rodeo, which is $10.00 for adults. Admission is free for children under 6 years of age. Other elements of the Rodeo event include several amusement park rides, games, and an arts and crafts contest.

Shuster Rides Again [P—Sheriff Shuster]

by G. Johnson

The Neighborhood's own Sheriff Mark Shuster will don his cowboy hat once again Thursday evening at 8:00 PM. Sheriff Shuster will be performing in a free concert as a fundraiser for the battered women's shelter. "By offering a free concert, we eliminate the need to feel troubled financially in order to have a good time," said Sheriff Shuster. The concert will also be accepting donations before and after the show. The Sheriff added that, "Most importantly, we want people to have a good time. If they can donate a dollar or two, we would be grateful, but we do not require it."

Police Report: Wife Formally Charged With Murder

by A. Lowell

As of last week, Karen Smith was being held on a $2 million bail, but she now has been formally charged with murder in the first degree. At a press conference earlier this week, Sheriff Mark Shuster announced that the Neighborhood Police Department has officially charged Mrs. Smith with first-degree murder in the death of her husband Jon Smith, a skilled mechanic at the Neighborhood Toyota dealership. Jon Smith died after eating a pie laced with poison—specifically, arsenic. At her arraignment, Mrs. Smith contended that the pie was bought at a local church bake sale and that any poison contained in the pie was in the pie when she purchased it. Smith also cites that the relationship with her husband had a plethora of abuse problems lasting for more than 2 years. According to her attorney, Nicholas Ocoada, Smith constantly feared for her life, and her reaction to her husband's death was misinterpreted.

See Report on page 3

EPISODE 7

Health Fair Welcomes All [P]

by A. Lowell

On Saturday, the Neighborhood Mall will be host to this year's Health Fair from 9:00 AM to 5:00 PM. This year's Health Fair will address a variety of issues, and all individuals are welcome. Programs at the fair are designed for individuals of every age group. Younger children can visit several information centers and participate in many programs, including one that helps inform the children how to avoid illness. The programs designed for teens and young adults focus specifically on sex education, including signs of sexually transmitted diseases and how to protect themselves. Programs for adults focus on health issues such as high cholesterol levels, elevated blood pressure, and obesity.

Emergency Department Sees Critical Capacities [P—Dr. Gordon]

by G. Johnson

Neighborhood Hospital is reportedly over capacity, and staffers are citing unsafe conditions. James Gordon, MD, physician director of the Neighborhood Hospital emergency department (ED), reports that the ED has become inundated with individuals seeking health care. Most of these individuals do not have emergency conditions but are unable to access health care through other means. Dr. Gordon stated that, "This city has a lack of adequate medical facilities, especially for low-income individuals or indigents." Gordon also suggested that people need to be educated about particular symptoms, because most of the time, an injury or sickness can be treated at home. Increasing hospital capacities force individuals to come to the ED for basic health care and a waiting period that can exceed 6 hours.

See ER on page 3

Cavities at All-Time Low, According to Dentists

by N. Mckinney

Dental professionals say that recent advances in dental care have resulted in a decrease in the incidence of cavities in children and adolescents. Improvements such as sealants and fluoridated water have contributed to such successes, say dentists. Sealants have become routine, being found so effective that such treatments are now offered at no cost to children of low-income households. Individuals interested in having sealant treatments for their children should stop by the Health Fair on Saturday. A booth titled "Healthy Teeth for Tomorrow" will be present at the event, sponsored by the local chapter of the American Dental Association.

See Dentist on page 4

EPISODE 8

Health Career Fair This Weekend [P]

by G. Johnson

Inspired by a recent interest of the general population in health care–related careers, there will be a Health Career Fair held at the Neighborhood High School on Saturday from 9:00 AM to 5:00 PM. The career fair is not only for students but also for the entire community. The careers that will be discussed and on display during the fair include those in medicine, nursing, radiologic sciences, dentistry, and medical technologies, among others. Various local health care centers are sponsoring the event, including the Neighborhood Hospital Association, State Nursing Association, Ruralton College, and the local chapter of the American Dental Association.

Gun Scare at Elementary School Ends in Expulsion

by N. Mckinney

Earlier this week, a young student was expelled from Neighborhood Elementary School for bringing a gun to school. The third-grader, whose name remains unreleased, claimed to be angry at another student after being teased at school. Being too young to own a firearm legally, the child claims he stole his father's handgun and brought it to school in order to scare the other student and not to hurt him. Police have yet to make an official announcement on the details of the case, and have only confirmed the information that other departments have released—essentially, that a child brought a gun to school and was expelled after being apprehended. In response to the incident, parents have expressed great concern with the age of the individual, expressing concern that if a child this young can commit this crime, the odds of a teen or young adult committing the same crime at the high school are even greater.

See Gun on page 2

Nurses Leave Due to Poor Work Conditions

by A. Lowell

An increasing number of nurses are leaving health-related facilities across the Neighborhood, citing difficult working conditions and low wages. However, this is not only a local problem. Across the state, nurses have been leaving positions faster than the positions can be filled—a trend that has been maintained for the past 3 years. Although new nurses are hired, medical facilities have been unable to attract applicants at the same rate that positions are being vacated. Employment centers have said that over the past 3 years, the state has seen job openings in nursing positions rise by 8%. "This situation is completely unacceptable," stated lawmaker Howard Rome. "The people of our state deserve to be cared for by competent health care professionals, and something needs to be done." Locally, government and health care officials hope that the recent Health Career Fair will inspire more students to pursue a career in health care. However, considering the length of schooling required, such hopes would take years to be fulfilled.

See Nurses on page 2

EPISODE 9

Kicking the Habit

by N. Mckinney

A group that meets weekly is offering more options for people trying to quit smoking. The Neighborhood Community Center will be host to the Smoking Cessation Class that will start meeting this week and every week (for 8 weeks) on Wednesday evenings at 7:00 PM. Although the fee for the class is $30.00 per person, those organizing the class insist that the price is negligible compared with the price of cigarettes. "People should think of the cost over the long term," said program head Katherine Hirschfield. "The program costs about the same as six packs of cigarettes, and once the class concludes, the money saved from not having to buy cigarettes anymore will be a great benefit," she added. **[P]**

Drug Use on the Rise

by G. Johnson

The Neighborhood Police Department claims that drug use in the Neighborhood is on the rise. This year the Neighborhood saw not only its first methamphetamine lab bust, but three subsequent lab busts succeeding the first. The elderly community is blaming the rise of drugs on the growth of the community. "I do not know what has happened to this community. When I was young, drugs were nonexistent in this community," said Rayleen Cordova. The increase of drug use is due to increases in the general population.

See Drugs on page 2

Smoking Breaks a Thing of the Past?

by A. Lowell

Smoking bans at large companies around the country have risen to a new level. A reported nine large U.S. companies have enacted policies to stamp out smoking among workers. Beginning next year, employees who smoke will potentially lose their jobs if they refuse to quit smoking. A spokesperson for the National Work-Right Association states that this ban is an infringement of worker rights and that such a policy is illegal, citing that an employer cannot force its employees to quit smoking altogether because employers do not have control of their workers outside of the workplace. Supporters of the proposal say the bans are about the health and well-being of nonsmokers in the work environment and the rising cost on insurance for individuals who smoke.

See Ban on page 6

EPISODE 10

Express Yourself at Art Fair [P]

by A. Lowell

Starting this Friday and lasting all weekend, the Neighborhood Community Center will be host to the Neighborhood Art Fair. The fair will feature a multitude of artistry works, including ceramics, water colors, oils, woodwork, and quilting, among others. Although the fair will feature works by several well-known artists, local artists are encouraged to attend and display their own work. "Art is not limited to only those regarded with fame," said the art fair's host, Marvin Rourke. "[Art] is also not limited to painting, so we encourage people to bring in any of their works."

Pit Bull Attacks Child [P—Dr. Gordon]

by G. Johnson

A Pit Bull attack this week has placed a 3-year-old child in critical condition. In order to maintain the privacy of all individuals involved, police have not revealed the names of the victims or the owner of the dog, by the wishes of the latter party. The details that are available about the incident are that the child was attacked while playing in the backyard sandbox opposite the yard where the dog was kept. The dog's owner claims that the dog was gentle and has never been violent before, claiming that the attack must have been provoked. James Gordon, MD, an emergency department physician at Neighborhood Hospital, was quoted saying that the incident was the worst he has ever seen and that the child will be lucky to recover without any facial scarring or lifelong trauma. The incident has ended tragically for both sides; when responding to the call, Sheriff Mark Shuster shot and killed the dog.

See Attack on page 3

Trial Report: Smith Murder Trial Begins Next Week [P—Jon Smith] [P—Karen Smith]

by L. Deacon

Karen Smith's murder trial is scheduled to begin next week with opening arguments. She is charged with first-degree murder of her husband Jon Smith, and is entering a plea of not guilty. Many already feel the trial will be an open-and-shut case. The defense team's strategy for Mrs. Smith is to sway the jury with allegations that the defendant suffered great physical and emotional abuse from her husband prior to his death. The prosecution team believes they have a stronger case because the defense's entire case depends on Mrs. Smith's allegations but is not supported by hard evidence. Supporters of the defendant in this case suggest that Mrs. Smith should have pleaded temporary insanity, which would have yielded a lighter sentence if she is convicted.

See Report on page 4

EPISODE 11

Flu Shots Encouraged [P]

by G. Johnson

This week, the Neighborhood Senior Center will offer flu shots daily from 1:00 PM to 4:00 PM. Health officials recommend citizens receive the vaccinations while it is still early in the flu season. The price of the shot is $20.00 for all ages except for those older han age 65, for whom the vaccination is free. This year, health officials hope to see a high turnout for the event as part of a long string of events that have taken place over the past few months to promote health and health-care careers.

Flu Deaths Expected to Rise

by N. Mckinney

Health officials are preparing for the worst this flu season, claiming that they expect flu-related deaths will increase. Officials maintain that the groups most at risk for contracting the flu and dying from the illness are elderly individuals, those with chronic health conditions, and infants. Last year, numerous people died from the flu statewide, and five from the surrounding area alone. Health professionals have tried to increase immunizations through health fairs, but they fear it will not be enough to curb flu-related deaths.

See Rise on page 2

Homeless Man Found Dead

by A. Lowell

"It is hard to believe anyone would hurt him," said director of the homeless shelter Carol Maddox. Yesterday, homeless man Lionel Daily, 62, was found dead next to a dumpster in the downtown Neighborhood area. According to the police report, Daily was found by a passerby around 7:00 AM, and an investigation is currently underway. Daily's death came as a shock for many of the homeless population in the Neighborhood. Daily was a well-known transient to the downtown area. "He frequented the homeless shelters and was very sociable," said Maddox.

See Homeless on page 3

EPISODE 12

Domestic Violence Hotline Established [P]

by A. Lowell

A community-based project to protect citizens from domestic violence situations will enter its second phase starting next month with the establishment of a domestic violence hotline. The first phase of the project, a safe house, was completed last year, but the implementation of a hotline serves as a means for victims of violence to call in privacy and confidence. The operators are trained to detail clients with information on how to prevent domestic violence and what to do to escape an abusive relationship. The toll-free number for the service is 1-800-111-1112 and is initially opening with a total of 20 operators.

Citizens Seek Pit Bull Ban

by G. Johnson

In the wake of a near-fatal Pit Bull Terrier attack on a 3-year-old Neighborhood boy, citizens are scouring the community for the necessary petition signatures to propose a ban on the dog breed. Those who are against the ban claim that the community is jumping the gun on banning an entire breed of dog based on one bad incident. However, supporters respond by saying that Pit Bull attacks are not isolated incidents, which is why several states maintain bans on ownership of these dogs. Nationwide, no dog breed is more legislated against than the Pit Bull (referring to American Pit Bull Terriers, American Staffordshire Terriers, and Staffordshire Bull Terriers), and several states hold bans on owning Pit Bulls.

See Pit Bull on page 4

Trial Report: Defense Comes Out Strong

by L. Deacon

The second week of the Karen Smith trial began this week. Karen Smith stands charged for first-degree murder by serving and baking a poison-laced pie for her husband Jon Smith. This week, the defense presented a strong case for Mrs. Smith. According to the defense attorney, Nicholas Ocoada, Smith's action was solely based on self-defense. Jon Smith was portrayed as a controlling man with a vicious temperament. Karen Smith described years of abuse by his hand and allegedly killed him to escape the abuse. Prosecutors pointed out that the defendant never made attempts to seek help and believe her story to be made up simply to gain sympathy from the press, women's groups, and the jury. Police reports revealed, in favor of the prosecution, that Jon Smith did not have a criminal history.

See Report on page 7

EPISODE 13

Take Me Out to the Ball Game [P]

by F. Odell

This weekend, the Neighborhood Sports Stadium will sponsor a baseball tournament for any to attend. Several teams from across the state are expected to compete for a total of six games. All children aged 6 and younger, as well as individuals older than 65, will be allowed admittance free of charge. For those of all other ages, the price of admission is discounted to $5.00 per person, per game, or one can buy one ticket for the entire tournament at the discounted price of $30.00. The reason for the free admittance and discounted tickets (usual price is $8.00 per person, per game) is due to a slow sports season. Compared with previous seasons, the stadium has not been selling as many tickets as they would like, and the organizers of the tournament hope that attendance will inspire audiences to return to the sports pastime.

Officials Hopeful for Governor Award

by G. Johnson

The residents of the Neighborhood are being encouraged by their local officials to participate in the upcoming "America on the Move" beginning next month. "America on the Move" is a nationwide effort to increase activity levels of its citizens. Communities who make the most progress are eligible for a Governor's award at the completion of the activity. "Even if the town does not end up being eligible for the award, it still inspires people to become physically active, something that is very important in a time when obesity is becoming widespread," said Councilman Richard Bradley.

See Award on page 2

Childhood Obesity Rises

by A. Lowell

Proportional to the increase state and nationwide, the obesity rates continue to rise in the Neighborhood among children as well as adults. It is estimated that 15% of youth under the age of 18 are obese. State and local authorities have called for a reinstitution for mandated physical education programs and a ban of soda and candy machines in all state-funded K-12 schools. Health officials say that the lack of physical exercise coupled with changes in dietary habits of school children are obvious contributors to the obesity trend. Another issue that has developed—and a common excuse used by the obese—is that junk food is cheaper than healthy food, prompting a movement to put a "fat tax" on unhealthy foods. Parents are urged to consider foods eaten by their children and to get their children involved in regular physical activity.

See Obesity on page 3

EPISODE 14

Directive Seminar This Week [P]

Announcement

The local Hospital Ethics Review Board of the Neighborhood will host an Advance Directive Seminar for community members on Friday at 7:00 PM in the Neighborhood Community Center.

Family Sues Hospital

by N. Mckinney

A local family has sued the Neighborhood Hospital over visitation rules in the intensive care unit. A Neighborhood man, Chad Winchester, has filed a lawsuit against the hospital over what has been labeled by some as a case of insensitivity. According to the affidavit, Winchester was not allowed into the intensive care unit to see his mother during what is described as the morning shift change. According to hospital policy, restrictions in the number of visitors and the hours of visitation are made in order to ensure quality of care for the patient. The allegation stated that Winchester left the hospital at that time and his mother, Mary Winchester, died unexpectedly later that day. Winchester contends that the nursing staff prevented him from seeing his mother one last time prior to her passing.

See Lawsuit on page 3

Trial Report: Murder Trial Ends in Conviction

by L. Deacon

Lasting a little less than 4 weeks, the trial of Karen Smith in relation to the murder of her husband Jon Smith could be considered an open-and-shut case. While the defense made a strong opening, its case depended greatly on emotional appeals, which in turn depend highly on the type of jury hearing the case. The trial ended this week with the jury delivering a guilty verdict for the first-degree murder charge against Karen Smith. Sentencing is scheduled for next week, and Smith has the possibility of being sentenced to a term of 50 years to life in prison. Prosecutors praised jurors for making the right decision in this case. "Individuals cannot take the law into their own hands," said lead prosecutor Jessie Corona.

EPISODE 15

Band Competition This Weekend [P]

by F. Odell

The Neighborhood high school will host the annual Regional Band Concert. Bands from all regions of the state will be competing, with participants ranging from grades K–12. The competition will be held on Friday and Saturday on the following schedule: Friday, 8:00 AM to 6:00 PM; Saturday, 8:00 AM to 3:00 PM. At 4:00 PM on Saturday, following the competition, an awards ceremony will commence. The event is available to all Neighborhood and state citizens free of charge. Last year, Neighborhood High School received the highest honor for performing an excerpt from Vivaldi's "The Four Seasons."

Local Instructor Honored [P—Ramona Rivera]

by A. Lowell

This week, Ramona Rivera, a lifelong resident of the Neighborhood, will be honored for her undying devotion and instruction of the arts, specifically the piano. The local piano teacher has been revered for exposing the area's youth to music education. Rivera has taught piano lessons to children of the community for more than 30 years. Regarded as one of the best piano teachers in the area, Rivera explains that she loves what she does, believing that music is an important developmental component to reach children. Recent scientific studies appear to agree with Rivera's viewpoint, showing that children exposed to music education have greater academic success and critical thinking skills compared with those who are not exposed to music education.

New Treatment Facility Planned

by G. Johnson

State lawmakers recently approved a multimillion-dollar bond to be used in developing a modern treatment center for cancer in the Neighborhood. Plans are to build the facility adjacent to the Neighborhood Hospital. However, the facility will not be a subdivision of the hospital, as it is funded independently by several charities and philanthropists. The facility will branch off from several other cancer treatment centers nationally and internationally in order to conduct research related to finding a cure for the disease. Construction on this project is set to commence in about 3 months.

SEASON 2 NEWS

EPISODE 1

Childbirth Classes to Begin This Week [P]

by N. Mckinney

Are you or someone you know expecting? The birth of a child is regarded as a joyous occasion by most, but the months before the delivery can be marked as an emotional rollercoaster. A new class hopes to dispel fears regarding adverse effects of pregnancy. The class covers the childbirth process as well as caring for an infant, including such topics as breastfeeding. Childbirth classes can ease the anxiety associated with childbirth, making the experience much more pleasurable for the mother, father, and infant. The organizers have informed that time is still available to sign up for the program before it starts this week. Classes will be held on Wednesday evenings from 7:00 PM to 9:00 PM for 6 weeks. To register, call the Neighborhood Hospital at 844-1000.

Child Seat Manufacturers Given a Crash Course in Safety

by A. Lowell

The National Highway Traffic Safety Administration's Ease of Use Ratings Program has delivered an ultimatum to child restraint device manufacturers—improve their products or incur legal action. These improvements are not just restricted to the realm of safety, but ease of use. Joel Zweick of the ratings program said, "An essential component in making a product truly safe is how easy it is to employ. One can make an infallible product, but its useless if the consumer does not know how to use it correctly." According to Neighborhood Sheriff Mark Shuster, the real benefit of the ratings program is to educate parents and caregivers about child safety seat features, and to assist them in finding the appropriate child safety seat for their needs. Under the new ratings system, child restraints are given an overall ease-of-use rating at defined levels of A, B, or C. The rating, however, does not apply to the performance of the restraint in the event of a crash. "Child restraints are most effective if the device is correctly installed," said the sheriff. "A child restraint that is easier to use should have a lower misuse rate, thus

See Safety on page 4

Domestic Violence Top Cause of Death for Pregnant Women

by L. Murrow

Pregnancy it is usually associated with thoughts of a coming together of family and friends in the form of showers and well-wishes in eager anticipation of a new life. For many women, however, pregnancy is marked as the beginning of a violent time in their lives. Surfacing evidence reports that pregnant women are more likely to die at the hand of their partner than from complications associated with the pregnancy and childbirth process. According to Mira Roberts, director of the Neighborhood Women's Shelter, incidents of abuse are underreported, and it is estimated that one in five women are abused during the course of a pregnancy. "Pregnancy is often a time when physical abuse begins," said Roberts. "When the abuse begins, many women are in denial, having difficulty coming to terms with the dangers involved." Dangers to a battered women and child during pregnancy include blunt trauma to the abdomen, hemorrhaging, uterine rupture, premature rupture of the membranes, miscarriage, and preterm labor. Such statistics support the need for a greater emphasis on screening and prevention as part of prenatal care.

See Domestic on page 2

EPISODE 2

Members of Senior Center to Visit National Park

by J. Harris

For a minimalist fee, seniors can join the local Senior Center for a 3-day weekend trip, by bus, to one of the Neighborhood's many nearby National Parks. Karen Williams, the geriatric nurse specialist at the Senior Center encourages those interested to attend. "Contrary to the image portrayed by the media, a large number of seniors are very active in the community but simply lack the means to travel," said Williams. Registration for the 3-day trip ends mid-week so it is recommended that seniors visit the center earlier this week to ensure that they can attend.

Senior Center Visits on the Rise, Say Employees

by G. Johnson

According to Karen Williams, a nurse at the Senior Center Clinic, visits to the center have been on a steady increase for the past few quarters, making the need for an expansion to the center a reality. Williams said that she has seen not only an increase in those using the facility, but also an increase in those seeking basic medical care. "It used to be that I might see a few people each day. Now I see at least one person every hour. That's quite an increase," said Williams. Williams has worked at the clinic for 5 years and says the increased use has been steady. A recent surge of use has been asserted to be related to the recent addition of a lunch program to the center.

See Visits on page 5

Furry Friends, Healers? [P]

by A. Lowell

Sometimes people can be healed by more than just medicine—or at least that's the mindset centers in the Neighborhood seem to be adopting with the incorporation of pet therapy into their respective programs. The therapeutic use of pets as companions has gained increasing attention in recent years and has made its way into health care. Studies have shown that pets are beneficial for a wide variety of patients—people with AIDS or cancer, the elderly, children with disabilities, and the mentally ill. Centers across the Neighborhood that are adopting pet therapy as a means of treatment include the Neighborhood Senior Center and the Neighborhood Nursing Home.

EPISODE 3

Cancer Awareness Fundraiser [P]

by N. Mckinney

Neighborhood residents are gearing up for the local "Walk for Life" fundraiser. The fundraiser will support efforts for the Neighborhood Cancer Treatment Facility, which was recently approved by the state. Participants for the event will walk a 10K course that begins and ends at the site of the future facility. Given the overwhelming support for the facility as well as the dire need for it, those who wish to participate can refer to any of the health-related centers in the Neighborhood for more information. The fundraiser will be held this weekend, and free beverages will be provided to those who participate in the walk.

See Fundraiser on page 3

Nursing Shortage Critical, Say Hospital Officials

by J. Harris

If you have grown concerned about the apparent lack of nurses in Neighborhood Hospital, your fears are neither alone nor unfounded. In fact, communities are suffering from nursing shortages on a national level—and the situa-

tion is expected to only get worse. According to Pam Lowell, Director of Nursing at the Neighborhood Hospital, health care professionals are bracing for a uncertain future. "It is like watching the destructive path of a hurricane coming right at you—there is nothing you can do to stop it, but you can only hope to ride out the storm," said Lowell. The number of unfilled positions at the Neighborhood Hospital has sharply risen, and shortages are seen on all patient care units. "The best we can do is try to minimize the damage before

See Shortage on page 4

Size Matters

by L. Sibray

Health care officials are concerned about the ever-increasing size of the college football athlete. The name of the game for front linemen is size and speed—but what are the long-term costs? Neighborhood fans were disappointed to see their beloved Maverick football team defeated by the top-ranked team in the conference this week. For Johnny Sands, center for the Mavericks, he lost more than just the game—he lost his mobility. A severe, career-ending knee injury sustained in the third quarter was made worse because of his 280-lb. frame. Sports nutritionist expert Tom Randall says scientific research concerning the nutritional needs of football players has been scant. Fortunately, new investigations are being conducted, and the up-to-date research suggests that football players should eat and drink like marathon runners, not like wrestlers.

See Athletes on page 6

EPISODE 4

"Two Green Thumbs Up" for Community Garden [P]

by G. Johnson

Neighborhood City Council this week announced the dedication of roughly 2 acres for a community garden. The goal of the garden is not to have it maintained by the state, but by the citizens. Individuals can apply for a plot within the garden and join other community members learning how to grow nutritious foods. Focus will be on healthy eating and exercise. All are invited to participate, and parents with children are encouraged to make visiting the garden a weekly family activity. City counselors are hoping that the garden not only brings community members together to form closer ties, but also brings diverse forms of plant life to the Neighborhood that are aesthetically pleasing.

See Garden on page 7

Studies Show Inadequate Diets in Americans

by N. Mckinney

It should not be surprising news to any American that diets are increasingly becoming worse related to yet another category—fruits and vegetables. The average person rarely eats adequate portions of fruits or vegetables in each daily meal, or for the entire day. However, many claim that dietary habits are simply too hard to change. There have been several attempts by the government to update the food pyramid to make it more understandable to Americans, but as shown by the results of new studies, these ventures have ultimately failed in changing the way Americans eat. Now, governments are adopting a more grassroots attempt at improving diet, by starting with families and changing regular habits within the home.

See Diets on page 3

Support Group Benefits Dieters

by A. Lowell

Whether the weight-gain culprit is food for comfort, the freshman fifteen, or holiday splurging, working together with another person who is interested in losing weight might improve chances for weight loss. Recent research has shown that having the help of a support group may be beneficial to individuals participating in a weight-loss program. Results of the Maryland-based study showed that dieters who have the help of a support group experience less stress and less "brainpower drain" than those individuals who are undertaking a weight loss program alone. In the study, dieters who dieted alone had increases in the stress-associated hormone cortisol; those who attended weekly support-group sessions did not. Those dieting alone demonstrated lower working memory capacity than did those in support groups. These findings may be helpful in understanding the high incidence of diet failure among those who need to lose weight.

See Group on page 4

EPISODE 5

Middle School to Host Science Fair [P]

by A. Lowell

Join the community's best and brightest this weekend for an event that is sure to please, inspire, and educate. This weekend the Neighborhood Middle School will host the annual Science Fair. More than 50 children from the school will participate in the event, with projects ranging from theoretical to those that can be applied in everyday life. Prizes will also be awarded to those projects deemed the best of show by the judges. Prizes include gift certificates and the chance to enter projects into higher-level regional, statewide, or nationwide science fairs.

Forest Fire Continues to Burn

by J. Harris

A forest fire that has been ravaging the forest west of the Neighborhood has still not been contained. For more than 5 days, the blaze has been destroying an uncalculated number of acres, and for each day the fire continues, it is causing irreversible damage. Initially, firefighters thought the fire would be easy to contain, but the windy season has started earlier than expected, causing the fire to be less predictable and to consume more rapidly. Although the fire is not contained, city officials urge that the citizens are not in any direct danger and will be notified in advance if there is any chance the fire's direction will shift toward the town.

See Fire on page 2

Smoky Air Fills Health Care Facilities With Patients

by N. Mckinney

While firefighters battle to bring the forest fire west of the Neighborhood under control, health care workers battle to keep patients breathing. "The smoky air conditions affect everyone, but especially those with pre-existing lung problems, such as chronic lung conditions," said Neighborhood Hospital emergency department (ED) physician James Gordon, MD. Increases in patient numbers can be seen in the ED and local physician offices. City officials have warned that while not life-threatening, the haze should still be regarded as a risk and has urged all citizens—particularly those with chronic respiratory conditions—to stay indoors unless a trip outside is absolutely necessary.

See Smoky on page 3

EPISODE 6

Task Force to Tackle Nursing Shortage

by J. Harris

If you have noticed an apparent lack of nurses in the Neighborhood, you are not alone. This week, leaders from across the state will convene in the Neighborhood to address the alarming shortage of nurses available to meet the health care needs of area and state residents. The issue comes as a response to the rising scarcity not just statewide, but nationwide.

See Shortage on page 2

Mandatory Overtime Angers Nurses, Cite Unsafe Work Conditions

by A. Lowell

A recently-proposed method to maintain adequate staffing at Neighborhood Hospital has ended with angering many nurses. "The increasing shortage of nurses across the nation has caused all hospitals to re-evaluate the way they operate," said Dan Packard, MD, a physician at the hospital. One of these re-evaluations resulted in the possibility of mandatory overtime—the legality of which is currently under question. Nurse Janice Calgary said, "If this measure is allowed, then the hospital is taking away a large portion of our private time." Hospital officials have claimed that mandatory overtime is only one of the proposed ideas; other alternatives include closing hospital beds. "We enjoy the prospect of overtime if we find ourselves strapped for cash, but forcing employees to work overtime is surely illegal," Nurse Calgary added.

See Overtime on page 5

Nursing Shortage Begins Before the Classroom
[P Note: add "Virginia Wade, left with best friend and nursing student, Mila Tajen" under the photo]

by N. Mckinney

Imagine wanting to enter the nursing profession in an attempt to curb a critical shortage. Imagine having a 3.7 grade point average, or GPA, and being denied admission to nursing school, while your best friend—who has a 3.76 GPA—is granted admission. This scenario is exactly what happened to Virginia Wade and her best friend Mila Tajen. Wade and Tajen, like thousands of individuals in the nation, are responding to the call to enter the nursing profession. "We certainly don't have a shortage of qualified applicants," says Dean Doris Mitchell. The problem of admissions has been tacked onto the issue of adequate funding. Mitchell added that, "What we have is a limitation on the number of students we are able to accommodate." Petitioning several state officials for more funding has been under way since before the shortage began, but the number of students seeking entrance into the nursing programs outstrips the funding.

See Applicants on page 3

EPISODE 7

City Hears From Parents on Proposed Music Ban [P]

by G. Johnson

A public forum has been opened for parents to participate in response to the recently proposed ban on the use of personal music players on school grounds by students and faculty. The proposed ban comes in reaction to the increasing popularity of the devices among teens, and in response to recent reports stating that the players contribute to hearing loss. Students have protested the idea since its inception, arguing that adults represent a very small percentage of individuals who own the players, thus they should not be allowed to ban the devices.

See Ban on page 5

Local Teen Pregnancy Numbers Down

by J. Harris

While the state is seeing an ever-increasing rate of teen pregnancy, numbers of teen pregnancies in the Neighborhood have dropped significantly. Implementation of a school-based sex education class is cited for this difference. School nurse Connie Ruiz says, "If you want rates to drop even further, condoms should be made available to kids in the high school—free of charge." Many members of the community feel the same way and have tried to implement Ruiz's ideas to lower the pregnancy rate, but are met by opposition from parents. "Most parents are unable to admit that their children are sexually active, when in fact, a majority of them are," Ruiz added.

Signal to Noise

by A. Lowell

Neighborhood school and city officials are urging parents to reconsider buying an MP3 player for their child, in response to results of a recent study indicating that a high percentage of young people have damaged their ears by playing the devices too loudly. Further dangers suggested by the study include activities in which music can cause distraction, such as driving. School officials have made efforts to ban the players from school campuses to reduce potential liability in the event a child's parents wishes to press charges against the school for not acknowledging such dangers. "We are covering our own back, that is true, but we also care about the well-being of our students," said Principal Adam Hurwitz. Several lawsuits have been filed nationwide against music-player companies despite warnings printed in the device user manuals.

EPISODE 8

Campaign Puts Smiles on Faces

by G. Johnson

This weekend, children ages 5-11 will have the opportunity to receive a free dental screening at the Neighborhood Dental Office. The offer is in response to the statewide campaign, "Healthy Teeth," which was recently approved by the governor last month. The campaign is working with local dentists, schools, and parents to improve the overall dental health of the community.

Editorial: Gay and Lesbian Couples, Fit to Be Parents?

by A. Beckett

Indeed, this is the question finding its way into every facet of society. Whether in the lobby of Congress, or in the professional office, one cannot help but hear the debate and have his or her own opinion. A growing issue on the national front is the increasing trend of extending adoption privileges to gay couples. Surely, such a trend cannot be harmful—what do children need but loving parents, regardless of sexual orientation? Granted, opinions in this issue are so strong that some stopped reading merely at the concept put forth in the headline; so in essence, this editorial is most likely preaching to the choir. This trend has certain individuals worried about the impact that being raised by gay or lesbian parents has on children, suggesting that being raised by someone who is gay may, in turn, make that individual gay. Others say that the sexual orientation of the parents has nothing to do with that of the child—for instance, many homosexual individuals were raised by heterosexual parents. People must consider this issue for a considerable amount of time and with great rationality in order to answer the question—what situation is better, a child with or without parents?

Think Twice About That Tan, Say Scientists [P]

by N. Mckinney

Skin cancer rates are on the rise. This comes at a shock to scientists, considering the multitude of warnings given every year regarding the risk of prolonged exposure to the sun. "Personally, I feel the disregard to the warnings is the obsession of vanity superseding one's health concern," says research scientist Steven Pearson, PhD. Doctors say exposure to the sun is not the threat, but exposure to the sun without protection is. Individuals are spending more time outside but are not wearing hats, sunglasses, sunscreen or other products designed to protect against the risk of prolonged exposure to sunlight.

EPISODE 9

Changing Semantics

by A. Lowell

As the care-giving population has grown over the years, the definition of "caregiver" has taken on many meanings. The San Francisco–based Family Caregiver Alliance describes caregivers as, "family, friends, and neighbors who stand by those whom they love as they face chronic illness, disability, or death. Caregivers are a diverse group of people from all walks of life—some new to care-giving, some anticipating becoming caregivers, and others for whom providing care has become a way of life." In the United States alone, caregivers provide more than 20 hours of care each week, accounting for an estimated $257 billion in unpaid services annually. This is double the amount spent on nursing home placement and paid home-care combined.

See Caregivers on page 3

Nursing Home Abuse and Neglect Widespread [P]

by J. Harris

According to results of new studies that have been surfacing over the past few months, a new epidemic has affected medical facilities. While the cause of this epidemic is neither bacteria nor virus, it is nevertheless as deadly. Nursing home abuse and neglect has become a widespread, growing epidemic, affecting thousands of nursing home residents who are dependent on nursing homes for care. Abuse and neglect can be difficult to recognize and are often covered up by nursing home staff. It is suggested that individuals who have a relative in a nursing home should search certified sites for key warning signs of nursing home abuse and neglect. It is estimated that as many as two million elderly patients are victims of nursing home abuse each year, a number that is projected to increase.

See Epidemic on page 2

Group Wants to Hear Your Troubles

by N. Mckinney

Later this week, the Neighborhood will sponsor support group leadership training in hopes of providing a mechanism for the formation of many support groups. Support groups have been found to be an effective way to manage problems, whether these problems stem from divorce, coping with a chronic illness, anxiety, or other aspect. Support groups are more effective than trying to manage problems independently. The purpose of the leadership training is to teach individuals how to effectively lead a support group. The meeting will be held at the Neighborhood Community Center, Thursday evening at 7 p.m.

EPISODE 10

Hospital to Offer Life-Saving Course [P]

by G. Johnson

The Neighborhood Hospital will be host to a 5-day cardiopulmonary resuscitation, or CPR, class open to all citizens of the Neighborhood. Completion of the 2-hour class in one evening results in qualification to administer

CPR, but the hospital is leaving the program open for 5 days in hopes that it will fit everyone's schedule sometime during the week. Hospital officials have suggested that a lot can be accomplished by grasping the concepts taught in this program, including saving a trip to the hospital, and maybe, someone's life. For more information call 881-1000.

Local Pathologist Dies [P—Danilo Ocampo]

by A. Lowell

Death always has wide-reaching affects, and this remains true for pathologist Danilo Ocampo, MD, PhD, who died suddenly this week after an apparent heart attack. Dr. Ocampo is best known for his contributions to law enforcement agencies during his career as the medical investigator for the Neighborhood County. In recent years, Dr. Ocampo assisted in gathering the evidence that was a key factor in the conviction of Harlan Randolph for the crime of murdering his wife with arsenic; a crime many believe was an influencing factor to the Karen Smith case in which she murdered her husband with an arsenic-laden pie. "His ability to determine specific details involving the deaths of crime victims was astounding and invaluable to our department," said Sheriff Mark Shuster following the announcement of the pathologist's death. "The amount of attention he gave to even the most minute detail of a case is only one of remarkable qualities of this man, and he will be sorely missed," added Shuster.

See Pathologist on page 2

Profile Sites Appeal to Teens [P—Your Zone]

by J. Harris

To say that Internet use is on the rise is an understatement—if Internet use were a disease, we would all be doomed. One of the most popular fascinations with the Internet is the ability to set up a personal Web site, a feature that has become overwhelmingly popular among teens. Teens can build a Web site from scratch or use a site with predefined templates to input personalized content. However, a tool most-used by teens is the personal profile. Thousands of individuals have posted personal information on such places as YourZone, which has the tagline "A Place for You." These sites are popular, but caution must be used regarding the type of personal information divulged. Although these sites promote socialization among youths, they also unintentionally invite the dangerous members of society—sexual predators and pedophiles have been documented in using the sites to gain access to and attract young, unassuming victims.

See Profiles on page 2

Event May Make People Play a Different Tune [P]

by N. Mckinney

Musicians from across the city are coming together in conjunction with the local Neighborhood Community Arts Program to sponsor a music appreciation workshop, open to children and adults. The workshop will be held each afternoon and evening this week and into Saturday, and will cover subjects both vocal and instrumental. Event organizer Ramona Rivera, well known to the community through her tireless efforts as a piano teacher, says that "Not enough children are given an opportunity to explore music has a hobby." The event marks the first exclusively oriented music workshop staged for the community in what Mrs. Rivera hopes to be a "recurring, if not continuous, event."

See Music on page 3

Sleep Depravity Is No Dream

by A. Lowell

Have trouble sleeping at night? You are not alone. In a recent national report, health experts seem to agree that most adults do not obtain enough sleep each night and are indeed suffering from sleep deprivation. Sleep deprivation is a rising cause of concern among the health community due to the adverse effects it can have on all levels of society—a ripple effect that experts agree may have already started. Health officials say that in order to prevent sleep deprivation, one must get at least 8 hours of sleep per night. Symptoms of sleep deprivation include irritability, blurred vision, slurred speech, memory lapses, and hallucinations, among others.

See Sleep on page 5

Road Construction Woes

by G. Johnson

Residents of the west side of the Neighborhood are complaining about the consistent, bombarding sound coming from an ongoing construction project. Construction superintendent Stephen Morton claims his company and workers are not violating any sound ordinance, as the Neighborhood has yet to sign legislation on such an ordinance. To stimulate the issue further than just noise complaints, issues have been raised with the construction crews also working at night to avoid problems with daytime traffic. "As if the noise weren't problem enough, I've got bright, halogen construction lights shining in my bedroom every night just because these people want to avoid a few cars," said resident Joseph Marrs.

See Construction on page 2

EPISODE 12

Adopt a Pet [P]

by G. Johnson

Everyone wants a loving family, and these desires are not exclusive those who walk on two feet. The local animal shelter is continually looking for homes for many of the community's abandoned animals. A free pet adoption clinic will be held each day this week from 9:00 AM to 3:00 PM, open to individuals who are 18 years of age or older. Types of pets that can be adopted include birds, cats, and especially dogs. Dogs remain the most-abandoned pets in the Neighborhood, and the heads of the animal shelter are trying to insure that their animals end up in the hands of a loving family so they are not abandoned again. All the animals that are available for adoption will have the appropriate vaccinations at no extra cost to the patrons.

Cancer Center Construction Halted

by J. Harris

In what appears to be one in a series of setbacks, the future site of the regional Cancer Center has once again been halted, with planners blocking proposed changes. City engineers and traffic experts say the current plan will create traffic flow problems within a 2-mile radius of the construction site. The problem of traffic does not seem to be a primary concern with the citizens who will be traveling these routes, however. Many area residents are angered by the ongoing delays to begin construction, citing the center is desperately needed by the community.

Cutting Through the Smoke

by A. Lowell

Neighborhood Council members are meeting this week to deliberate on the recently proposed citywide smoking ban. The ban is one in which the only gray area is maintaining the current ban on smoking in public areas, such as restaurants and city buildings. One side of the debate claims that limiting smoking to private residences is restricting freedom and making those who smoke less equal than nonsmokers. Conversely, anti-smoking advocates claim the general health of the community is at greater stake if people are allowed to smoke in public.

See Proposal on page 2

EPISODE 13

Special Olympics Golf Tournament Next Week [P]

by N. Mckinney

Late next week, the Neighborhood Golf Course will play host to a statewide Special Olympics golf tourna-ment. The event organizers expect anywhere between 50 and 75 participants for the tournament and over 100 spectators. Admission is free, as is participation. The golf course will be closed to open play between 7:00 AM and 3:00 PM on Saturday and Sunday due to the event.

Exposing Fears

by G. Johnson

This week, a local college experienced a crime that is making female students wary of their walks to class. According to a police report, two female students were walking to class on campus when they spotted a man lying naked on the grass. Claiming they had no idea what the man's intentions were, whether he was injured or planning to attack them, the women called the campus police, who arrested 18-year-old Anthony Martin for indecent exposure. Martin reportedly became combative when officers arrived on the scene, although no one was hurt during the incident. Martin was transported to a local hospital for a psychiatric evaluation.

Nest Eggs Hardly "Grade-A"

by J. Harris

How well have you prepared for your golden years? This question was addressed in a recent national survey—and as it turns out, the most common answers to the question did not bode well. The report showed that only 25% of Americans believe they will have enough money to pay for long-term care when they are elderly. The concern for inadequate finances increases with age; those who are between 50 and 60 years of age have far greater concerns than do younger adults. Adding to this a concern, less than half of adults have reportedly taken steps to prepare for their retirement. Many younger adults are concerned about financing their own long-term care in addition to the cost of caring for their aging parents.

See Finances on page 5

EPISODE 14

Pedaling to Safety [P]

by J. Harris

The Neighborhood Elementary School will be the host of an annual Bicycle Safety Awareness Fair this weekend for children ages 6–12. The purpose of the fair is to ensure that children are educated regarding danger prevention for riders. In addition to educating children, bicycle professionals will be attending the fair to make sure that children who already employ safety into their riding are also employing the right techniques and equipment. These professionals will also inspect a child's bicycle if the child brings his or her bicycle to the fair. Among the lectures on bicycle safety, agility tests and games will be conducted to reinforce safe riding practices and the use of helmets. Prizes will be awarded for the best riders in various age categories.

Angered Golfers Hit Back at Olympics

by N. Mckinney

Many area golfers were angered this week when no tee times were available because the golf course had chosen to sponsor the Special Olympics rather than remain open on its regular schedule. "It amazes me that event organizers were not sensitive to the routines of the serious golfers in this community—to give the Special Olympics the preferred tee times on the busiest golf days of the week was poor planning on the part of the golf club," says Neighborhood Golf Association (NGA) president Lee Malcoeur. "These individuals can play anytime, and the ones who support this golf course should always be given priority over others—after all, we're paying members." The recent Special Olympics event drew over 60 participants and over 100 spectators.

Vending Frustration

by G. Johnson

A recent school-board decision has angered many parents and students regarding the Neighborhood High School vending machines. The recent decision determined that "junk food" would no longer be served in the school's vending machines to curb the national obesity trend. Parents and students of the high school are claiming that by limiting what the students can purchase, the school is limiting the teenager's free choice. Parents and students assert that by the time an individual enters high school, he or she is capable of making food choices, and the school system should not be making decisions about what is appropriate to eat and what is unhealthy for students.

See Vending on page 4

Vending Viewpoints [P]

by G. Johnson

This week, parents who are against the recent School Board decision to ban junk food from high school vending machines will be given a chance to voice their concerns. The school was compelled to offer a public forum to debate the issue after the decision was met with such outrage the previous week. The event will be held Wednesday at 7:00 PM in the Neighborhood High School auditorium.

Theft, Narcotic Use on the Rise[P—Sheriff Shuster]

by L. Deacon

The recent emergence of a string of unsolved car thefts has prompted fears and apprehension in the Neighborhood. Many believe the thefts are a result of the influence of drug-related activity in the community. The series of thefts began around the residential and apartment district of the downtown area of the Neighborhood, but has since moved into the wealthier and seemingly more protected areas of the town. While theft of the vehicles seems the more salient trait of these crimes, other reports state that cars are also being vandalized, and car stereos are being stolen. Sheriff Mark Shuster believes the thefts are related to the recent rise in drug-related activity in the town, a view shared by a majority of the Neighborhood. "It is not my job to point the finger, but statistically, high school and college students are the most likely subjects for these crimes and they remain our primary focus point," said Shuster at a recent press conference.

See Theft on page 3

Crafting a Community

by J. Harris

Like a quilt is a combination of many types of fabric, this past weekend's Arts and Crafts Fair drew a diverse population as well. Drawing hundreds from around the state, the fair, held at the Neighborhood Community Center, drew both competition and spectators. Neighborhood resident Pam Allen won the grand prize for the best quilt, which was sold to local businessman Greg Ross for an astonishing $1,500. The opinion of many quilt experts was that the quilt was well inspired and worth the cost.

SEASON 3 NEWS

EPISODE 1

Seminar Offers Closure [P]

by N. Mckinney

Death symbolizes the final transition in life, but this transition does not just bring the end to one life—the grief inflicted by a loved one's death can affect anyone. A Neighborhood nurse hopes to change the long-term effects of death by offering a Grief and Bereavement Seminar titled, "Don't Let Death Ruin Your Life: Reclaiming Happiness After the Death of Your Loved One." The seminar will take place every night this week at 7:00 PM. Admission is free. Call 555-947-6341 for more information.

Local Man Dies in "Freak Accident"

by A. Lowell

"It happened so fast," commented assembly-line worker Adam Delpy on the death of his coworker, James Palmer. Palmer met a tragic end 3 days ago in an accident at a local automobile production annex. The reports gathered indicate that Palmer died while moving a set of car doors that were suspended from the roof by several chains. "We were behind on production, and we thought the chains could support the extra weight," stated Palmer's supervisor Alan Sharp. The chains, however, did not support the added weight and subsequently snapped, with the falling parts causing severe head trauma to Palmer, killing him before the ambulance could arrive. The Occupational Safety and Health Administration (OSHA) is investigating the incident; Sharp has been put on paid administrative leave during the investigation. A closed memorial service and mass, said by Fr. John Olivia, will be held at the Neighborhood Catholic Church on Saturday.

'Roid Ruckus

by F. Odell

Nathan Roberts, widely held as Neighborhood's star high school football player, was accused last week of the use and possession of steroids. The 17-year-old football player admitted to steroid use, stating he wanted to get a full-paid scholarship to a prestigious university and knew he would be overlooked by Division I scouts without the enhancement. Roberts, a linebacker, was known for his ability to hold a strong defense in any situation, and was a standout athlete this past season. "It is too bad," says Coach Anderson. "Kids these days have just gotten so competitive," he added. Roberts did not disclose the source of the steroids, but it is speculated that his father, Randall Roberts, was not only was aware of his son's steroid use, but was also the supplier. Nathan denies the former allegation. Steroid use is known to be harmful because it causes high blood pressure, edema, unwanted hair growth, and menstrual cycle disruption.

EPISODE 2

Changing Eating Habits [P]

by G. Johnson

Starting next week, the Neighborhood Community Center will be offering a cooking class for individuals aged 15–18. The class is designed to modify current diets through healthy eating. It is being offered in response to the growing obesity trend in the Neighborhood, and nationwide. "Our children need to learn what they are putting into their bodies, and that eating healthily does not mean just eating rabbit food," said class sponsor Damien Nichols. The course is set to focus on nutrition, risk assessment, dietary modification, and meal preparation using all four food groups.

Tragedy Strikes Family, Community[P—Sheriff Shuster]

by L. Deacon

Yesterday morning, the body of Allison Bloom was found in a field near the outskirts of the Neighborhood following an extensive all-night search. The 6-year-old girl was reported missing the preceding morning after Bloom's playmate reported seeing Bloom leave with an adult white man from the front yard of Bloom's household. The report was corroborated by a neighbor, who said he saw the two leaving in a white sedan. Initial findings showed the girl had been raped before being killed and dropped in the field where she was found. Sheriff Mark Shuster reported that a manhunt is in progress and that there are no concrete suspects as of yet.

See Tragedy on page 3

Food Fight [P- Jenna Riley]

by A. Lowell

Kentucky Fried Chicken, the nation's largest fried chicken restaurant, has again been put in the deep fryer by food activists' complaints regarding the chain's use of unhealthy trans-fatty acids in food preparation. "Americans are demanding healthier eating conditions," said food activist Gene Westchester. "It is fast food business such as KFC that benefits from obesity. They don't care what they feed us, they are only out to make a buck," added activist Jaren Dolland. KFC company spokesperson Gerald Rossum said that the company was "willing to adopt and explore alternative cooking preparation, but not at the expense of changing the recipe." Neighborhood customers continue to gobble (no pun intended) the fried chicken during the lunch and evening hours. "I don't want some political dude telling me that I can't eat KFC—I happen to like it," says local citizen Jenna Riley.

See Chicken on page 4

EPISODE 3

Conference Focuses on Substance Abuse [P]
Announcement

This weekend, the Neighborhood Community Center and Neighborhood Medical Association are coming together to host an event titled, "Multidisciplinary Health Providers Conference: Approaches to Treating Substance Abuse." Approved by the National Association of Substance Abuse Treatment, the conference will focus primarily on drug abuse, with a secondary focus on alcoholism. The event will be held at the Neighborhood Community Center on Saturday from 1:00 to 4:00 p.m.

Drug Use Rise Continues
by N. Mckinney

There has been an alarming rise in the rate of drug use and addiction in the Neighborhood. The culprit? Methamphetamines, otherwise known as "meth." Communities nationwide are seeing a sharp increase in meth houses, and an increase has also been seen in use among youth attending Neighborhood schools. It has become commonplace for students to know someone who uses in the school setting, where drug deals are being conducted in classes, between classes, and during lunch breaks under the eyes of teachers and administration. "It has become as frequent as passing a note in class," said a student from the high school.

See Drug Use on page 2

Suspect in Rape Case Injured During Chase [P—Alvin Cromwell]
by L. Deacon

Alvin Cromwell, suspected child rapist and murderer was injured following a brief chase with police. Cromwell, who is wanted in connection with the rape and murder of 6-year-old Allison Bloom was the target of a week-long manhunt. Police began to associate the 38-year-old Cromwell with the rape and murder of Bloom after a DNA test returned with Cromwell's profile based on samples taken from previous crimes. The chase began when Cromwell saw police approaching his one-bedroom apartment downtown, at which time he escaped out a back window of the apartment. While running from police, Cromwell broke his femur and sustained internal injuries when he jumped from a 30-foot cliff in attempts to elude authorities. Currently conscious and in the Neighborhood Hospital for treatment, Cromwell has been undergoing questioning by Sheriff Mark Shuster and other members of law enforcement.

See Suspect on page 4

EPISODE 4

Run, Neighborhood, Run! [P]
Announcement

Why walk when you can run? The Neighborhood is forming a running club for its residents. An information and organizational meeting for the runners club will be held next week at the Neighborhood Community Center. "Most communities our size have running clubs," says event organizer Ron Williams. The purpose of the club is to motivate individuals to improve their health through running, and to provide a mechanism for individuals with mutual interests to meet. In order to kindle social interaction, the primary location where the running club will meet for their runs is the Neighborhood Community Garden. The club is welcome for individuals of all ages at no cost. "We just want people to be healthy and have a fun time achieving that goal," concluded Williams.

See Running on page 6

Suspected Rapist Complains of Poor Medical Treatment [P—Alvin Cromwell]
by L. Deacon

In what appears to be an ethical battle waiting to boil over, Alvin Cromwell, the suspected rapist and murderer of 6-year-old Allison Bloom, is claiming he received poor and substandard treatment at Neighborhood Hospital while recovering from injuries sustained during chase with authorities. According to hospital officials, Cromwell, 38, claims that nurses at Neighborhood Hospital were withholding pain medications from him as punishment for the crime of which he is accused. Cromwell also cited rude comments and being referred to as a child killer by some of the nurses. Neighborhood Hospital spokeswoman Elizabeth Blanchett would not comment other than to say that an investigation is currently under way and that any incidence of confirmed abuse will be disclosed.

See Treatment on page 2

Auto Accident Leaves Local Man in Critical Condition; Nursing Staff Insensitive [P—Mark Martin]

by G. Johnson

Last night, local Mark Martin rolled his vehicle after failing to negotiate a turn. Martin was taken to Neighborhood Hospital, where he remains in critical condition with spinal cord injuries. According to bystanders and those who interacted with him before the crash, Martin had been drinking heavily all evening and was drunk when the accident occurred. Martin will not face jail time, since the only person he hurt was himself and there was no property damage. "In a way, given his current state, he has already received punishment for his actions. We are just happy no one else was hurt," said Sheriff Mark Shuster. Martin's father, Gil Martin, has accused the Neighborhood Hospital emergency department nursing staff of being insensitive and uncaring because they refused to allow family members to see Mark while he was being treated in the emergency department. Hospital spokesperson Beverly Mayer refused to comment on the situation.

EPISODE 5

Senior Center Set to Host Talk [P]

by N. Mckinney

Medication management can be a problem for even the young, and it is needless to say that as an individual ages and the number of required medications increases, the hassle of managing these medications also increases. Karen Williams, local gerontology nurse, hopes to change this fact of life. This Thursday afternoon at 1:00 PM, Williams will present a local talk on "Medication Management for the Elderly." The talk will be presented in the Neighborhood Senior Center. "We chose this location because the elderly are accustomed to visiting here, and a comfortable locale provides a better atmosphere to help people change," said Williams. The presentation will focus on issues elderly individuals face when taking medications. The talk is free and will be open to the general public.

Nursing Strike Imminent?

by A. Lowell

Just when you thought it could not get any worse. In a time when the crisis of nursing shortages is still a palpable taste on the tongues of those in need of medical assistance, now there is the possibility for the nursing community in the Neighborhood to strike. However, this concern is not merely a local one, as many nursing unions have reported such possibility in their area. The nursing union announced demands for better working conditions. "Ultimately this will impact the quality of care for patients," said nurse Marie Weldon. One of the leaders of the nursing union in the Neighborhood added that, "The public needs to know this is not about wanting to be paid more. It means expecting and allowing us to provide the level of care we have an obligation to provide." Community members have found themselves in an impossible situation—accept a tax increase to fund the nurses or try to cope with potentially substandard care. Hospitals and health care agencies are searching hard for alternatives, but a clear answer has yet to present itself.

See Strike on page 2

Pedestrian Involved in Accident, Remains in Hospital [P—Marcus Young]

by G. Johnson

"Speed and inattention were the leading causes for the accident," said Sheriff Mark Shuster in response to the accident. Yesterday, a car struck 7-year-old Marcus Young while he was riding his bike near home. The car, driven by 16-year-old Charles Dirk, was traveling at a high rate of speed through a residential neighborhood. The car sideswiped Young was he was riding back and forth from his yard to the street. "Had he been in the street, he would have been killed" said Shuster. Young remains at the Neighborhood Hospital.

EPISODE 6

Forum Open to Discuss Proposed Community [P]

by A. Lowell

Next Tuesday, discussion will be open on the topic of a recently proposed large-scale retirement community. The meeting, hosted at the Neighborhood Community Center will begin with a focus on the common questions regarding the proposed construction—cost to townspeople and the effects it will have on the community. The proposed community, referred to as The Mature Oasis expects to break ground on a 17-acre facility in the northwest part of the city late this season.

Water Supply Breached—Broken Water Line?

by G. Johnson

When a natural resource is a basic necessity for life, one would expect pandemonium and chaos to erupt in its absence. Such has not appeared to be the case with the Neighborhood's recent water crisis. Many Neighborhood residents have no access to water due to a broken water line. Affected residents are expected to be without water for at least the next 48 hours. Officials have jumped on the issue immediately, by having the National Guard dispense water bottles to all citizens in need. Residents are also urged to use water conservatively if they have a separate supply of water. Facilities such as the Neighborhood Hospital have assured patients that the current situation will not affect their care; the hospital keeps large caches of water for such incidences.

See Shortage on page 2

March MADDness

by N. Mckinney

This week, the group Mothers Against Drunk Driving, or MADD, marched outside of City Hall calling for tougher laws in the Neighborhood for drunk driving offenses. The immediacy and catalyst for this march came in response to an alcohol-related accident involving Mark Martin of the Neighborhood a few weeks ago. While the members of MADD admit that no one else but Martin was hurt in the accident, there is always the chance someone else could have been hurt. In addition, MADD holds the position that since Martin himself was hurt, it was not a victimless crime. "We must protect the drunk drivers from themselves as much as we must protect innocent bystanders," said a member of MADD.

See March on page 6

EPISODE 7

Anti-violence Organization Holds Festival

by G. Johnson

Staring Friday, and lasting until the end of the weekend, the organization Safe Haven will be sponsoring its second annual River Jazz Fest. The statewide organization is one that speaks out against domestic violence, and the proceeds from the festival will go toward this cause and to support shelters and counseling for battered women and children. Individuals who attend the event will find music, food, arts and crafts, and carnival games. The event is scheduled to start Friday, and Safe Haven is looking for anyone who would offer a hand in setting up for the festival. Hours for the festival will be Friday and Saturday, 12:00 PM to 11:00 PM, and Sunday, 12:00 PM to 5:00 PM.

Negligence Cited in Amputation Mishap

by A. Lowell

Earlier this week, 62-year-old Joseph Benson underwent an amputation of his leg just below the left knee and only suffered one complication—the wrong leg was amputated. Benson, a diabetic who suffered from poor circulation for the past 5 years, was shocked to wake up after his surgery and learn of the mishap. "I kept hoping that I was just dreaming, but I kept waking up to the same thing," said Benson. Staff at Neighborhood Hospital have not officially commented on the case, but this incident comes at a dire time for the hospital, which has experienced quite an assortment of problems lately, including union problems and nursing shortages.

Teenage Girls Lead in Smoking, Drug Use [P]

by G. Johnson

According to a recently released health report, teenage girls have surpassed their male counterparts in smoking and prescription drug abuse. In the past 2 years, more young women than men started using marijuana, alcohol, and cigarettes. In correlation to these findings, Sheriff Mark Shuster reported that most of the drug violations at the local high school involve female suspects. Given the recent rise in methamphetamines in Neighborhood schools, the sheriff only sees this number rising. High school student Jenna Riley told reporters, "Girls want to do what older guys are doing—they want to be cool." Riley denied using drugs herself, but admits that some of her friends do. Carol Ramsey, a nurse midwife who also works at the Neighborhood Public Health Department finds the results disturbing. "Adolescent girls who consume illicit substances are at a higher risk for depression, addiction, and stunted growth," said Ramsey. Those who were surveyed reported that they felt peer pressure was more common among female cliques than male ones, stating that the chances of becoming an outcast are more likely for female students than for male students. "Because substance abuse goes hand-in-hand with risky sexual behavior, these females are more likely to contract a sexually transmitted disease or become pregnant," warned Ramsey. The surveys that led to the reported results canvassed over 70,000 households in the nation.

EPISODE 8

Lecture to Help People See Danger [P]

by N. Mckinney

Peter Raush, MD, a Neighborhood ophthalmologist, will present a lecture, "Things You Should Know About Macular Degeneration," on Thursday at 7:00 P.M. at the Neighborhood Community Center. Raush explains that the purpose of the lecture is to inform individuals of a relatively common and significant eye disorder among elderly individuals. Macular degeneration is a disease of the eye in which the light-sensing cells of the macula mysteriously malfunction and cease to work over time. While the lecture does not offer ways of preventing the disease, early signs and symptoms will be discussed with the hopes that individuals will recognize a need for medical treatment. Macular degeneration occurs most often in people older than 60 years of age. Estimates indicate that one in six Americans between the ages of 55 and 64 are afflicted with the disease; the incidence rises to one in four Americans between ages 64 and 74, and one in three over the age of 75. It is also estimated that about 1.2 million of the estimated 12 million people with macular degeneration suffer severe central vision loss each year—200,000 individuals will lose all central vision in one or both eyes. The talk is open to the public, and individuals of all ages.

Nurses Walk Out, Cite Poor Working Conditions [P—Dr. Gordon]

by A. Lowell

In what seems to be a series of unfortunate events, nurses at the Neighborhood Hospital staged a walkout yesterday. While the hospital responded to this problem immediately by recruiting nurses from several communities, the impact on the psyche of the community is not so easily mended. Several nursing units have been closed, and only the sickest of patients are being kept for treatment. Patients involved in trauma cases have been diverted to other hospitals until the strike is resolved. James Gordon, MD, an emergency department (ED) physician at Neighborhood Hospital says that the effects are devastating. Dr. Gordon estimates that only a few nurses in his department are involved in the strike, but that his department is not immune from the effects. "Even if we keep our nurses from walking off the job in the ED, we have no place to send patients who need to be admitted," says Gordon.

See Strike on page 4

Teen Charged With Murder of Infant

by L. Deacon

This week, Reyna Clarkson was formally charged with murder after leaving a newborn infant in a toilet at Neighborhood High School. Clarkson, a junior, first claimed she did not know she was pregnant and thought she was simply having bad menstrual cramping and heavy bleeding—claiming that she did not know the infant was in the toilet. The story garnered her a great amount of sympathy in the community, but with each recantation her story changed, and the truth finally emerged. Clarkson later admitted that she had the baby and attempted to dispose of it by flushing the infant down the toilet. Sheriff Mark Shuster took the teen into custody following the confession Tuesday night. Her parents posted the $100,000 bail.

EPISODE 9

Meditation Group Forming [P]

Announcement

Do you often feel irritable? Do you have trouble sleeping? Do you have difficulty focusing? No, this is not an advertisement for Geritol, but if you have answered yes to any of these questions, you might be experiencing stress. Meditation has been shown to be an effective method to manage and curb stress levels. A meditation group is forming in the Neighborhood, and if you or someone you know might be interested in joining, then come to the information meeting at the Neighborhood Community Center, Wednesday night at 7:00 P.M.

Local Woman Loses Battle With Cancer [P—Pamela Allen]

by A. Lowell

The Neighborhood lost one of their finest residents this week. Pam Allen, a woman known for her highly sought-after homemade quilts, died this week following a long battle with cancer. Allen leaves behind a husband, Clifford, and son, Gary. "One cannot say that she merely left a family behind, she left a legacy. Everyone in the community got some sense of comfort by owning or even looking at one of her quilts," said Greg Ross, who owns a quilt made by Allen. Father John Olivas will lead a funeral mass in dedication to Allen this Friday, with a private memorial service the night before.

Nursing Strike Enters Second Week

by G. Johnson

Neighborhood Hospital administrators and nurses remain in a deadlock over the ongoing nursing strike. "The hospital is still open and serving patients," says hospital spokesperson Raymond Fletcher. "It is true, however, that the number of admissions is significantly down, and we are not admitting any new patients," added Fletcher. Fletcher says new admissions are being diverted to other hospitals in nearby communities, but patients who are hospitalized are being cared for by a group of temporary workforce nurses from other states. Meanwhile, strike organizers say hospital administrators are not cooperating in talks to bring closure to the dispute as the strike enters its second week. "We are striking so we can ensure safe conditions for our patients," reports nurse Cheryl Keller. "The media is trying to make us look like the bad guys," she added.

See Strike on page 4

EPISODE 10

Swimming Classes to Be Offered [P]

Announcement

The local pool will begin to offer swimming classes to young children as early next week. The Neighborhood Community Parks and Recreation is offering free swimming classes to Neighborhood children in three age-separated classes: 4–6, 7–9, 10–12. Classes will be available on a first-come, first-served basis. Signups begin this weekend at the Community Center.

Sexual Predator Apprehended in Sting

by L. Deacon

As social networking sites become as large as societies themselves, it is obvious that the indecency that comes with reality will migrate into these digital media. Such was the case last weekend when a sting operation lead to the arrest of a 42-year-old man in his attempt to meet with an underage female. The man, Bryan Phillips, was apprehended when he used the popular Your Zone online communication site to arrange a meeting with a girl whom he thought was 13 years old, but in fact was an undercover police officer posing as the girl.

See Sting on page 2

Hospital Strike Ends

by G. Johnson

To the relief of Neighborhood residents, the nursing strike at the Neighborhood Hospital has come to an end, and nurses have returned to their jobs in full force. Hospital Administrators agreed to reduce the patient load and hire more nurses as opposed to non-licensed staff. "This is not a win for nurses as much as it is a victory for patients," says local nurse Cheryl Keller. Nurses who had been pulled from other communities in order to assist in the shortage during the strike have also returned to their local areas. Some patients who were redirected to these areas are being moved back to Neighborhood Hospital in order to help some patients' mental recovery as well as their physical recovery—by seeing doctors to whom they are accustomed.

See Strike on page 8

EPISODE 11

Bin Burning Ban to Begin

Announcement

Local government officials want to remind citizens of the new trash burning ban that is set to begin this week following a 6–2 vote in favor of the ban at the last City Council meeting. The council was quick to approve the ban in light of the negative effects on the air quality in the city from the recent forest fire. Councilman Ray Santori stated that if production of manmade pollutants could be curbed, the adverse effects of things such as forest fires would be slightly less severe.

Robbing Spree Ends in Deadly Crash [P-Casey Holmes] [P-Robert Bandish]

by L. Deacon

What started as a robbery ended in a death this weekend in the Neighborhood when two individuals, Casey Holmes and Robert Bandish, caused a collision with another vehicle while fleeing the scene of a robbery they had committed earlier. The names of the two victims have not been released, but it is known that one was an honor student at Neighborhood High School. Holmes and Bandish have been arrested and charged with armed robbery and vehicular homicide. Current reports state that the robbery was conducted in the interest of the two young men supporting a long-standing drug habit.

See Crash on page 3

Bumping Up Safety [P]

by G. Johnson

A local woman is circulating a petition to install speed bumps around residential areas. Angie Young, whose son Marcus was seriously injured several months ago by a speeding car, is attempting to get enough signatures on a petition for a proposal to install speed bumps in a majority of the family areas around the Neighborhood. It is Young's opinion that the streets are unsafe for children because speed limits are not enforced by the local police. If she is able to collect enough signatures, Young plans to take up the issue with city officials.

EPISODE 12

Scout Food Drive [P]

Announcement

Girl and Boy Scouts in the area are joining forces to increase food donations for the Neighborhood homeless shelter. Boy Scout official Gary Eddy states the combined efforts of Girl and Boy Scouts within the community are expected to yield large donations desperately needed by the shelters. Scouts will be going door-to-door asking for donations. Alternatively, food donations can be dropped off at any of the four local Stanley Food Market locations.

Black Widow Outbreak Worries Residents

by N. Mckinney

Residents of certain areas of the Neighborhood are reporting large number of Black Widow spiders in recent weeks. James Gordon, MD, director of the Neighborhood Hospital emergency department, confirmed there have been several individuals treated in recent weeks following an alleged black widow bite. According to Dr. Gordon, the female black widow spider is the most venomous spider in North America, although it rarely causes death to humans. The male black widow spider is relatively tame by comparison and will not bite unless intensively provoked—the female is far more territorial and vicious. National statistics indicate that human mortality is less than 1% from black widow spider bites. The bite itself is often not painful and may go unnoticed, but the poison can cause abdominal pain similar to that associated with appendicitis as well as pain to muscles or the soles of the feet. Other symptoms include alternating salivation and dry-mouth, paralysis of the diaphragm, profuse sweating, and swollen eyelids. If bitten, it is recommended to apply ice to the bite and contact a local poison control center.

Homeless Shelters Running at Critical Capacity [P—Sheriff Shuster]

by G. Johnson

The city homeless shelter manager cannot explain the increase in the homeless population, but the numbers are expected to increase further as winter approaches. Many of those staying in shelters are those who are mentally ill and those suffering from severe drug and alcohol dependencies. Sheriff Mark Shuster confirms that along with the increases in shelter guests, there has also been a sharp increase in local area crime rates.

See Homeless on page 4

EPISODE 13

Encouraging the Elderly to Exercise [P]

by N. Mckinney

When thinking of aging, some envision the cliché of an elderly person in a rocking chair, waiting for the inevitable. Fitness Guru Jack Blaine hopes to change this. Blaine, who in previous years performed endurance feats such as participating in a triathlon and participating in the Tour de France, has been well known throughout the country as an expert in exercise regimens for elderly individuals. Blaine will be hosting a free seminar at the Neighborhood Senior Center this coming week. The seminar will focus on exercise, fitness, and aging, although all ages are welcome. Call the Neighborhood Senior Center at 260-4400 for more information.

Safety Crusader Met With Mixed Reception

by L. Davis

This week at city hall, a local woman was greeted with both praise and complaints regarding her movement to install speed bumps into all residential areas. The woman, Angie Young, took her petition with 500 signatures to the City Council meeting this week. Although there were many people at the meeting complaining about the speeding, speaking in favor of installing speed bumps on all the streets, there were many more opposed to the idea, citing damage to the suspension of vehicles and huge impairment of traffic flow. City counselors voted down the motion in order to appease the majority against the speed bumps. Others claim, however, that the movement is not over, stating that Young inspired them to pursue action at higher levels of government.

See Petition on page 2

Breast Cancer Mortality Continues Rise

by A. Lowell

Breast cancer mortality among women of ethnic minorities is continuing to increase. The National Cancer Institute reports that over the past 10 years, approximately 500,000 American women have died from breast cancer. The lifetime risk of breast cancer has almost tripled in the United States, and currently, a woman has a one-in-eight lifetime risk of being diagnosed with breast cancer. Hispanic women have lower breast cancer screening rates than do non-Hispanic White women, and tend to seek and obtain health care services less frequently than individuals of other ethnicities. The report also indicates that although the lifetime risk of developing breast cancer is higher for White women than for African American and Hispanic women, African American women and subgroups of Hispanic women continue to have a lower breast cancer survival rate.

EPISODE 14

Pride Parade Addresses Inequities [P]

Announcement

Local chapters of gay and lesbian support groups are sponsoring a Gay and Lesbian Awareness Parade Saturday in the Neighborhood Community Garden. The parade will begin in the Neighborhood's downtown district, at the city government offices, and then work its way up to the garden, where there will be a multitude of booths available to attendees, which will provide information on equality groups, safe sex, and disease prevention. Event sponsors say the goal of the parade is to raise awareness of the societal inequities experienced by gay and lesbian citizens. The event will begin at 9:00 AM Saturday, and attendance is free. All are encouraged to spectate or participate in the parade.

Hospital to Go Under the Microscope

by G. Johnson

The Joint Commission, formerly the Joint Commission on Accreditation of Healthcare Organizations, will be making an accreditation site visit next week to Neighborhood Hospital. The organization sets standards for health care organizations to meet for accreditation purposes. The accreditation essentially serves as a nationwide "seal of approval" that indicates a hospital meets high performance standards for patient care. Many are concerned about the visit, given the recent controversies that the hospital has endured, including the nursing strike that was only recently resolved. However, hospital spokeswoman Mimi

Patterson is optimistic, and shared with reporters that the hospital is more than ready for the visit, despite setbacks to planning in recent months.

See Accreditation on page 6

Student Nurse Selected to Aid in Alleviating Nurse Shortage

by N. Mckinney

This week, a student nurse was selected to the Governor's Task Force to increase the number of nurses in the state. State Governor Joe Desmedt is forming a task force to look at ways to increase the number of nurses in the state. Local student nurse Jill Harris has been selected to participate on the task force with the hopes that she might be able to offer insight as to how to increase the number of students that are accepted to and graduate from nursing programs. Desmedt thought that adding a student to the task force would provide an inside look at the shortcomings and benefits of particular nursing programs so that the state knows exactly what areas to address in order to remedy the shortage.

See Shortage on page 5

Benner, P. & Sutphen, M. (2007). Learning across the professions: The clergy, a case in point. *Journal of Nursing Education, 46,*103–108.

Charon, R. (2004). Narrative and medicine. *New England Journal of Medicine, 350*(9), 862–864.

Davidhizar, R. & Lonser, G. (2003). Storytelling as a teaching technique. *Nurse Educator, 28*(5), 217–221.

Diekelmann, N. (2005). Engaging the students and the teacher: Co-creating substantive reform with narrative pedagogy. *Journal of Nursing Education, 44*(6), 249–252.

Durgahee, T. (1997). Reflective practice: Nursing ethics through story telling. *Nursing Ethics, 4*(2), 135–146.

Ebbert, D. W. & Connors, H. (2004). Standardized patient experiences: Evaluation of clinical performance and nurse practitioner satisfaction. *Nursing Education Perspectives, 25,* 12–15.

Hodge, F. S., Pasqua, A., Marquez, C. A., & Geishirt-Cantrell, B. (2002). Utilizing traditional storytelling to promote wellness in American Indian communities. *Journal of Transcultural Nursing, 13*(1), 6–11.

Ibarra, R. (2001). *Beyond Affirmative Action: Reframing the Context of Higher Education.* Madison, WI: University of Wisconsin Press.

Ironside, P. M. (2005). Teaching thinking and reaching the limits of memorization: Enacting new pedagogies. *Journal of Nursing Education, 44*(10), 441–449.

Milton, C. L. (2004). Stories: Implications for nursing ethics and respect for another. *Nursing Science Quarterly, 17*(3), 208–211.

Rutledge, C. M., Garzon, L., Scott, M., & Karlowicz, K. (2004). Using standardized patients to teach and evaluate nurse practitioner students on cultural competency. *International Journal of Nursing Education Scholarship, 1.* Article 17.

Shawler, C. (2008). Standardized patients: A creative teaching strategy for psychiatric mental-health nurse practitioner students. *Journal of Nursing Education, 47*(11), 528–531.

Siebert, D. C., Guthrie, J. T., & Adamo, G. (2004). Improving learning outcomes: Integration of standardized patients and telemedicine technology. *Nursing Education Perspectives, 25,* 232–237.

Thomas, M. D., O'Conner, F. W., Albert, M. L., Boutain, D., & Brandt, P. A. (2001). Case-based teaching and learning experiences. *Issues in Mental Health Nursing, 22,* 517–531.

Vessey, J. A. & Huss, K. (2002). Using standardized patients in advanced practice nursing education. *Journal of Professional Nursing, 18,* 29–35.

ADHD, 184, 188, 199

Adoption, 176, 220, 222, 228–30, 275–77, 297, 299, 302

Advanced practice nursing, 266, 272

Allergic reaction, 28, 120, 159

Anemia, 20, 22–23, 27, 33–34, 160, 166–67

Angina, 161–64

Alzheimer disease, 19, 32, 34–35, 165–68, 255

Anxiety, 32, 92, 119–20, 130–32, 148, 263, 293, 297

Asthma, 18, 28, 30, 173, 231, 239, 242, 246–47, 256, 267

Atrial fibrillation, 23, 34, 99, 102, 104

Back pain, 18, 23, 119, 121–29

Board of Nursing, 39, 254, 264–65

Benign prostatic hypertrophy, 16, 24, 70–71, 77

Burnout, nursing, 255–58

Chlamydia, 27, 120, 147–52, 176, 272, 276

Cancer, 16–17, 23–25, 38, 45, 70–74, 76–80, 133–38, 224, 233, 259, 261, 263, 272–73, 292, 294, 297, 299, 305, 307

Cataract, 25, 34, 36, 119, 125, 133–38, 266, 269

Caregiver, 17, 19, 23, 32, 34–35, 37–38, 104–6, 138, 160–65, 168, 293, 297

Chemotherapy, 16–18, 20, 70, 72–75, 78–81

Childbirth education, 27, 42–43, 45, 174, 179–80, 205, 234, 239, 274, 293

Cholecystitis, 20–21, 119, 129, 131

Colitis, 17, 19, 220–25

Conjunctivitis, 17, 29, 30, 238,

Community services, 38, 42, 224

Dental caries, 29, 120, 158, 288

Diabetes mellitus
type 1, 24, 169–76, 266–67
type 2, 24, 29, 34, 99–106, 184, 189–96, 200, 279

Decubitus ulcer, 19, 21, 23, 120, 156–57, 160, 168

Dehydration, 25, 29,173, 201, 204, 215, 241

Depression , 23, 32, 34, 35, 70–76, 79, 92–93, 99, 103, 111, 120, 125, 132, 143, 153, 156–57, 264–65, 304

Diarrhea, 17, 19, 29, 70, 77–81, 103, 222, 225, 227, 232, 241, 252

Diversion program, 32, 39, 254, 260, 264–65

Domestic violence, 26, 27, 30, 32, 33, 38, 201, 203–19, 266, 272, 290, 293, 304

Down syndrome, 70–86, 224

Drunk driving, 32, 33, 120, 131, 156, 287, 303–4

Eating disorder, 32, 120, 144–48

Emphysema, 22, 25, 34, 35, 87–93, 256, 268

Elder abuse, 36, 37, 40, 266–68, 297

End of life, 17, 21, 70–86, 160–68

Erectile dysfunction, 220–25

Ethics, 39, 43, 254–77, 291

Health care funding, 39, 266–71, 296

Health promotion 28, 36, 43–45, 278–83, 285

Failure to thrive, 18, 29, 201, 204, 214–17

Fatigue, 17, 24, 70, 78–82, 107–14, 160–64, 173, 179–81, 203–4, 223, 254–56, 274

Fracture
Femur, 199–200
Hip, 17, 18, 23, 25, 34, 163–68
Pelvis, 26, 29, 250–51, 255

Growth and development, 28, 107, 114–18, 157–59, 182–83, 190–96, 196–200, 201–4, 214–17, 218–19, 251–53

Infertility, 27, 169–75, 176–82

Internet, 30, 31, 38, 87–91, 107, 111, 170, 176, 193–96, 221, 223, 239, 258, 298

Ketoacidosis, 20, 24, 25, 169, 173–75, 179

Hearing loss, 22, 25, 26, 31, 34, 45, 87–93, 93–97

HELLP syndrome, 26, 169, 181

Heart failure, 17, 19, 22, 23, 33, 34, 160–64

Homeless, 33, 38, 97, 119, 126, 132, 138, 290, 306, 307

Homosexuality, 220–30, 297, 307–8

Hospital visitation, 26, 308

Hypertension, 23, 24, 34, 99–106, 107–13, 156, 161–64, 220–25, 266–70, 274

Immunizations, 20, 21, 28, 30, 31, 37, 38, 44, 45, 120, 154–55, 157–59, 182–83, 186, 203, 214–17, 218–19, 235, 240–53, 255, 280, 282, 284, 286, 290

Mandatory overtime, 40, 43, 254, 256–58, 259–61, 263, 296

Medication management, 21, 36, 37, 38, 44, 45, 266, 270, 303

Myocardial infarction, 20, 33, 160–64

Nausea and vomiting, 18, 77–81, 119, 128–32

New graduate experience, 254–58, 296

Nursing management, 30, 254, 258–61

Nursing shortage, 40, 43, 156, 254–83, 294–96, 303–4, 308

Nursing strike, 40, 43, 98, 254, 258, 261, 282, 285, 303, 305, 306

Nutrition, 18, 19, 21, 24, 26, 29, 31, 34, 44, 45, 70, 78–81, 92, 99, 103–5, 127–28, 165–68, 190–96, 201, 214–15, 218–19, 226, 237, 281–82, 294, 301

Obesity, 18, 24, 29, 31, 38, 127–32, 190–96, 279, 282, 288, 291, 300–2

Occupational safety, 301

Oral care, 31, 45, 120, 123, 130, 135, 151, 154–55, 157–59, 243–44, 246, 247–48, 250, 288, 296

Osteoarthritis, 18, 24, 34, 87, 93–98

Osteoporosis, 24, 34, 36, 94, 119, 133–37, 268

Otitis media, 17, 29, 201, 208, 219

Pain, 18–19, 23, 24, 34, 70, 72, 75, 77, 81, 87, 90, 93–97, 99–100, 107–13, 115, 119–26, 127–32, 136–37, 151, 160, 165–66, 178, 184, 206–8, 222, 225, 227, 230, 231, 250–53, 256–58, 269, 277, 307

Pneumonia, 22, 23, 35, 91–93

Poisoning, 31, 38, 141–42, 166, 286, 287, 288, 291, 307

Power of attorney, 36, 39, 161, 168

Prematurity, 26, 29, 169, 175, 180–83, 293

Preeclampsia, 26, 29, 169, 180–82, 272, 274

Pregnancy, 17, 18, 26–27, 31, 33, 146, 169–82, 201, 203–6, 233, 237–40, 272–77, 282, 293, 296, 304, 305

Reactive airway disease, 239, 243–47

Renal insufficiency, 24, 107, 112–14

Restraints, 19, 21, 39, 142, 161–62, 293

Respiratory failure, 18, 20, 22, 23, 25, 35, 87–93

Respiratory syncytial virus, 17, 204, 215

Schizophrenia, 32, 119, 139–43

Senior care, 17, 19, 23, 33, 36, 37, 38, 40, 41, 42, 87–98, 99–106, 133–38, 160–68, 266–71

Sexual discrimination, 220–30, 277, 297, 307–8

Sex education, 27, 31, 42, 44, 278, 282, 288, 296,

Sexual violence, 31, 33, 38, 257–58, 261, 301, 302

Sleep deprivation, 19, 38, 73–75, 127–30, 132, 162–67, 181, 189, 202, 240, 298

Smoking cessation, 26, 44, 45, 87–94, 98, 104–5, 181, 203–4, 233–38, 267, 289

Social services, 30, 36, 40, 41, 201, 215, 275

Spinal cord injury, 23, 26, 35, 120, 125, 156–57

Stroke, 16, 17, 18, 20, 21, 23, 24, 32, 34, 35, 99–106, 266, 269

Substance abuse, 31, 32, 33, 38, 201–14, 254, 262–65, 302, 304

Systemic lupus erythematosus, 17, 25, 107, 112–13

Transitional care, 34, 36, 42, 92–93, 98, 102–3, 166–68

Trauma, 26, 29, 30, 31, 32, 125, 201, 206, 218, 231, 235, 242, 285, 290, 293, 301, 305

Upper respiratory infection, 22, 30, 35, 216, 232, 253

Urinary tract infection, 17, 24, 103

Vitreous hemorrhage, 19, 25, 169, 171